616.0478

# About the author

Dr Charles Shepherd qualified in me
Hospital in 1974, where he initially spec
ally transmitted diseases. He then held
a number of specialities including casualty, infectious diseases,
paediatrics and psychiatry before becoming Resident Medical Officer at
Cirencester Hospital, Gloucestershire. Charles Shepherd has also
worked in general practice and the pharmaceutical industry. Since
becoming ill with ME/CFS, he has reluctantly had to leave the NHS and
now works privately from his home in Gloucestershire.

His involvement with the ME Association led him to become its first
Medical Director and Secretary to the Scientific and Medical Advisory
Panel. In his role as Medical Director, Charles Shepherd is involved in
promoting a better public understanding of this illness through contact
with the media, politicians, benefit agencies and health professionals. He
has also been involved in a number of research projects, and in 1990 was
co-organiser of the first international symposium on ME/CFS at
Cambridge University.

Charles Shepherd maintains a keen interest in the area of alternative
medicine and health fraud. His public campaigning for better public protection in these areas has resulted in a number of dubious forms of treatment aimed at people with ME/CFS being banned or severely
restricted.

He has made numerous contributions to the scientific literature on
the subject of ME/CFS and is author of *Guidelines for the Care of
Patients:* a standard source of management advice for doctors which is
now being used in many parts of the world.

YEOVIL COLLEGE
LIBRARY

Yeovil College

Y0070137

# LIVING WITH ME

*The Chronic/Post-Viral Fatigue Syndrome*

Dr Charles Shepherd

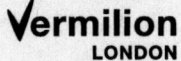

**Vermilion**
**LONDON**

15 17 19 20 18 16 14

Published in 1999 by Vermilion, an imprint of Ebury Publishing
First published in the United Kingdom by Cedar in 1989

Ebury Publishing is a Random House Group company

Copyright © Charles Shepherd 1989, 1992, 1998

Charles Shepherd has asserted his right to be identified as the author of this
Work in accordance with the Copyright, Designs and Patents Act 1988.

All rights reserved. No part of this publication may be reproduced, stored in a
retrieval system, or transmitted in any form or by any means, electronic,
mechanical, photocopying, recording or otherwise, without the prior permission of the copyright owner.

The Random House Group Limited Reg. No. 954009

Addresses for companies within the Random House Group can be found at
www.randomhouse.co.uk

A CIP catalogue record for this book is available from the British Library

The Random House Group Limited supports the Forest Stewardship
Council® (FSC®), the leading international forest certification organisation.
All our titles that are printed on Greenpeace approved FSC® certified paper
carry the FSC® logo. Our paper procurement policy can be found at
www.randomhouse.co.uk/environment

Printed in the UK by CPI Antony Rowe, Chippenham, Wiltshire

ISBN 9780091816797

Copies are available at special rates for bulk orders. Contact the sales development team on 020 7840 8487 or visit www.booksforpromotions.co.uk for
more information.

To buy books by your favourite authors and register for offers, visit
www.randomhouse.co.uk

# Contents

## Part 4: Appendices

# Acknowledgements

I should like to acknowledge the help of Dr Melvin Ramsay, who diagnosed my own illness back in 1980.

Dr Ramsay was consultant physician at the Royal Free Hospital in London during the time of an outbreak of an infectious illness that became known as 'the Royal Free disease' and subsequently myalgic encephalomyelitis (ME). He did more than anybody else to legitimize this devastating illness, and was prepared to stand up for his patients against a background of controversy and cynicism from the medical establishment. In the end his theories have been shown to be correct.

Sadly, Melvin Ramsay died on 29 March 1990, just a matter of days before he was to be the first speaker at the Cambridge University International Symposium on ME, where he would have presented the culmination of 35 years of painstaking work.

I must also acknowledge the assistance of my son, Patrick, with his computer skills. Finally, I would like to thank my wife, Pam, who has stuck by me through all the difficult times.

# Foreword

Dr Melvin Ramsay, the first doctor to recognise ME in the UK, wrote this foreword for the first edition of this book, in 1988.

There is still a great deal of confusion in the mind of the medical profession regarding the precise clinical identity of myalgic encephalomyelitis and this can, in great measure, be attributed to the current belief that ME and the many post-viral fatigue states are synonymous. Far from being synonymous they are distinguishable, in the first place, by the long delay in the restoration of muscle power after even a minor degree of physical effort; secondly, by the extraordinary variability of symptoms even in the course of one day; and finally, by the alarming tendency of the disease to become chronic. On the other hand, the fatigue factor in the post-viral states is merely part of a general fatigue, shows no daily variability and the condition is unlikely to last longer than two years.

The incidence of ME among doctors is out of all proportion to their numbers in the general population. Dr Charles Shepherd has now had the disease for over ten years [now 20 years]. His experience of the vagaries of the disease – alternating periods of remission and relapse since the diagnosis was confirmed in 1980 – puts him in an ideal position to help other victims of this distressing complaint.

The chronic ME sufferer faces a condition of constant muscle fatigue, often severe muscle pain and discomfort as a result of spasm and twitchings. This is accompanied by cerebral dysfunction in the form of impairment of memory and powers of concentration, emotional liability, disturbed sleep rhythm, vivid dreams and lack of muscle co-ordination that renders the patient incapable of carrying out simple manoeuvres. This is all too often accompanied by a sense of rejection by friends and relatives as a hopeless neurotic. Dr Shepherd can give these pitiful victims of a disease that is still imperfectly understood, invaluable assistance in the planning of their lives, on a basis that can afford them a sense of purpose in combating what would otherwise be a drab and pointless existence. I thoroughly commend his excellent treatise.

*Dr A Melvin Ramsay*
Died 29 March 1990

# Introduction: How I Became Involved with a Very Controversial Illness

*'You'll never ever see another case of ME in your lifetime. Go away and forget about this illness – it's all hysterical nonsense.'*

These words of wisdom were delivered by an eminent consultant standing at the bedside of a young woman who'd been admitted to my London teaching hospital with a possible diagnosis of ME. I was still only an impressionable young medical student, but the consultant's insensitive and dogmatic remarks summed up the views of most doctors at this time.

For the next few years I did forget about ME. I'm not sure whether I did even see another patient with it. Like many young doctors straight out of medical school, I became increasingly sceptical (and sometimes rather hostile) towards patients who had a variety of symptoms, yet nothing was obviously wrong when they were examined, and all their various laboratory results were reported as perfectly normal.

Then came the summer of 1978. This was a time of great happiness in my life. I'd recently been married and bought a cottage in the Cotswolds. All the hard work of being a junior hospital doctor had finally paid off. At long last I was at a point in my career where I could settle down and fulfil my ambition to become a general practitioner.

One summer weekend, something very strange began to happen. On the Saturday morning I woke up feeling as though I was about to go down with a dose of 'flu. My weekend off was spent in London, where I became increasingly tired, unwell and slightly confused – a combination of symptoms which are very similar to those I still experience some 20 years later!

The real explanation had to wait till I rather stupidly decided to go back to work on Monday morning. By then I'd developed a fever, and at lunch I was told to go home as my face was starting to develop spots. The diagnosis was chicken-pox – caught from one of my elderly patients with shingles.

After ten days' sick leave, mainly resting in bed, I still felt weary, slightly disorientated and unsteady on my feet. But junior doctors aren't allowed to be ill – this was my first ever period of sick leave since leaving school – so it was time to return to work, even though I was far from well.

To cut a long story short, an attack of chicken-pox had triggered ME. Returning to a full-time demanding job and then struggling on to the point of exhaustion was a daft thing to do in the circumstances.

Having been sent home, and told not to return till I was fully better again, I began a fruitless succession of appointments with various respected consultants. Some believed I was genuinely ill and did all they could to help, but none could provide an explanation or diagnosis. Others were far less sympathetic and advised me that it was time to 'pull yourself together' or 'get back to work before you become a chronic invalid'. Not surprisingly, my DSS benefits were stopped and some of my colleagues began to conclude that I was either mad or malingering.

What followed was the unhappiest period in my life. Not being believed and running into serious financial difficulties was bad enough. Even worse was having no option but to keep going back to work for short periods and not being able to look after my patients in a proper manner. The final straw came when late one night I very nearly made a serious drug-dose error whilst treating someone who was seriously ill with asthma. There was no alternative but to resign from general practice and, once again, try to discover why I felt so ill.

Nearly two years after originally becoming ill with chicken-pox, I finally obtained a diagnosis of ME. This was initially from Dr Melvin Ramsay, the infectious disease physician at London's Royal Free Hospital who'd reported on a famous outbreak back in 1955, and later from Professor Peter Behan at the University of Glasgow. Receiving an explanation about what was going wrong, and then being able to plan an appropriate course of management, came as a tremendous relief. There wasn't any 'cure' for the illness – there still isn't – but having a diagnosis provided a basis for improvement rather than continuing to drift in a state of uncertainty.

Fortunately, the story of ME, and the people it affects, isn't all doom and gloom. Doctors like Peter Behan, Betty Dowsett and the late Melvin Ramsay here in the UK; David Bell, Paul Cheney and Tony Komaroff in America; and John Dwyer, Andrew Lloyd and Denis Wakefield in Australia all believed their ME patients were genuinely ill. And despite encountering scepticism and sometimes unpleasant hostility from medical colleagues, they undoubtedly acted as catalysts in opening up a scientific debate into both cause and management.

As a result, most doctors do now accept that this illness exists, even though they may not like the name ME or the way in which sufferers have campaigned for recognition and research. The ME debate is now moving on to discuss a more suitable name, the possible causes and how patients should best be managed – some very important questions, but no easy answers.

The negative side is that many doctors, whilst being sympathetic to the problems faced by people with ME, remain confused about both diagnosis and management. And this is the prime purpose of my book: to provide comprehensive up-to-date information on all aspects of this illness. By learning about the range of treatment options – both orthodox and alternative – currently available, appropriate changes in lifestyle, benefit provision, and all the practical and emotional aspects of coping with a long-term illness, I hope that you, too, can now make a start on the road to recovery from ME.

*Charles Shepherd*

# PART ONE
# WHAT IS ME/CFS?

# Names, Definitions and Numbers

## A Disease of Many Names

Although most doctors do now accept that ME/CFS is a genuine and disabling illness, an intense debate continues over what it should be called, how it should be defined and how many people are affected. In the next chapter, I look at the history of myalgic encephalomyelitis/chronic fatigue syndrome (ME/CFS) in various parts of the world and explain how early outbreaks led to a confusing variety of names and definitions being adopted – most of which were almost certainly describing people with a very similar illness.

Many of these names – 'Icelandic disease' in Iceland, 'Royal Free disease' in Britain, 'Tapanui flu' in New Zealand – were linked to the geographical locations where relatively small outbreaks took place and which often attracted extensive media publicity. More recently, as it became clear that the vast majority of people with ME/CFS become ill in isolation, yet another set of names began to appear. These have tended to concentrate on describing either the presumed cause (myalgic encephalomyelitis), main symptom (chronic fatigue syndrome) or a combination of both (chronic fatigue and immune dysfunction syndrome or post-viral fatigue syndrome).

### ME (myalgic encephalomyelitis)

This term has become widely accepted in the UK, Canada, Australia, New Zealand, South Africa and some parts of Europe. It is not generally used in America. The World Health Organisation also uses the term 'benign myalgic encephalomyelitis' in its most recent *International Classification of Diseases*, which includes it in the section on 'diseases of the nervous system' (reference: ICD10, G93.3).

ME was originally introduced into medical language by an editorial in *The Lancet* back in 1956 (reference 36) in an attempt to explain the cause of an outbreak at London's Royal Free Hospital the previous year. 'Myalgic' refers to muscle symptoms (fatigue, pain, twitching); 'encephalomyelitis' to brain symptoms (problems with speech, memory, concentration, balance, etc), but the major problem with the term ME is that encephalomyelitis really means inflammation (-itis) within the brain (encephalo-) and spinal cord (myelo-). In fact, very little scientific evidence has emerged over the past 40 years to confirm that any form of ongoing inflammation in the nervous system is actually taking place in ME/CFS. A far more likely explanation of what may be happening in the brain involves alterations to the levels of chemical transmitters, hormones such as cortisol, and blood flow. Consequently, the medical profession is almost unanimous in believing that the name myalgic encephalomyelitis should have a red line placed through it and be abandoned completely – a view which received further strong endorsement in the 1996 Royal Colleges' report into CFS (see pages 438–9).

## CFS (chronic fatigue syndrome)

This description came into common use during the mid-1980s. It is the term currently favoured by most doctors and researchers. Unlike ME, CFS makes no formal assumption about the cause. Instead, it emphasises the chronicity of an illness whose principle symptom is assumed to be fatigue. Almost all the mainstream medical journals and research papers now refer to CFS when describing anyone with this illness.

However, labels are important to patients as well as doctors. Self-help support groups throughout the world have been unanimous in agreeing that the term CFS is neither helpful nor appropriate.

The principle disagreement with CFS is that it is a *totally inadequate description* for the complex range of symptoms and resulting level of disability experienced by most sufferers. Second is the fact that CFS concentrates on only one symptom – fatigue – which is common to a whole range of physical and psychiatric conditions. Many people with ME/CFS state that *fatigue is not their most troublesome or disabling symptom*; they have far greater problems as a result of ongoing "flu-like symptoms or difficulties with normal mental functioning. Third is the way in which CFS is increasingly being used by doctors as a convenient 'dustbin diagnosis' for anyone who comes to the surgery feeling 'tired and unwell' – symptoms which are extremely common amongst the normal adult population and have nothing to do with this illness.

## PVFS (post-viral fatigue syndrome)

This term was introduced during the early 1980s in Britain as an alternative to ME. It remains a useful description for anyone whose illness can clearly be traced back to an acute viral infection. The drawback to PVFS is that it cannot be used to describe cases where some other factor (e.g. vaccination or pesticide) acted as the principal trigger.

## CFIDS (chronic fatigue and immune dysfunction syndrome)

This name has become increasingly popular in America, mainly as a result of it being used by the principal self-help organisation (CFIDS Association). As a longer variant of CFS, it tends to dilute the unpopular 'F' word (fatigue). Although most doctors do now accept that abnormalities in the body's immune response occur quite frequently in ME/CFS, they are neither consistent enough nor sufficiently severe to be incorporated into an official name. CFIDS is seldom used outside America and is rarely mentioned in scientific literature.

## A completely new name?

The present situation, where doctors and their patients are using a variety of different names, is clearly unsatisfactory. Neither is the compromise solution of ME/CFS – the one I intend to use throughout the rest of this book. *A new name, on which everyone can agree, desperately needs to be found.*

Reaching some form of compromise on a new name isn't going to be easy. Some patient support groups have suggested that an eponym (i.e. naming an illness after a well-known person) should be used to recognise the outstanding contribution made by doctors such as Melvin Ramsay, Peter Behan or David Bell, who have done so much to fight for proper recognition and research. Although popular with those who have ME/CFS, such an idea is unlikely to be supported by the medical establishment. Another alternative – the one I currently prefer – is to wait until we know more about what is going wrong in the brain and then see if the resulting pathology suggests a more appropriate name (e.g. a neuroendocrine fatigue syndrome). If, as appears likely, there are consistent abnormalities in the way the brain is functioning in ME/CFS, these findings could be incorporated into a name that attracts widespread support. We could even end up by retaining the name ME, so long as encephalomyelitis is replaced by encephalopathy (which means 'brain disease' to American doctors but has rather more serious implications to their British colleagues).

# Definitions and Diagnostic Criteria

A description of the type of illness seen during the Royal Free outbreak – where some of those affected had obvious neurological symptoms and signs when examined – formed the basis of Dr Melvin Ramsay's definition of ME. He believed that this rested on three main clinical features, namely:

- A unique form of *muscle fatiguability* whereby, even after a minor degree of physical effort, three, four, or five days, or even longer can elapse before full muscle power is restored. Tenderness in the muscle, along with spasms or twitchings, also occurs quite frequently.

- *Circulatory impairment* involving cold extremities (hands and feet), increased sensitivity to climatic change, and episodes of sweating (which can occasionally necessitate a complete change of bedding when they occur at night).
- *Cerebral dysfunction* involving impairment of memory and powers of concentration. Other typical symptoms include difficulties in completing a line of thought, mixing up words (e.g. saying 'hot' when the correct word is 'cold'), sleep disturbances (including a complete reversal of normal sleep patterns) and emotional lability.

In addition, Dr Ramsay noted that all his patients would report on a characteristic variability and fluctuation of symptoms during the course

---

### Table 1: Oxford Criteria (see page 8)

CFS is a syndrome that is characterised by:
- a definite onset
- fatigue as the principal symptom
- fatigue which is severe, disabling and affects both physical and mental functioning
- fatigue which has been present for a minimum of six months during which it was present for more than 50 per cent of the time
- other symptoms which may be present, particularly myalgia (muscle pain), mood and sleep disturbances.

Specific exclusion criteria include:
- an established medical condition known to produce chronic fatigue (e.g. severe anaemia, hypothyroidism)
- a current diagnosis of schizophrenia, manic depression, substance abuse, eating disorder or proven organic brain disease. Other psychiatric disorders (including depressive illness, anxiety disorders and hyperventilation) are not necessarily reasons for exclusion.

Post-infectious fatigue syndrome (PIFS) is defined as:
- a subset of CFS which either follows an infection or is associated with a current infection
- an illness which fulfils the above criteria for CFS.

of a day along with the very strong possibility of the illness becoming chronic and disabling.

Other doctors and academics then went on to develop their own definitions as to what they felt constituted ME/CFS/PVFS/CFIDS, etc, which only added to the confusion. *I still believe that Dr Melvin Ramsay's original definition is the best clinical description of the lot!* (See also Further Reading on page 438.)

The first internationally agreed definition of CFS emerged following publicity associated with the outbreak at Lake Tahoe in the state of

---

**Table 2: CDC Criteria (see above)**

CFS is a syndrome characterised by fatigue that is:
- medically unexplained (i.e. not caused by conditions such as anaemia)
- of new onset (i.e. not life-long)
- of at least six months' duration
- not the result of ongoing exertion (e.g. overwork or athletic over-training)
- not substantially relieved by rest
- causing a substantial reduction in previous levels of occupational, educational, social or personal activities.

In addition, there must be *four or more* of the following symptoms:
- self-reported problems with short-term memory or concentration (cognitive defects)
- sore throats
- tender neck (cervical) or armpit (axillary) glands
- muscle pain (myalgia)
- headaches of a new type, pattern or severity
- unrefreshing sleep
- post-exertional malaise lasting more than 24 hours
- multi-joint pain (arthralgia) without swelling or redness.

Conditions which would *exclude* a diagnosis of CFS include:
- established medical disorders known to cause chronic fatigue
- major depressive illness with psychotic or melancholic features (but *not* anxiety states, somatisation disorder or non-melancholic/psychotic depression)
- any medication which causes fatigue as a side-effect
- eating disorders – anorexia, bulimia or severe obesity
- alcohol or substance abuse.

Nevada, USA (see pages 15–17). This was produced by a group of doctors meeting at the Centre for Disease Control in Atlanta in 1987 (reference 2).

Around the same time, a group of Australian researchers, headed by Professor Andrew Lloyd, published their CFS diagnostic criteria, which contained an added emphasis on neuropsychological symptoms (references 5 and 23).

In 1990, a group of UK experts devised the so-called 'Oxford criteria' which included a specific subgroup whose illness had clearly been triggered by some form of infection (reference 6).

The recently updated version of the CDC criteria was developed by the International CFS Study Group meeting in America and published in the *Annals of Internal Medicine* in December 1994 (reference 1). This has now become the most widely used and accepted definition for anyone carrying out research.

Unfortunately, just as with the *name* CFS, there are also a number of major disadvantages to the way current diagnostic criteria are used to *define* the illness.

First is the fact that CFS has become an umbrella term covering a number of different conditions in which fatigue is a prominent feature. Second is the way in which CFS fails to satisfactorily exclude people whose fatigue is the most prominent symptom of a pre-existing psychiatric problem such as depression or somatisation (physical symptoms being caused by a psychological illness). In cases such as this, making a diagnosis of CFS becomes superfluous and may well produce major problems for the person concerned. Third is the fact that a diagnosis of CFS cannot be made until the symptom complex has been present for at least six months. This is fine when it comes to selecting patients for research studies, but is of no practical value to ordinary working doctors who should be making the diagnosis well before six months have elapsed and initiating an appropriate plan of management.

We may well have to wait several years before the name CFS is changed to something more acceptable. Further revisions to the way CFS is currently defined clearly need to be made much more rapidly. For more detailed discussion on the current CDC definition see reference 4.

## How Many People Have ME/CFS?

Epidemiology – the study of epidemics and how many people are affected by a particular illness, along with details of their age, sex and social class – forms a vital part of trying to understand something as complex as ME/CFS. Not surprisingly, this is yet another area in which there is considerable confusion and disagreement.

One of the main problems in the past has been that data have largely been obtained from people who were involved in minor outbreaks of ME/CFS and this information is different from that seen in individual cases – these who now form the vast majority of people with this illness.

Despite the fact that the media often portray people with ME/CFS as being white, female, middle class and middle aged, the truth is that this illness affects both sexes and occurs across a wide spectrum of age, race and social class.

There are currently around 20 different published research studies which have looked at various aspects of ME/CFS epidemiology (references 7–28). Some of these studies contain a number of highly questionable conclusions about ME/CFS, particularly those which have failed to properly distinguish between people who are just suffering from some degree of chronic fatigue and those who have well-defined Chronic Fatigue Syndrome.

One undisputed fact that has emerged from studies carried out in America, Australia and the UK is that chronic fatigue – as opposed to ME/CFS – is an extremely common problem in the community. Somewhere between 10 and 20 per cent of all adults visiting a GP admit to feeling more tired than they should. For a significant minority this is the principal reason for their visit to the doctor. There is an almost endless list of physical and psychological illnesses that produce chronic fatigue as the first or main complaint. Some of the more important ones, which are frequently confused with ME/CFS, are considered in more detail in Chapter 6. Only a very small percentage of people visiting their doctor complaining of fatigue actually turn out to have ME/CFS.

## Prevalence* of ME/CFS

Research studies which have attempted to estimate the true prevalence of ME/CFS in the adult population have produced a wide range of results. In America, the CDC currently estimates a *minimum figure* of 4 to 10 cases for every 100,000 adults over the age of 18. In Britain, the 1996 Royal Colleges' report into CFS concluded that the illness was far more widespread and quoted a figure of between 1 and 2 per cent of the population. In Australia, a survey of people living in the Richmond Valley area of New South Wales, which was carried out in 1988, produced a figure of 37 cases per 100,000 (reference 23).

My own view, based on a critical analysis of all the published infor- mation to date, as well as speaking to large numbers of doctors who

* The total number of cases of an illness at a given time in a given area

recognise ME/CFS when they see it, is that this illness affects around 1 to 2 per thousand of the population. This produces a total figure of between 50,000 and 100,000 here in the UK. In the continuing absence of good-quality epidemiological studies, the true figure remains uncertain.

Other important information to emerge from epidemiological studies concerns the age, sex and social class of people with ME/CFS.

## Age at onset

A number of studies (references 16, 17 and 137) suggest that the commonest age of onset lies between 20 and 40, with the most frequent starting-point being in the early thirties. Possible explanations as to why age may be a factor in the development of ME/CFS are discussed on pages 27–28.

## Sex differences

Almost all published studies show that females are more likely to develop ME/CFS than males although there doesn't appear to be any significant difference when it comes to the type of symptoms experienced (reference 9). The overall conclusion is that around 60 to 70 per cent of people with ME/CFS are female, but one important study from Belfast, Northern Ireland (reference 16), noted that in those under the age of 20 there was no difference at all. Some of the possible reasons why women appear to be more susceptible to developing ME/CFS are discussed on pages 29–30.

## Social class

Despite the media's obsession with the derogatory term 'Yuppie 'flu', the evidence is that this is an illness which affects all social classes and occupational groups (references 14 and 17).

Health workers and teachers do, however, appear to be over-represented in some of the studies carried out on patients attending specialist referral centres. This probably reflects the fact that there are two groups of people who are unlikely to accept feeble explanations about why they feel so ill!

# The History of ME/CFS in Different Parts of the World

Before looking at some of the numerous outbreaks of ME/CFS that have hit the headlines over the past 70 years, it is worth noting that this is not a new illness confined to the twentieth century. The combination of diverse neurological and muscular symptoms which follow an infective illness has almost certainly been around for very much longer. As early as 1750, Sir Richard Manningham described a syndrome he termed *febricula*, or 'little fever', which presented with numerous physical symptoms but few objective clinical signs (reference 38). There have also been suggestions in medical literature that Florence Nightingale (reference 46), Elizabeth Barrett Browning (reference 47) and Charles Darwin (reference 32) were all early victims of the illness we now call ME/CFS.

'Neurasthenia' was a term that was commonly used in America during the mid-nineteenth century to describe an illness that mainly affected young women. It was often preceded by an infection and thought at the time to be due to some form of 'weakness' in the nervous system. The term neurasthenia gradually went out of fashion, and although some of these young women probably had what we now call ME/CFS, in others the diagnosis was far less certain.

It wasn't until 1934 (in America) and 1955 (in the UK) that the medical profession started to give this subject any serious attention. Following publicity surrounding two famous outbreaks it soon became apparent that ME/CFS wasn't just confined to these two countries. Similar reports of an ME/CFS-like illness started to emerge from other parts of Europe, Australia and South Africa. As a result the illness acquired a confusing variety of names along the way: 'Chronic Fatigue and Immune Dysfunction Syndrome' in the USA, 'Icelandic disease' in Iceland, 'Tapanui 'flu' in New Zealand and 'Low Natural Killer Cell Syndrome' in Japan.

## The Royal Free Disease

In the late spring of 1955, the infectious disease unit at London's Royal Free Hospital began admitting patients from all over north London with an unusual collection of symptoms (reference 41).

Initially the illness was unremarkable, with respiratory symptoms, sore throat, enlarged lymph glands and a slight fever. Some patients had a gastric upset and a few had marked dizziness (vertigo). Then, instead of slowly improving, new symptoms started to appear – headaches, blurred or even double vision (diplopia) and abnormal sensations in the skin (paraesthesiae). All the patients had difficulties with brain functioning, particularly short-term memory and concentration, but the most striking feature was the severity of muscle fatigue caused by even the most limited exercise. Many patients also had cold hands and feet, were troubled by bladder disturbances and were extremely sensitive to any change in external temperatures.

Doctors at the Royal Free were in no doubt: their patients had an infection that the body's front line of defence – the lymphatic glands – seemed unable to filter out, and it was spreading to the nerves and muscles. However, no such illness had been clearly defined in the textbooks.

The degree of muscle weakness initially suggested polio – still a possibility in those days – but there was no muscle wasting taking place, which is one of polio's most characteristic features. Investigations failed to confirm the presence of polio, so the doctors were left with an infection looking for a cause.

Some patients were given an EEG (electroencephalogram) to measure brain activity. A few showed abnormalities, and an assumption was made that they were experiencing a form of brain inflammation (encephalitis), probably caused by a virus, but not the polio virus.

The most dramatic events of that year involved the Royal Free's own medical and nursing staff. An outbreak of infective illness started on 13 July, and over the following 12 days, 70 doctors and nurses were taken ill. So many staff became involved that the hospital was forced to close, and remained so until 5 October. In all, there were 292 cases, but only 12 of the hospital's patients – who were resting in bed – were taken ill.

Just like the cases admitted earlier, the hospital staff's illness followed a characteristic pattern of symptoms we now associate with ME/CFS. First came the non-specific 'flu-like illness with the sort of symptoms that can occur in any viral infection. Following this acute onset some of the staff had a short period of remission during which they began to improve. Then it became obvious that their defence mechanisms had failed to limit the spread of the presumed infection, and that it was now affecting their brain, nerves and muscles. They all started to feel ill again with the characteristic features of brain malfunction, nervous disturbances and overwhelming muscular fatigue.

Unlike most people who now develop ME/CFS following an infection, many of those involved at the Royal Free had definite abnormalities in their nerves, which could be demonstrated on clinical examination. Nearly 20 per cent developed a paralysis of the facial nerve – the one which controls our facial expressions – and 11 had paralysis of swallowing, even having to be tube-fed. Clinical examination showed that the nervous system had been affected in 74 per cent of cases.

Two other important features of the illness that emerged from this outbreak were muscle pain (sometimes intense) and changes in skin sensations. Doctors found that the slightest movement of one of the weakened limbs could result in severe pain, and there was often pain below the ribs which coincided with extreme tenderness in the corresponding muscles. Other patients had significant areas where skin sensation was lost (hypoaesthesiae); in some cases this involved half the body. Twenty-eight of the cases were investigated with electromyograms (EMG), which show how messages are transmitted from the brain via the nerves to the muscles. The results suggested that there were definite abnormalities in the way these messages were being transmitted at the level of the spinal cord. This led to the suggestion that inflammation in this part of the nervous system (= myelitis) could be responsible.

The dramatic way in which this mystery illness closed a major hospital made headline news; the papers called it 'the Royal Free disease'. But the inconclusive nature of the tests, which failed to isolate the cause, left many members of the medical profession sceptical and they soon lost interest in further research. Some patients quickly improved but others have remained permanently disabled. One person who did not forget their plight was Dr Melvin Ramsay, consultant physician in the infectious diseases unit. He published a report in *The Lancet* on some of the cases at the Royal Free the year after the outbreak, in which a leading article described the disease as 'A New Clinical Entity?', and suggested it be named 'benign myalgic encephalomyelitis' (reference 36).

What happened at the Royal Free made ME/CFS briefly famous, but there have been other, less spectacular outbreaks – over 70 in fact – reported world-wide, particularly in affluent countries with temperate climates. Outbreaks seem to occur more frequently in closed communities such as schools, hospitals and barracks, where an infectious disease can spread quickly.

## Other Outbreaks of ME/CFS in Britain

In 1952, an infectious disease, never identified, but which appeared to be similar to ME/CFS, broke out at the Middlesex Hospital in London. In 1955, just before the Royal Free outbreak, there was a cluster of cases with classic ME/CFS symptoms at a primary school in Cumbria in the north of England. A small outbreak in a teacher-training college in Newcastle-upon-Tyne occurred in 1959. The cases here supported the theory that – as with polio – physical stress during the acute infection was an important co-factor in the development of ME/CFS. The student teachers shared their accommodation with a group of nuns; the students developed ME/CFS, but the nuns, who were naturally leading a very quiet life, did not.

During 1964–6 a large number of cases was reported from the north London practice of Dr Betty Scott, who observed that many of her patients had low levels of blood sugar (hypoglycaemia).

One further outbreak of interest occurred during 1970–1 at London's Great Ormond Street Children's Hospital. Once again, those affected were mainly nursing staff, and none of the children on the wards at the time succumbed. There were nearly 150 cases in all. The Great Ormond Street nurses had a list of almost identical symptoms to those experienced at the Royal Free, and again went on to follow the familiar pattern of remission followed by relapse or continuing disability.

In 1970, the *British Medical Journal* published a paper by two psychiatrists, Drs McEvedy and Beard (reference 40), which concluded that the Royal Free outbreak had been due to mass hysteria. The effect on medical opinion was profound – ME/CFS became a 'dustbin diagnosis' and a subject that few doctors were prepared to take seriously.

One prominent physician who went against the tide of medical opinion was Peter Behan, Professor of Neurology at the Institute of Neurological Sciences in Glasgow. During the late 1970s and early 1980s he started to see a growing number of ME/CFS patients from all over the country who were being referred to his neurological clinic. Professor Behan became more and more convinced that they had a genuine organic disorder affecting their brain, muscles and immune system. He also became involved with the local general practitioners such as Drs Keighley, Calder and Warnock, who had witnessed minor outbreaks in their practices in Balfron and Helensburgh on the Clyde (references 322, 323 and 326).

In 1985, Professor Behan's first major research paper on the subject was published in the *Journal of Infection* (reference 131), documenting clear abnormalities which were not psychologically based. This was soon followed by steadily increasing interest from both the medical and lay media. In the UK, the diagnosis once again became 'acceptable' and before long an almost unknown illness became one on which all doctors had strong opinions – even if some weren't all that complimentary!

And, as you will read in the following chapters, the debate, at last, opened up as to what was really going wrong in ME/CFS.

# ME/CFS in the USA

In the United States, the condition has been referred to as 'neurasthenia' (reference 31), 'epidemic neuromyasthenia' (reference 34), 'chronic Epstein-Barr virus disease' and 'CFIDS' – the Chronic Fatigue and Immune Dysfunction Syndrome. The first ever recorded outbreak involved doctors and nurses at the Los Angeles County General Hospital in 1934. At first, the illness was thought to be due to polio, but although the patients' muscles remained weak they did not become wasted, so this explanation seemed unlikely (reference 33). Nearly 200 members of staff were affected and when they were thoroughly reviewed six months later half were still unwell. Further small outbreaks continued to be reported from various parts of the USA, but the American public did not really become aware of the condition until 1985, when following an outbreak at Lake Tahoe, Nevada, media attention became overwhelming (reference 30).

The shores of Lake Tahoe are a retreat for successful, active, professional 'high achievers' – the last type of person to stay away from work without good reason. Late in 1984 strange things started happening in the area – previously fit adults in their thirties and forties began to fall ill with a mysterious 'flu-like illness which was followed by the classic muscular fatigue and intellectual malfunction associated with ME/CFS. So many were involved that one magazine labelled the area 'Raggedy Ann Town', as the people involved said they felt like Raggedy Ann dolls. But with all their blood results being reported as normal, many doctors began to query whether these patients had a genuine physical illness.

Fortunately, two doctors, Dan Peterson and Paul Cheney, didn't share these doubts; they became increasingly convinced that the steady stream of patients arriving at their consulting rooms were genuinely ill. These patients had sore throats, glandular swellings and headaches, and the doctors wondered whether this might be glandular fever (called infectious mononucleosis in America).

The problem was that glandular fever is a teenage disease; patients in the age group affected should have developed antibodies and be immune to the virus by now. Nevertheless, the similarity with glandular fever led Peterson and Cheney to research Epstein-Barr virus (EBV) as a possible causative agent.

Epstein-Barr virus belongs to the herpes group of viruses, which causes cold sores, genital herpes and chicken-pox. EBV is passed on from person to person by saliva – hence the term 'kissing disease' for glandular fever. Carriers of the disease can even pass it on without developing it themselves. By the age of 30, nearly 90 per cent of all adults will have developed antibodies to EBV, indicating a full degree of immunity, so after this age an attack of glandular fever becomes increasingly rare.

All viruses in the herpes group have a capacity to stay on in the body after causing an initial infection, acting as a reservoir of dormant infection. So once a person has been infected by EBV, the virus doesn't go away. EBV remains for life, usually without causing any harm, in the salivary glands and the B cells of the immune system, which are responsible for antibody production. The virus is kept in check by other cells of the immune system known as natural killer cells.

What Doctors Peterson and Cheney began to wonder was whether the Epstein-Barr virus, lying dormant in the B cells, had been reactivated to produce symptoms of the unusual fatigue syndrome that they were witnessing at Lake Tahoe. In other words, was something weakening the body's immune system, which up until then had successfully prevented the dormant EBV from becoming active? Was EBV multiplying, and leaving the B cells to start a further episode of glandular fever, from an original infection which the patients had picked up during childhood? After all, other members of the herpes group of viruses can be reactivated from their dormant stage, given the right circumstances. Herpes cold sores will reappear at times of stress, during menstruation, in hot sun, or when someone is feeling run down – exactly the same sort of stimuli which can cause a relapse or exacerbation of ME/CFS.

Doctors Cheney and Peterson decided to look for evidence of Epstein-Barr virus in the Lake Tahoe patients. They found raised antibodies to EBV in about three-quarters, but this still left a quarter with normal levels and a small percentage with no antibodies at all. The hypothesis was further complicated by the fact that EBV antibody tests are difficult to interpret and that the Lake Tahoe patients produced a fairly similar spread of results to those which could be expected from a similar group of normal healthy controls.

In the meantime the American press and broadcasting media had become extremely interested in the 'mystery virus' and the outbreak was now receiving extensive publicity throughout the United States. The magazine *Newsweek* referred to it as 'the malaise of the 80s'. Other papers used the name 'yuppie 'flu', as so many of those affected were fit young professionals. Somewhat prematurely, the name chronic Epstein-Barr disease became the accepted term and a national self-help group was founded. It was soon receiving requests for information from all over the USA, and pressure was put on Congress for a proper research programme to be initiated.

Blood samples were sent to Robert Gallo, the scientist who had been working on the AIDS virus at the National Cancer Institute, and who had recently isolated the first 'new' herpes virus (human herpes virus type

6/HHV–6) for 20 years. As a result HHV–6 became the next 'culprit' virus to be linked to ME/CFS (see pages 128–9).

The Lake Tahoe outbreak eventually subsided, but as in all the other epidemics already described, many of those who were taken ill have still not recovered. It seems that about one third improved; about one half followed the familiar pattern of remission alternating with relapse; the rest remain chronically unwell.

## New Viruses Emerge

As the AIDS epidemic gathered pace during the late 1980s, enormous sums of money were spent in trying to identify the virus responsible for this devastating infection. The cause turned out to be HIV (human immunodeficiency virus), which belongs to a group known as retroviruses. All these viruses contain a unique fingerprint enzyme called reverse transcriptase, hence the name RE-TR-ovirus: RE for 'reverse' and TR for 'transcriptase'. The reverse transcriptase is a vital enzyme which is involved in the way the virus makes copies of itself once inside the cell. In the past, these retroviruses had been linked to rare cases of leukaemia in animals, but never to any form of human illness. In the case of HIV infection, a picture slowly emerged of a 'new' virus which was capable of attacking key parts of the human immune system – the T helper cells. Two other viruses in the same group, human T cell leukaemia viruses 1 and 2 (HTLV1 and HTLV2), also became linked with leukaemia and neurological diseases. Researchers in the States then began to query whether there could be a link between retroviruses and ME/CFS.

Dr Paul Cheney enlisted the help of Dr Elaine DeFreitas, a virologist, working on HTLV research at the prestigious Wistar Institute in Philadelphia. In March 1988, Dr Cheney sent six blood samples from ME/CFS patients to the Wistar – they all turned out to have antibodies to HTLV. During the summer of 1988 he widened the project by enlisting the help of Dr David Bell, a paediatrician from Lyndonville, New York, who had recently become involved in caring for children with ME/CFS. A larger batch of blood samples was then sent to Dr DeFreitas, including some from healthy people to act as controls.

Using a new technique for magnifying viral genetic codes (the polymerase chain reaction), Dr DeFreitas set about looking for evidence of retroviral infection. The study took her two years to complete, but the final results suggested that about 80 per cent of the adults and 70 per cent of the children did have evidence of genetic material from HTLV2 (reference 354).

However, other researchers, including those at the Centre for

Disease Control (CDC) in the States, and Professor Peter Behan in Glasgow were unable to replicate these findings. It is possible that the viral DNA sequences found by Dr DeFreitas are very similar to those which can be found in normal cells, and so a big question mark still hangs over any link between ME/CFS and retroviruses (references 355–357).

Further evidence to support a retroviral connection appeared shortly afterwards from Dr John Martin and his colleagues, working at the University of Southern California. Using a similar type of genetic probe, they claimed to have found a spumavirus – a subgroup of the retro- viruses – which had not been associated with any human disease.

The spumavirus is also known as a foamy virus because of the 'foamy' appearance it can create in infected cells. Dr Martin's claims about find- ing evidence of a spumavirus in more than 200 patients with ME/CFS were received with considerable scepticism when he presented them to a meeting at the CDC in September 1990. At the time they received con- siderable media publicity in *Newsweek* and the *New York Times* but not in the mainstream medical journals. Even so, reports continue to appear in the medical literature about possible links with this type of virus (ref- erences 314).

Further evidence of a link with herpes-type infections came in 1992 when Dr Dedra Buchwald and Professor Tony Komaroff's team reported in the *Annals of Internal Medicine* (reference 258) that two human her- pes viruses were *actively replicating* in a significant number of patients which they had examined – many of whom had first become ill in the communities around Lake Tahoe. The new evidence for an HHV–6 con- nection came from laboratory experiments in which the patients' white blood cells were placed in a special culture. The resulting cellular changes were highly characteristic of HHV–6 damage and further con- firmation of the presence of active HHV–6 came from the use of mono- clonal antibodies and polymerase chain reaction analysis.

As with Epstein-Barr virus infection, most adults come into contact with HHV–6 during childhood, after which the virus lies dormant. Dr Buchwald and Professor Komaroff's findings suggest that some external factor (infection, stress, toxin) has produced an upset in immune system regulation which, in turn, leads to a *reactivation* of HHV–6 from its dor- mant state. At the moment we can only speculate as to whether HHV–6 then goes on to affect nerve cells and produce symptoms, but the possi- bility is certainly there.

In America, the subject of ME/CFS is now being taken very seriously. The US Congress has granted a considerable sum of money to original research and a growing number of highly respected scientists are now becoming involved in looking at all aspects of the illness.

As in the UK, a number of self-help groups have emerged during the past 15 years. Undoubtedly the most influential is the CFIDS Association, whose headquarters are in Charlotte, North Carolina. Besides publishing the regular *CFIDS Chronicle* (a highly authoritative and comprehensive review of current medical research and treatment) this group has been responsible for stimulating and financing various research programmes in the United States. The CFIDS Association also organises regular conferences which involve clinicians, researchers and patient participation. Overseas membership is welcomed – see Useful Addresses, page 404.

# ME/CFS in Europe

## Denmark

Thanks to a small but extremely active self-help support group (see Useful Addresses, page 406), ME/CFS is now starting to be recognised by the medical profession and treated sympathetically by the media. However, some doctors still remain hostile to the idea that ME/CFS could be a genuine medical illness. There are a small number of specialists who are willing to offer help with diagnosis, but few doctors have managed to gain the necessary experience from seeing large numbers of patients to offer comprehensive advice on management. A number of small research projects have been carried out, but ME/CFS does not yet have the same research status as in either the UK or USA.

Despite these improvements, considerable problems still exist for many people with ME/CFS living in Denmark, especially in locations where there are no sympathetic doctors, and in the important area of pension provision.

## Iceland

An outbreak here during 1948 was of particular interest for a number of reasons. First, it followed several cases of polio around the small northern township of Akureyri. Altogether there were over 1,000 cases, mainly in high-school children. Second, when an epidemic of polio swept around the coastal areas of Iceland in 1955, the Akureyri township was unaffected. It appeared that the original infective agent (presumably a virus) had produced, just like a vaccination, a degree of immunity to polio. This strongly suggested that both infections were linked and possibly belonged to the enteroviral group. When these children were subsequently given their polio vaccination, they responded by producing unusually high levels of antibodies to polio, suggesting that they might have already been exposed to a similar infection. Last, when the

Akureyri patients were re-examined by a distinguished neurologist in 1955, only 25 per cent of them had gone on to make a complete recovery. The remainder still suffered from significant degrees of muscle fatigue and brain malfunction. A further assessment, carried out in May 1988, indicated that some of these patients continued to experience a considerable degree of disability (reference 35).

Incidentally, on a more positive note, there is apparently no hostility or scepticism about ME/CFS from the Icelandic medical profession!

## The Netherlands

It has been estimated that around 70 per cent of Dutch doctors do now recognise ME/CFS as a genuine illness, mainly as a result of campaigning by the Dutch self-help support group based in Amsterdam (see Useful Addresses, page 406) and the fact that Dutch medical journals contain regular contributions about the illness.

Apart from Italy and the UK, this is the only other European country where a significant amount of research is taking place into both cause and management of the illness. Much of this work is being carried out by Professor Van der Meer and colleagues at the University of Nijmegen.

Although the situation for patients in the Netherlands is steadily improving, some people are still experiencing difficulties in obtaining sickness benefits.

## Norway

Diagnosis and good management advice still present considerable difficulties for patients in several parts of Norway. However, the health authorities and a growing number of specialists are now taking the illness seriously. There are also plans to open a specialist centre in one of the main Bergen hospitals. An extremely effective self-help support group, organised by Mrs Ellen Piro, is based in Østeras (see Useful Addresses, page 406).

## Other European countries

Although there is growing recognition and a considerable amount of research activity taking place in the UK, Italy and the Netherlands, the same cannot be said for the rest of Europe.

A small number of research studies are underway in Belgium and Sweden, but the degree of interest and knowledge amongst the remainder of the medical profession remains extremely patchy. Almost all of the campaigning is, as usual, left to support groups, the most active of which are in Belgium, Germany, Italy, Norway and Switzerland (see Useful Addresses, pages 405–7).

In countries such as France (where ME/CFS is sometimes referred to as *spasmophile*), Portugal and Spain, there is little or no interest from the medical profession and there are no national self-help groups providing information or support.

# ME/CFS in Other Parts of the World

## *Australia*

The history of ME/CFS in Australia dates back to 1949, when a major epidemic occurred in Adelaide (reference 42). As with many of the other early outbreaks, there was a close and interesting link with poliomyelitis. The polio epidemic started in May of that year, but it wasn't till August that cases of ME/CFS started to appear. These continued right through until April 1951, by which time nearly 700 people had been admitted to hospital. No virus was ever isolated, but when material from two of the patients was inoculated into monkeys, damage to the sciatic nerve could clearly be seen under the microscope.

Since the late 1980s, doctors such as John Dwyer, Ian Hickie, Andrew Lloyd and Denis Wakefield, from the University of New South Wales CFS Research Team, have achieved international recognition for their important contributions towards our better understanding of this illness, particularly in the areas of immunology, infection and practical management. Doctors Hugh Dunstan, Neil MacGregor and colleagues at the University of Newcastle are also carrying out innovative research into the presence of what appears to be abnormal chemical markers (CFSUMs) in the urine of people with ME/CFS (see page 158).

Public understanding and awareness of ME/CFS have greatly improved during the same period, mainly due to the work of self-help groups in the various states (see Useful Addresses, pages 404–5), along with help from supportive doctors. Sadly, however, there is still a significant minority of Australian doctors who refuse to even accept that ME/CFS exists as an illness. As in the UK, funding of some of the most important research studies has only been achieved thanks to the work of self-help groups.

In 1998, a Working Group convened by the Royal Australian College of Physicians produced guidelines on the diagnosis and management of patients with ME/CFS (see page 439).

## *Canada*

Up until recently, recognition of ME/CFS by both the Canadian government and the medical profession has lagged behind that in the UK and USA. This has been partly due to the fact that there have never been any major outbreaks of ME/CFS in Canadian schools or hospitals to attract media attention.

The major force for change in Canada has been ME Canada, the principal self-help organisation based in Ottawa (see Useful Addresses, page 405). Besides producing an extremely informative magazine, *The Messenger*, ME Canada actively campaigns on a range of issues relating to research, benefit and welfare matters, and educational provision for children with ME/CFS.

Canadian doctors are also making some interesting contributions to research into ME/CFS. Among the most important is the work being carried out by Professor Harvey Moldofsky, from Toronto, into sleep disturbances in both fibromyalgia and ME/CFS (see page 156).

## Japan

Interest in immunological abnormalities associated with ME/CFS has led some Japanese doctors to refer to this illness as the 'low natural killer cell syndrome'. Others, such as Dr Hirohiko Kuratsune at Osaka University Medical School, have been involved in research into muscle abnormalities, particularly carnitine deficiency (see page 140). Research is also being carried out into a possible link with Borna virus, an infection which normally affects cattle and sheep. One report, again from the Osaka Medical School, indicated that genetic material from this virus was found in 32 per cent of a small group of ME/CFS patients (reference 316). However, Professor Behan's research group in Glasgow has been unable to find any evidence to support such a link in UK patients (reference 313).

Despite the obvious interest being shown by a small number of hospital researchers, there is very little information or advice available to members of the public in Japan. Consequently, many patients remain undiagnosed or misdiagnosed.

## New Zealand

A well-publicised outbreak of ME/CFS occurred during 1984 in a rural part of Western Otago in the South Island of New Zealand (reference 43). These patients developed extreme fatigue four to six weeks after an initial 'flu-like illness. It was quite clear that all of this group of patients were part of a very hard-working, conscientious community who had obviously succumbed to an illness which was not psychological. Not surprisingly, New Zealanders found their own name for ME/CFS at this time – 'Tapanui 'flu'.

In 1997, the results of a 10-year follow-up study on 21 of these Tapanui patients was published in the *Archives of Internal Medicine* (reference 37). Sixteen had managed to return to their normal level of functioning, although some needed to modify their lifestyle in order to prevent relapses. The relatively high proportion of patients showing full recovery suggests that epidemic-associated ME/CFS may have a better outlook than is seen in isolated cases.

Much of the early research work in New Zealand was carried out by Professor Campbell Murdoch and Dr Mike Holmes at the University of Otago Medical School. They, too, have looked at retroviruses as a possible cause and Dr Holmes is currently involved in a study into the immunological aspects, particularly natural killer (NK) cell activity.

Also working at the Otago Medical School is Dr Les Simpson, an expert in haematology (the study of blood). He has published some interesting findings on possible abnormalities in the shape of red blood cells in ME/CFS. Using a high-powered electron microscope, Dr Simpson has found that some red cells (which carry oxygen around the body) are not their usual shape. The result, he suggests, is that the cells are less able to pass down the smallest blood vessels (capillaries) which supply oxygen and vital nutrients to tissues such as brain and muscle (references: *New Zealand Medical Journal*, 1989, 102, 106–107; 1992, 105, 136 and 501).

Dr Ros Vallings, a general practitioner from Auckland, is also carrying out research into the epidemiology/outcome of ME/CFS and the role of hormonal disturbances.

Recognition of ME/CFS by both the public and medical profession is slowly becoming more widespread, but there are still some 'black holes' when it comes to finding a sympathetic doctor. Although most patients tend to be managed by general practitioners, there is an increasing number of specialists who are becoming interested in and knowledgeable about ME/CFS.

A very active support group called ANZMES (Associated New Zealand Myalgic Encephalomyelitis Societies Incorporated) is based in Auckland (see Useful Addresses, page 406). ANZMES is not only a campaigning and support organisation; it also raises a considerable amount of money for research activity. *Meeting Place*, its regular magazine, is an extremely useful source of information.

## South Africa

In 1955, a few months earlier than the Royal Free outbreak in London, an almost mirror-image situation occurred 6,000 miles away in Durban, South Africa. Once again, as in Iceland and Adelaide, there were close connections with an outbreak of polio. The South African cases occurred at the same time as polio was rife in Durban. In the beginning it was the nursing staff at Addington Hospital who were mainly affected, but as time went on, cases were admitted from the surrounding general population, just as happened in London. Many of these nurses quickly relapsed when they returned to work on the wards and several had to accept early retirement from nursing as a result of chronic disablement.

ME/CFS is slowly starting to be recognised by the medical profession in South Africa despite the fact that very little information appears in South African medical journals. Unfortunately, some of those doctors who do now accept that ME/CFS exists believe that it is simply a form of depression. The lack of reliable information means that inappropriate or even harmful approaches to treatment are sometimes recommended, especially in the case of children. Claims for long-term disability insurance benefits may also be turned down on the grounds that ME/CFS does not cause severe or permanent disability.

The ME Association of South Africa (MEASA) is based in Kwa Zulu Natal (see Useful Addresses, page 407). MEASA is working with a group of sympathetic doctors to improve medical recognition and stimulate research into ME/CFS (there are no accurate figures on how many people are affected in South Africa). They also maintain a close watch on new 'cures', which appear quite frequently in South Africa.

## Further Reading

*Myalgic Encephalomyelitis and Postviral Fatigue States: The Saga of Royal Free Disease* by Dr Melvin Ramsay (Gower Medical Publishing). A unique description of the history of ME/CFS, which includes detailed accounts of early outbreaks in various parts of the world along with the author's recollections of the events at the Royal Free Hospital during 1955. Copies are available from the ME Association (see Useful Addresses, page 399).

# What Causes ME/CFS?

'Why me?' is a question that anyone suffering from chronic disability wants an answer to. In the case of ME/CFS, why is it that large numbers of previously fit young adults and children should suddenly be struck down with such a devastating illness?

Following the outbreak at London's Royal Free Hospital back in 1955, doctors were left with more questions than answers. ME/CFS had all the characteristics of being triggered by an infection, presumably a virus, which didn't seem to have been dealt with by the body's immune system in a normal efficient manner. But which virus or viruses were responsible? Did a virus then persist and multiply inside the body to cause persisting symptoms? Or were there more complex reasons to explain the continuing ill health? Clearly a great deal of research needed to be carried out in the areas of virology, immunology, muscle function and brain abnormalities, to find out what was 'going wrong'.

Dr Melvin Ramsay, the Royal Free Hospital's infectious disease specialist, remained convinced that ME/CFS was a genuine organic illness. Sadly, many of his colleagues became increasingly sceptical, so it wasn't easy to persuade good-quality researchers to become involved in looking for a cause. And 15 years after the Royal Free outbreak, two psychiatrists dealt a severe blow to the credibility of ME/CFS when they published a paper in the *British Medical Journal* (reference 40) concluding that the illness was hysterical. The medical establishment didn't challenge this view and most doctors became convinced that ME/CFS was 'all in the mind'.

Despite all these setbacks, researchers such as Professor Behan at Glasgow University believed that their ME/CFS patients were genuinely ill. During the 1980s Professor Behan managed to once again stimulate real interest in finding the cause of ME/CFS.

It now appears that ME/CFS may be a three-stage illness involving: (a) predisposing factors which make people more susceptible; (b) events which then act as stressors on the immune system and so trigger the onset; and (c) factors which are then responsible for perpetuating the symptoms and resulting disability. In the remainder of this chapter I'll look at those factors which may *predispose* to or *precipitate* the onset of ME/CFS. Chapter 8, on current research, examines those factors which may *perpetuate* ME/CFS.

# What causes ME/CFS?

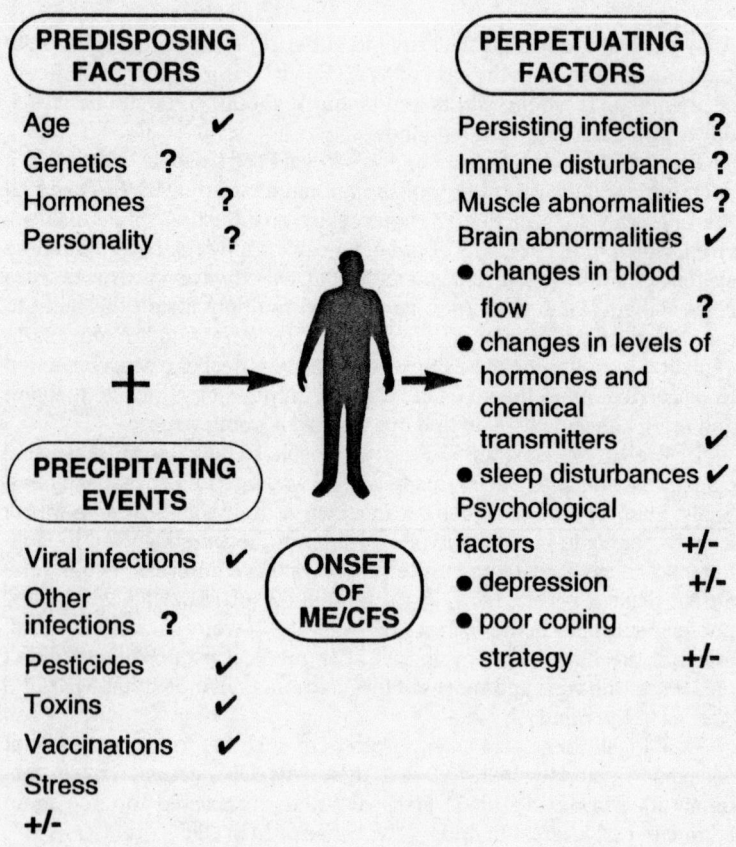

**PREDISPOSING FACTORS**

Age ✔
Genetics ?
Hormones ?
Personality ?

**PRECIPITATING EVENTS**

Viral infections ✔
Other infections ?
Pesticides ✔
Toxins ✔
Vaccinations ✔
Stress +/-

**ONSET OF ME/CFS**

**PERPETUATING FACTORS**

Persisting infection ?
Immune disturbance ?
Muscle abnormalities ?
Brain abnormalities ✔
● changes in blood flow ?
● changes in levels of hormones and chemical transmitters ✔
● sleep disturbances ✔
Psychological factors +/-
● depression +/-
● poor coping strategy +/-

? = role as yet uncertain
✔ = reliable research evidence now present
+/- = relevant in some cases

# Predisposing Factors

A number of different factors probably play a role in deciding who goes on to develop ME/CFS when the right 'trigger' – be it infection, vaccination, toxin or some other form of major stressful event – comes along. Among the more important are your age, your genetic make up, your sex, and psychological influences such as ongoing stress, personality and previous mental health problems.

## Age

This is already recognised to play an important role in how people react to a wide variety of infections. 'Childhood illnesses' such as rubella, mumps and chicken-pox often affect adults far more severely than they do children. And when children become infected with Epstein-Barr virus (the glandular fever virus) they don't usually develop much in the way of symptoms, just protective antibodies. When infected with an enteroviral infection, they likewise tend to have a minor self-limiting illness with no after-effects. But teenagers who haven't managed to develop immunity to Epstein-Barr virus infection may contract glandular fever, which leaves them debilitated for months.

### Table 3: Age at onset of ME

| Age group | Males | Females | Total | |
|-----------|-------|---------|-------|------|
| 10 years | 3 | 12 | 15 | (3.5%) |
| 11–15 | 5 | 14 | 19 | (4.5%) |
| 16–20 | 15 | 40 | 55 | (13%) |
| 21–25 | 12 | 26 | 38 | (9%) |
| 26–30 | 8 | 30 | 38 | (9%) |
| 31–35 | 22 | 58 | 80 | (19%) |
| 36–40 | 20 | 56 | 76 | (18%) |
| 41–45 | 13 | 33 | 46 | (11%) |
| 46–50 | 6 | 15 | 21 | (5%) |
| 51–55 | 3 | 9 | 12 | (3%) |
| 56–60 | 4 | 10 | 14 | (3.5%) |
| 60 | 2 | 4 | 6 | (1.5%) |
| | | | | |
| Total | 113 | 307 | 420 | |

From: E. G. Dowsett *et al.*, *Postgraduate Medical Journal*, 1990, 66, p. 527.
*Reproduced by kind permission of the* Journal.

In the survey by Drs Betty Dowsett and Melvin Ramsay of 420 ME/CFS patients, the average age of onset was 32 years. It could be that women of this age are more frequently in contact with young children and babies – prime sources of infections which can trigger ME/CFS. Altogether, about 75 per cent of people with ME/CFS first develop their illness at some time between their late teens and mid-forties, but there are also plenty of well-documented cases in children as young as seven, as well as more elderly people occasionally being affected.

## Genetic markers

It's possible that people with ME/CFS have an inherited defect in their ability to respond to infections and other immune system stressors. This is a similar situation to the way in which men with a genetic predisposition sometimes develop a severe rheumatic disease called ankylosing spondylitis following a gastrointestinal infection with a special type of bacteria.

Sometimes ME/CFS affects different members of the same family, with first-degree relatives developing the illness over a period of time. In order to explore a possible genetic link, researchers are now looking for evidence of common genetic markers called HLA antigens in the blood of people with ME/CFS. One such study, albeit small, looked at 12 patients, all of whom had significant sleep disturbances as well. Eleven of the 12 were found to be positive for a genetic marker known as DQw1. A second study, using 110 ME/CFS patients, suggested that three genetic markers (DQ3, DQ4 and DQ5) may be more common. The researchers went on to speculate that a combination of genetic predisposition plus an appropriate triggering event could result in an abnormal response by the body's immune system, followed by the development of ME/CFS. (Details of research into genetic factors can be found by consulting reference 52.)

## Mental health and personality

Many psychiatrists believe that certain aspects of your mental health, particularly having a perfectionist type of personality and/or a previous history of depression are important reasons for increasing your vulnerability to developing ME/CFS. I have yet to be convinced that this is the case and there are certainly some good research studies to show that the incidence of psychiatric disorders in people with ME/CFS before they become ill isn't all that different from the normal population (references 53 and 440). I also believe that most people with ME/CFS are conscientious individuals who have carried on at work or running a home when they're extremely unwell, rather than having any kind of personality defect. Unfortunately, very little research has been carried out into the possibility that people with certain types of personality may be more prone to developing ME/CFS. The only controlled study (reference 57) to look at this aspect found no evidence to suggest that people with ME/CFS are perfectionists or had unusually high levels of personal standards before the onset of their illness – findings which are clearly at odds with the way the illness is often portrayed in the media. (Differences of opinion on the way in which a past history of psychiatric or personality problems may predispose towards the development of ME/CFS are explored in more detail on pages 227–231.)

## Sex and hormonal status

There is a definite female:male sex bias to ME/CFS with a 3:1 ratio being reported by Drs Dowsett and Ramsay (reference 137) and a 1.8:1 ratio by Dr Darrel Ho-Yen (reference 17).

Outbreaks involving female nursing staff have been frequently reported in the medical literature over the years, though in other instances the sex ratio was more equal. But if women are more likely to be affected, could there be any logical reasons?

First is the fact that mothers of small children are in constant contact with sources of infection. Teachers and nurses are in a very similar position.

Second is that when women are ill and need to rest, their domestic and family arrangements make it very difficult to do so. Unless a partner takes time off work, or extra help is drafted in to look after the home and family, women are unable to rest, no matter how hard they try.

Third is the fact that women are more likely to know about ME/CFS and so obtain a correct diagnosis. Much of the publicity for this illness appears in women's magazines. Very little information of a similar nature is ever aimed at men, so they're far less likely to have read anything about ME/CFS.

Fourth is the question of hormone balance. There is already good scientific evidence to show that hormones can affect immune system functioning and the production of vital chemical transmitters in the brain. Women with ME/CFS often notice a considerable improvement in symptoms during pregnancy, when there is a major shift in hormone status taking place, especially a rise in the levels of oestrogen (see page 189).

In the laboratory, female mice may die young when introduced to a specific infection, but male mice tend to survive. If sex hormones are removed from the male mice they, too, die more quickly. And if the female mice are given the male sex hormone testosterone, their resistance to infection significantly improves. In scientific experimentation one has to be extremely careful about drawing conclusions that results in animals can automatically be applied to humans. However, these results give support to the theory that sex hormone status may be related to the risk of acquiring ME/CFS when you meet the right 'trigger' at the wrong time in your life.

## Stress

One of the most significant factors in increasing someone's vulnerability to developing ME/CFS around the time of whatever acts as the principle trigger is undue physical or mental stress. Time and again I hear the story of a conscientious individual who struggles on in a stressful work or home environment until they are finally forced to stop through sheer exhaustion. Back at the Royal Free Hospital in 1955, it was the doctors and nursing staff, constantly on their feet, and mentally and physically stressed, who were taken ill, while only 12 of the patients resting in bed were affected!

The way in which the human body reacts to stressful events is only just starting to be understood by research scientists. It may, however, be crucial to understanding part of theME/CFS 'jigsaw'.

Any kind of stress – and this can be an infection, an accident or an emotional reaction such as bereavement – is immediately recognised by a small gland in the brain called the hypothalamus. Brain cells inside the hypothalamus which are involved in responding to stress produce two important hormones called arginine vasopressin (AVP) and cortisol releasing factor (CRF).

The main effect of acute stress is to switch on a gene which controls production of the main stimulatory hormone for cortisol, corticotrophin releasing hormone (CRH). This then instructs the adrenal glands to rapidly increase their production of cortisol, a hormone which assists all parts of the body to respond to stress in an appropriate way. Levels of CRH and cortisol rise quite rapidly and then fall back to normal again. In contrast, something rather strange seems to happen in people whose lives are subjected to chronic levels of physical and mental stress. Instead of producing CRH and cortisol, the hypothalamus switches to making AVP and a normal positive response to stressful events no longer occurs.

It's now becoming clear that inappropriate reactions to stress may play a crucial role in the development of a number of serious illnesses. An underactive stress response has been shown to produce multiple sclerosis-like lesions in the nervous system in animal model experiments. An overactive stress response – which produces increased amounts of cortisol – results in depression. And it could well be that repeated episodes of acute stress or prolonged periods of stress are important risk factors in the development of ME/CFS. High levels of stress certainly seem to have a very negative impact on the chances of recovering from ME/CFS.

Research into the hypothalamus and the hormones it produces and controls – particularly AVP, CRH and cortisol – is now being carried out on people with ME/CFS. Abnormalities in AVP, CRH and cortisol are described in more detail on pages 146–50.

One other way in which stress could be playing a role in the development of ME/CFS is by increasing the permeability of what is known as the *blood–brain barrier*. This helps to prevent infections, toxins, drugs and other harmful substances which normally circulate around the body in the bloodstream, from 'leaking through' the blood vessel walls and entering tissues in the brain. Research by Israeli doctors on soldiers who were given the drug pyridostigmine during the Gulf War to protect them from chemical warfare attack has shown that the side-effects of this drug on the nervous system were significantly increased during periods of extreme stress. This suggests that stress was increasing 'leakage' of the drug from the blood into parts of the brain where it normally wouldn't penetrate. Studies involving animal experiments have also provided further evidence to support this view (reference 50).

Research into the way that various forms of physical and mental stress may be interacting with infections, vaccinations and toxins to increase the permeability of the blood–brain barrier and so trigger ME/CFS is currently being carried out in the UK.

It's also worth remembering that chronic stress – physical and/or mental – can result in a number of symptoms which are similar to those found in ME/CFS. Stress related 'burnout' and the subject of athletic overtraining syndrome are discussed in Chapter 6: Other Causes of Chronic Fatigue.

Although various other co-factors have been implicated as predisposing towards the development of ME/CFS, an American study involving 47 patients (reference 53) found no evidence for a link with sleep disorders, consumption of raw meat or milk, cigarette smoking, pet ownership or exposure to farm animals.

Interestingly, this study found a slightly higher incidence of allergies in the ME/CFS patients than in the controls (66%:51%); very similar rates of depression (15%:11%) and major life stresses in the previous year (47%:51%). The patient group also reported higher rates of regular exercise before onset of their ME/CFS than the controls (66%:40%) – a finding that could be of particular relevance to future research.

A more recent study from the UK (reference 49) asked people who had made claims on permanent health insurance policies about their previous health problems before the onset of ME/CFS. The results suggested that those with ME/CFS were more likely to have complained about a number of symptoms (e.g. headaches, infections, back problems) when compared to those of similar age/sex who had either developed multiple sclerosis or had not had to make a claim. The authors went on to make some very debatable conclusions about these results, including the view that their findings gave strong support to the idea that a psychological problem known as abnormal illness behaviour (see pages 229–230) was a major factor in deciding who might go on to develop ME/CFS.

# Precipitating Events

In many of the outbreaks described in the previous chapter it was clear that some form of infection had precipitated the onset of ME/CFS. Similarities with some of the symptoms of polio – still present in the UK and America before the arrival of widespread vaccination – led researchers to question whether viruses belonging to a group known as enteroviruses (which contain the three strains of polio) could be the principle viral culprits. In America, interest centred on the possible role of Epstein-Barr virus after the outbreak in the state of Nevada, but then moved on to look at various other infections associated with the herpes group of viruses.

As more and more cases of ME/CFS started to be recognised, it soon became apparent that a wide range of infections besides enteroviruses and Epstein-Barr virus could act as triggers. And although the vast majority of people predated the onset of ME/CFS to a vague 'flu-like illness, sore throat, chest infection or gastroenteritis, in others a specific (or occasionally bacterial) infection seemed to be the trigger. Even though infection still seems to be the major triggering event in ME/CFS, it is becoming clear that vaccinations, toxins, pesticides and some types of major stressful event or trauma can produce an ME/CFS-like illness.

## The enteroviral connection

Enteroviruses are a group of viruses which include polio, coxsackie, echoviruses and hepatitis A. Hippocrates first recognised hepatitis (inflammation of the liver) and carvings from the second millennium BC depict cases of polio – these infections have been around for a very long time. Today, enteroviruses have a world-wide distribution and are known to cause a variety of both common and rare conditions ranging from trivial sore throats through to life-threatening infections involving the heart and brain.

Even within the same family an enteroviral infection may have different effects according to age, sex and pre-existing immunity.

In underdeveloped tropical countries, enteroviral infections occur all the year round, so this population quickly builds up a strong degree of natural immunity from a very early age. In developed countries with cool temperate climates, enteroviral infections tend to flourish during the warm summer months, often in epidemics that occur every few years. Increased levels of hygiene mean that fewer enteroviral infections occur, possibly leading to a less efficient state of natural immunity.

The main carriers of enteroviral infections are children in the first few years of life – 'the nappy years'. Children can remain as carriers without any ill-effects, yet still be capable of passing on the infection to susceptible adults who come in close contact with nappies or excretia. Insects and cockroaches also act as reservoirs of infection, especially in unhygienic kitchens.

Enteroviruses survive in sewage because they are resistant to most chemical disinfectants used in its treatment. So, when contaminated water is disposed into sea water close to the beach, there is likely to be a large source of enteroviral infection awaiting unsuspecting bathers, surfers and eaters of shellfish. Perhaps this is why some people develop ME/CFS shortly after an attack of gastroenteritis contracted during their summer holiday. The use of sludge as a fertiliser may also be infecting fresh fruit and vegetables – a good reason for removing the peel.

Once an enterovirus enters the body via the mouth or nose it may do nothing more than cause a mild sore throat and a few enlarged glands. If the primary immune response fails, the virus can then spread to the lungs or intestines to produce a chest infection or gastroenteritis. Once inside the intestines, enteroviruses are capable of multiplying rapidly to form yet another reservoir of infection. From here they can spread via the bloodstream to various other tissues including nerve, muscle and hormone-producing glands.

A large number of illnesses have now been linked to enteroviral infection. These include summer 'flu (sore throat, headaches and diarrhoea), chest and throat infections, brain infections (meningitis and encephalitis), muscle disease (polymyositis and Bornholm's disease), heart inflammation (myositis and pericarditis) and glandular inflammation affecting the liver (hepatitis), pancreas, prostate and thyroid glands. Enteroviruses have recently been linked to childhood diabetes and, where they persist in heart muscle, to a life-threatening condition known as cardiomyopathy. This means it's possible that some cases of ME/CFS, which have *definitely been triggered by an enteroviral infection*, may start to produce symptoms in other parts of the body which wouldn't normally be seen in this illness.

Details of research into the link between enteroviral infection, including the possibility that persisting viral presence may be involved in ME/CFS, are contained in Chapter 8: Current Research. Methods of testing for the presence of enteroviral infection are given on page 168.

## Glandular fever (Epstein-Barr virus infection)

Doctors have always recognised that a small minority of teenagers and people in their early twenties who have glandular fever go on to develop a protracted ME/CFS-like illness.

The most comprehensive research on the fatigue syndrome that can follow glandular fever comes from Dr Peter White and his colleagues at Saint Bartholomew's Hospital in London (references 352 and 353). They followed a group of 191 young adults with glandular fever (108 with good laboratory evidence of Epstein-Barr virus infection and 83 with no laboratory evidence) for a period of six months and concluded that a distinct fatigue syndrome follows this particular infection.

Apart from physical fatigue, the most commonly reported symptoms were:

- mental fatigue
- emotional lability (more easily upset than normal)
- enlargement and tenderness of the neck glands
- sore throat
- alcohol intolerance
- increased sleep requirements

Other symptoms of ME/CFS which were less frequently reported by this group were:

- muscle pain
- dizziness
- headaches
- increased sweating

Further information on the role of Epstein-Barr virus infection in ME/CFS is contained in Chapter 8: Current Research.

## Other viruses which may be involved

Although enteroviral infections and glandular fever remain the two most commonly associated with the development of ME/CFS, there are plenty of well-documented cases where the illness has followed other types of specific viral infection. Examples include chicken-pox, herpes zoster (shingles), rubella and Ross River virus (in Australia).

Cases which are initiated by chicken-pox seem to be particularly severe and protracted, possibly because this infection is capable of causing problems in both the liver and brain (Reye's syndrome), as well as persisting within the central nervous system.

Encephalitis (inflammation of the brain tissues) and meningitis (inflammation of the lining membrane that covers the brain) are both serious infections, frequently caused by viruses, which occasionally lead on to ME/CFS. A small research study found that around 12 per cent of a group of hospital patients with meningitis had ME/CFS symptoms eight months later (reference 51).

Other viral infections which can produce an ME/CFS-like illness include cytomegalovirus, hepatitis B and C, HIV and parvovirus. These illnesses are described in more detail in Chapter 6. (For a general review of the association between viral infections and ME/CFS see reference 56.)

Despite all the above evidence, some doctors still refuse to accept that common or uncommon infections play any role in the onset of ME/CFS. They maintain that everyone picks up several such infections in the course of a year and so any clear association is impossible to prove. They will also quote a research paper from *The Lancet* (reference 55) to back up their case against infection.

## Non-viral infections

A number of important infections which are not viruses – and so can sometimes be very successfully treated with antibiotics – are also quite capable of causing an ME/CFS-like illness. Examples include brucellosis, campylobacter, clostridium (botulism), giardia, leptospirosis, Lyme disease, mycoplasma, Q fever and toxocara. These conditions are covered in more detail in Chapter 6.

## Pesticides and toxins

Agricultural and farm pesticides, especially the organophosphate compounds used in sheep dips and some household pest control products, can no longer be dismissed as possible trigger factors in the development of ME/CFS.

It has also become apparent that chemical toxins produced by bacteria such as clostridium or ciguatera fish poisoning can produce an ME/CFS-like illness. All these conditions are discussed in Chapter 6.

## Vaccinations

Although uncommon, I have no doubt that a number of commonly used vaccinations are capable of triggering ME/CFS. This is hardly surprising considering the fact that vaccines are designed to act by mimicking the effect of an infection on the immune system in order to produce protective antibodies.

My own data on such cases indicates that the most commonly implicated vaccines are those designed to protect against tetanus, typhoid and hepatitis B. I have very few reports linking vaccination against hepatitis A (using immunoglobulin), polio, rubella or those which are predominantly given during childhood. Almost all of my 150-plus cases involve adults and in a significant number of instances the vaccine in question was given at a time when the person involved may not have fully recovered from an infection.

My particular interest in the area of vaccine-induced ME/CFS involves the possible role of *hepatitis B vaccination* as around half of all reported cases involve the use of this vaccine. The vast majority are health workers, particularly nurses, but there are others who have been given hepatitis B vaccine for occupational health purposes (e.g. policemen and teachers) or for foreign travel. Overall, the outlook in this group has been poor, with very few patients reporting any significant degree of recovery. A considerable number have had to terminate their employment (or even been dismissed) and apply for early retirement. In a few instances the illness has been accepted as an industrial injury, but only after a long battle with officialdom.

Of particular concern is the way in which several of these health workers were persuaded to continue a course of hepatitis B vaccine even though they were feeling unwell or had failed to fully recover from an adverse reaction to the first or second dose. A small number were vaccinated whilst recovering from a glandular fever-like illness – something which could have important implications when hepatitis B vaccine is automatically being given to student nurses and doctors in the 17 to 25 year age group.

Although chronic debilitating fatigue is the most commonly mentioned symptom, a minority also complain of joint pains, a finding which is consistent with several reports in the medical literature linking hepatitis B vaccine to arthritis. It is also interesting to note that a number of other more serious reactions have been linked to this vaccine in the medical journals. These include autoimmune disorders (e.g. systemic lupus erythematosus) and neurological disease (Guillain-Barré syndrome and multiple sclerosis-type symptoms). A number of doctors, including myself, believe that that incidence of such reactions could be higher than is officially thought and that there is an urgent need to carry out a large long-term follow-up study of people who have been vaccinated against hepatitis B.

One possible explanation as to why hepatitis B vaccine seems more likely to trigger ME/CFS may be some form of genetic susceptibility to a particular immunisation which has a powerful stimulatory effect on the body's immune system response. There is already some evidence to suggest that people who fail to produce an effective antibody response following hepatitis B vaccination may have common genetic markers which affect their immune response. The same genetic explanation could also apply to those who develop severe adverse reactions to the vaccine. If such markers (HLA antigens) could be clearly identified, then it's possible that both groups of people could be identified before being given this extremely useful form of protection against a potentially fatal liver disease.

If it can be shown that certain individuals are at increased risk because of an inherited genetic defect, then serious thought would need to be given as to whether they should be vaccinated in the first place.

At present, there is no official acceptance from either the manufacturers, the Department of Health (UK) or the Food and Drug Administration (USA) that hepatitis B (or any other vaccination) can trigger ME/CFS. The manufacturers of hepatitis B vaccine acknowledge that adverse reactions may include fatigue, muscle pain, arthritis, headaches and enlarged glands. However, they do not as yet mention the possibility of Chronic Fatigue Syndrome in their data sheets. The only published report on the possible link between this vaccine and ME/CFS comes from Canada (reference 48). Unfortunately, it came to the conclusion that no such association exists. Despite this lack of official acceptance, a growing number of specialists who see ME/CFS patients do support my view and research is now underway in the UK to explore this further.

Please note:

- If you believe that your illness has been triggered or significantly exacerbated by a vaccine, then do make sure that your doctor has notified this adverse reaction to both the manufacturer and the Committee on Safety of Medicines (Department of Health) using a Yellow Card.
- Eligibility for vaccine damage payments is discussed on pages 393–4.
- The use of vaccinations in people who already have ME/CFS is discussed on pages 219–20.

## A Western disease?

Some scientists believe that environmental pollution, along with a 'Western way of life', with its junk food, additives, cigarettes and excessive alcohol intake, may be steadily weakening the body's immune system over a long period of time. Then, when a particular infection or stressor comes along, the immune system has become so 'overloaded' that it can no longer cope. Conditions such as ME/CFS, Gulf War Syndrome and allergies are the result.

Allergic illnesses, particularly asthma and hayfever, do certainly seem to increase when a Western way of life is introduced into more primitive communities, so it may be that the way we respond to environmental change has important implications for human health. It's also possible that some cases of ME/CFS may be the result of allergic reactions or environmental chemicals, and I have no doubt that organophosphate pesticides are implicated in this illness. However, the scientific evidence to support other popular theories linking specific environmental factors in the development of ME/CFS is not quite so convincing.

# ME/CFS – The Cardinal Symptoms

## How ME/CFS Starts

Having seen well over 800 people with a suspected diagnosis of ME/CFS, I've come to the conclusion that although they all have two key symptoms in common – namely fatigue and problems with normal mental functioning – there are a number of important differences in the way this illness starts and progresses.

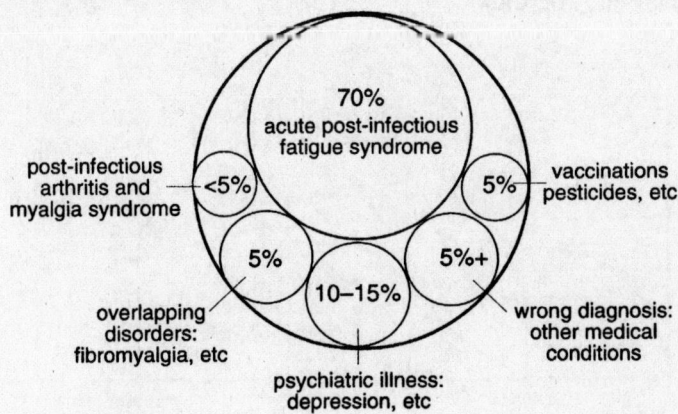

*Infectious onset*

Around 70 per cent of the patients I see describe an acute onset linked to some form of infection. Before this, they invariably describe themselves as being fit and healthy, with no previous history of emotional problems or psychiatric illness.

Common precipitating infections include a vague 'flu-like illness, tonsillitis, chest infection or gastroenteritis. Sometimes the onset coincides with a more specific infection such as chicken-pox.

The initial symptoms are generally consistent with a pattern that is seen in many acute infections. There may be swollen and tender lymph glands in the neck or armpit, loss of appetite, mild fever, generalised aches and pains. Marked dizziness and vomiting are an occasional presenting feature, in which case a diagnosis of labyrinthitis – infection involving the inner ear – may be the cause. Severe chest pain is occasionally reported and the person concerned may then be rushed into hospital with a suspected heart attack. Here the explanation may be that a viral infection has affected either the lining of the heart (pericarditis), the heart muscle itself (myocarditis) or the muscles of the ribcage (Bornholm's disease). A few predate the onset of their ME/CFS to either meningitis (inflammation of the membrane covering the brain) or encephalitis (actual brain tissue).

As these infective symptoms gradually start to subside, there may be a short period of return to relatively normal health. Most people, however, continue to feel generally unwell 'flu-like, fatigued and unable to make their brains work properly. No matter how hard they try to resume a normal way of life, their muscle fatigue and brain malfunction become increasingly prominent and disabling – simple post-viral debility is now turning into ME/CFS.

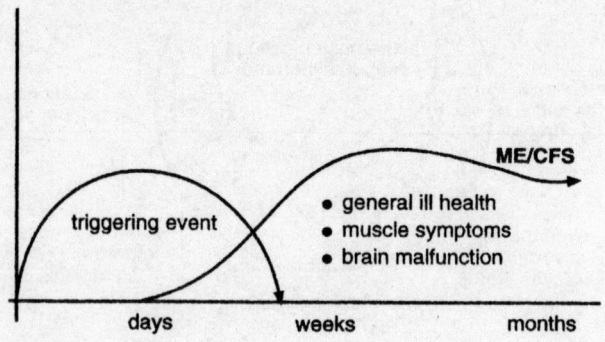

## Vaccinations, pesticides and toxins

Around 5 per cent of my patients predate the onset of ME/CFS to either a vaccination (particularly hepatitis B), exposure to pesticides (mainly organophosphate ones) or some form of chemical toxin (e.g. ciguatera fish poisoning). The role of vaccinations in ME/CFS is discussed on pages 34–37 and an ME/CFS-like illness resulting from exposure to organophosphate pesticides is discussed on pages 110–112. Ciguatera fish poisoning is discussed on page 106.

## The post-infectious arthralgia and myalgia fatigue syndrome

A small number of patients present with a condition which principally involves joint pain (arthralgia), muscle pain (myalgia) and severe fatigue.

If the onset is clearly linked to an acute infection, then it's important to rule out conditions such as brucellosis, leptospirosis, Lyme disease, parvovirus and yersinia, some of which can be successfully treated with antibiotics.

If there is no clear-cut infection, then rheumatic disorders such as Sjögren's syndrome and systemic lupus erythematosus (SLE) ought to be excluded.

All these rheumatic conditions are covered in more detail in Chapter 6: Other Causes of Chronic Fatigue.

## ME/CFS and psychiatric illness

About 10–15 per cent of patients I see have no clear onset to their illness and although they may fit with the internationally agreed diagnostic criteria for CFS described in Chapter 1, their underlying problem is some form of psychiatric illness. The most common explanations here are either severe depression, somatisation disorder (where a multitude of physical symptoms have a purely psychological origin) or a stress-related illness. As I'm not a psychiatrist, I would accept that this percentage figure is somewhat distorted and that there is probably a much higher percentage of people suffering from chronic fatigue where the main cause is psychiatric. Such cases are best dealt with by psychiatrists and psychologists using the sort of management approaches described in Chapter 12: Mind and Body.

## Overlapping conditions

In another 5 per cent the real diagnosis turns out to be a condition such as fibromyalgia or athletic overtraining syndrome. These conditions have a number of features in common with ME/CFS, but there are also some important differences. These are described in more detail on pages 105–13.

## The wrong diagnosis

A final 5–10 per cent turn out to have an entirely different diagnostic explanation for their chronic fatigue. Sometimes this is a perfectly treatable condition such as an underactive thyroid gland (hypothyroidism) – a fact which emphasises the need for doctors to make sure that all other causes of chronic fatigue have been eliminated before diagnosing ME/CFS. This means taking a good clinical history and arranging the correct blood tests. The many other causes of chronic fatigue are discussed in Chapter 6. Blood tests and other investigations are covered on pages 163–9.

Whatever event seems to have triggered your ME/CFS, there are three groups of symptoms which are nearly always present in various degrees of severity. These are:

- general ill health
- muscle symptoms (fatigue, pain, twitching, post-exertional malaise)
- brain malfunction (problems with memory, concentration, balance, etc).

For some people, the muscle symptoms are most disabling. Others consider brain malfunction to be a far greater problem. A third group find both sets of symptoms are either equally disabling or they fluctuate between the two.

# General Ill Health

Although this aspect of ME/CFS isn't referred to in any international definition, it's something that almost all my patients comment on. They frequently refer to a constant feeling of just 'not being well' or describe a general malaise that is very similar to how normal healthy people feel when they're about to fall ill with a bout of 'flu. This just 'not being well' is one of the main reasons why people with ME/CFS find it so hard to cope with normal aspects of everyday living. They can make lifestyle adjustments to cope with fatigue and brain malfunction, but there doesn't seem to be any way of alleviating the constant state of feeling so ill.

# Muscle Symptoms

## Muscle Fatigue

Although the term chronic fatigue syndrome places great emphasis on just one symptom, namely fatigue, this body sensation can have a number of different meanings. For some people, fatigue simply refers to problems associated with lack of sleep. For others, it's much more to do with failing to have enough energy to start or complete mental or physical activities. In a third group, it's more applicable to muscles which soon become 'tired and weak'.

In the case of ME/CFS, there is often a feeling of not having enough energy to carry on with normal everyday tasks, but the most characteristic description of physical fatigue relates to the adverse effects of exercise on muscles.

Rapid fatiguability of muscle is often first noticed during the triggering infection or very early on during convalescence. The load-bearing muscles of the legs are predominantly affected and many people with ME/CFS find that the effort required to stand up for long periods of time is far more tiring than going for a walk.

Arm muscles may become fatigued after lifting heavy objects or reaching up to place things on a high shelf. Any repetitive activity using these muscles quickly results in weakness. Even a simple task such as washing hair can leave some people with ME/CFS feeling exhausted.

Sometimes the small muscles of the eye are involved, so that vision becomes progressively blurred after reading.

The activity required to bring on muscle fatigue may be negligible – walking a few hundred yards, say, or just doing some light gardening. Any further activity after the onset of fatigue will then cause weakness and sometimes complete exhaustion. For the more severely affected, even minimal amounts of physical exertion may seem impossible and as a result they find themselves wheelchair-bound or confined to the house.

Muscle fatigue is also made worse following prolonged mental activity, and patients frequently mention how they find it extremely difficult to carry out mental and physical activities at the same time. This is partly why teachers, hairdressers and nurses invariably find returning to work so difficult, and why a weekly shop around the supermarket is such a debilitating experience. Equally, any form of sporting activity which combines rapid mental judgements and stamina becomes impossible.

Anyone with ME/CFS soon learns to recognise their limitations when it comes to physical activity and the dangers of 'pushing on' beyond such limits. Once the point of weakness or near exhaustion has been reached, the only solution is to stop, rest and recover – just like recharging a flat battery!

The highly characteristic recovery period can take minutes, hours, even days – it all depends on how far you've exceeded your limitations. Exercising well beyond the point of fatigue can result in a prolonged period of relapse (see pages 209–10).

Despite being less active, *actual muscle wasting is unusual* in ME/CFS. This usually only occurs following prolonged periods of immobility from being in bed or in a wheelchair. If you're still mobile and progressive muscle wasting is occurring, then I would strongly advise referral to a neurologist to rule out the possibility of some other muscle disorder being present.

The practical approach to management involving rest and activity is described on pages 203–9.

## Post-Extertional Malaise

This medical term, which is now incorporated into the CDC definition, describes the way in which excessive exercise results in an exacerbation of fatigue and other muscular symptoms. It can also cause exacerbation of fever, gland enlargement, sore throats and problems with mental functioning. Interestingly, this exacerbation of various ME/CFS symptoms doesn't usually occur within minutes or hours following a period of over-exertion; it is often not apparent until the following day.

## Muscle Pain (Myalgia)

Around 75 per cent of people with ME/CFS experience some degree of muscle pain. At one end of the spectrum are those who only have mild or intermittent pain. A small minority at the other end experience far more severe and sometimes persistent pain, which disrupts sleep and can become the most disabling part of the illness.

Muscle pain may be generalised throughout the body, but is more usually confined to the shoulders, neck, chest and thigh muscles. It tends to fluctuate in severity and is often made worse by exercise. There can also be small areas of increased tenderness – 'tender spots' – in the muscles which are affected.

The cause of muscle pain in ME/CFS remains uncertain. Psychiatrists frequently claim that it is due to physical inactivity (deconditioning), but some of the most inactive patients I see experience no pain whatsoever. However, muscle pain occurs in a number of infectious diseases (see pages 88–96) and research into muscle physiology in ME/CFS suggests that there could be a biochemical explanation, possibly involving the accumulation of lactic acid (see pages 141–3). (The practical management of muscle pain is reviewed on pages 194–8.)

## Muscle Twitching (Fasciculation)

The third quite common muscle symptom is twitching of the muscles, known to doctors as 'fasciculation'. This abnormality occurs in quite normal people who are feeling run down, but its frequency in ME/CFS, especially early on in the illness, suggests that it may be related to abnormal co-ordination between nerve messages and contraction of the muscle fibres they supply (reference 233). These fasciculations may just be fine ripples under the skin or they can be much more obvious. They appear almost anywhere in the body from the large muscle groups in the thigh to the tiny muscles controlling movement of the eyelids.

Involuntary flickering of the eyelids is called blepharospasm. This tends to vary in intensity from day to day and throughout the day, often being less marked in the morning or when concentrating. It also tends to be associated with sensitivity to bright light. Blepharospasm occasionally becomes more severe and may even start to affect the vision. In such cases opthalmologists are now using injections containing minute amounts of botulinum toxin to paralyse the tiny muscles around the eyelids. This particular form of treatment is very costly and has to be repeated every ten weeks or so. It is only available from a limited number of specialist centres, but would need to be used with care in someone with ME/CFS as this type of toxin has been implicated as a possible trigger factor in the development of ME/CFS (references 77 and 78).

Fasciculations are usually only a temporary problem in ME/CFS, appearing early on in the illness or at times of relapse. They quite often disappear completely over a period of time.

# Brain Symptoms

Brain fatigue and malfunction can become a major cause of disability in ME/CFS. Just like muscle fatigue, brain symptoms tend to fluctuate throughout the day and also on a day-to-day basis. They are often made worse by excessive physical or mental activity, stress, alcohol, or another infection. Surgical operations and anaesthetics also seem to cause a major exacerbation in brain malfunction. For many people, the fact that their brains have stopped functioning correctly is the most distressing feature of this illness. And for those whose employment depends on sustained mental activity throughout the day, the results can be devastating.

## *Memory and concentration*

Mental exertion from academic work, reading, attending meetings or any other activity requiring a prolonged period of concentration soon produces a gradual deterioration in normal brain activity. People with ME/CFS frequently described how a cloud or fog seems to descend over their brain as attention span and concentration rapidly decline. Phrases such as 'a brain full of cotton wool' are often used to describe the frustrations. It's interesting to note that excessive physical activity has a very similar adverse effect on mental activity as it does on muscle performance, so that at the end of a walk or a spell in the garden, not only are the muscles feeling fatigued but also the brain is no longer functioning properly.

The two commonest symptoms to be reported are loss of concentration and short-term memory. This latter symptom refers to any information which has entered the brain within the past few seconds, minutes or hours. Longer-term memory loss for events in the more distant past isn't usually affected in ME/CFS. This frustrating inability to keep the mind operating, and at the same time store and process new incoming information makes it almost impossible to try and carry out two tasks at the same time. It also means that few people with ME/CFS are capable of carrying on with demanding mental activity for more than half an hour; for some the period is even shorter (see also page 155).

## Speech and language

Once the ability to concentrate has deteriorated, it's not uncommon to discover that you can no longer find the correct name for everyday objects (dysnomia in medical jargon) or familiar faces. Others find that they are at a complete loss to find the right word (anomia). A few even find that their speech becomes temporarily slurred and difficult (dysphonia), but when this occurs the diagnosis of myasthenia gravis should always be considered (see pages 97–8).

## Co-ordination

The ability to carry out familiar routines – even knotting a tie or shoelace – may become impossible during a period of brain malfunction. It's only following a period of rest, when energy levels seem to slowly return, that brain function once again reaches relative normality.

Clumsiness, especially when carrying out fine tasks such as threading a needle, is extremely common – something which can lead to a great deal of broken crockery in the kitchen. Trying to co-ordinate leg movements on moving escalators is a frequently mentioned problem – provided you dare step on in the first place!

Although a considerable minority of people who are severely affected by ME/CFS report that they 'no longer walk properly', very little research has been carried out into this particular disability. The only published research report (reference 60) confirmed that *walking (gait) abnormalities* do, in fact, exist, and that they are probably caused by a combination of balance problems, muscle weakness and malfunction in the central nervous system.

## Handwriting

Deterioration in the quality of handwriting is sometimes noticed by people who have had ME/CFS for a long period of time. If handwriting becomes progressively smaller, then the possibility of Parkinson's disease should be queried (see page 99). Hypergraphia – the tendency to write extremely long letters – is an unusual neurological feature that is occasionally found in people with ME/CFS.

## Transient neurological events

A small number of people with ME/CFS have what Professor Tony Komaroff, a physician at Harvard Medical School in Boston, USA, who has a special interest in ME/CFS, describes as 'transient neurological events'. These can include small *seizures* ('fits'), profound *ataxia* (severe problems with balance, walking and co-ordination), temporary *visual loss* and *sensory disturbances* in the skin (paraesthesiae). These are unusual symptoms which suggest that a rather more serious disturbance in brain function is taking place in this group of patients. If such symptoms occur, they almost certainly require further assessment and investigation by a neurologist with experience of ME/CFS.

Whatever part or parts of the brain are involved in ME/CFS, no form of progressive dementing process appears to be taking place. Fortunately, there is no evidence of loss of intelligence over a long period of time.

A large amount of research data has recently been published on aspects of cognitive functioning (memory, concentration, etc) in ME/CFS. This work is described on page 155.

# Management of Brain Malfunction

This second cardinal feature of ME/CFS invariably becomes an extremely disabling and frustrating part of everyday life. However, on a more positive note, it's something that can definitely improve as time goes on, as I'm able to testify from personal experience. For some people though, their frequent and often severe episodes of mental incapacity bring sheer despair.

At present, there is no drug therapy that can be routinely recommended to help this particular aspect of the illness. *Antidepressants* may improve memory and concentration where there is co-existent depression, but I am not convinced of their value in its absence. The use of *galanthamine* and other new drugs which affect chemical transmitters in the brain looks more promising (see page 187), but we must await the results of proper clinical trials before coming to any firm conclusions. In America, some doctors are using drugs such as *calcium blockers*, which may increase blood flow to the brain, but these claims are largely anecdotal (see page 186). This type of approach does have some theoretical advantages if the results from SPECT scans (see pages 152–3) really do mean that there are significant reductions in blood flow and oxygenation to certain parts of the brain.

## Self-help

One of the biggest problems for anyone with ME/CFS is sustaining any

form of intellectual or mental activity. Here are a few practical suggestions which may help you to improve your coping strategies:

- Start off by splitting your mental activity into small regular amounts,
  say five or ten minutes every hour, rather than trying to carry on as
  long as possible for two or three times a day.
- Accept that mental activity is going to fluctuate widely from day to
  day, even from hour to hour. Tasks which could be easily accomplished on one day may not be possible on the next.
- Totally abstaining from any kind of mental activity isn't a good idea,
  even if your brain function may only feel like 20 per cent of normal.
- Even when you are coping quite well with mental tasks, it's still a
  good idea to 'switch off' and relax completely for a set period each
  hour rather than pushing on to the point of mental exhaustion and
  confusion.
- Most people with ME/CFS tend to feel better at fairly predictable
  times during the day, so try to schedule activities which can be
  planned in advance to fit in with those times.
- As with physical activity, try to *gradually* increase mental activity on a
  day-to-day basis and accept that progress may be two steps forward
  followed by one step back.
- Make use of memory aids by keeping a pocket notebook to record a
  daily list of activities which need to be attended to, phone calls to be
  made, etc. Tick them off as they're completed. It's also a good idea to
  use a Filofax or keep a careful diary of forthcoming events.
- Mental confusion is always made considerably worse when there's
  too much activity going on around. Try to do the shopping at quieter
  times of the day and if you do have to concentrate on a mental task,
  then do it in a quiet environment.
- If you need to memorise some really important information, it can
  help by reading it out aloud. Seeing, hearing and reading something
  will reinforce your chances of retaining it.
- As far as leisure activities are concerned, if you can't concentrate on
  a favourite television programme at its scheduled time, consider hiring a video recorder rather than missing out on what may be one of
  your few sources of pleasure. Active sports and hobbies which have
  been abandoned should ideally be replaced by something passive
  rather than doing nothing at all.
- If you're having severe difficulties with mental functioning, it may be
  worth asking to be referred to a clinical psychologist for an opinion
  and advice. These psychologists are often attached to neurological
  departments in hospitals or centres specialising in rehabilitation of
  stroke or head-injury patients.

- Lastly, it's worth remembering that the brain needs feeding just like the rest of the body, so people with ME/CFS must take care to eat regular nutritious meals.

## Headaches

This symptom occurs in about 75 per cent of people with ME/CFS. My personal experience is of headaches which appear intermittently, but which are of sufficient severity to prevent any meaningful mental activity for a considerable part of the day.

If you have persisting or severe headaches it is always a good idea to check with your GP as they could be due to high blood pressure, a sinus problem or something called temporal arteritis in the elderly age group. This latter condition is often accompanied by visual disturbances and quite severe muscle pain. It *must* be treated urgently with high doses of steroids to reduce inflammation in the blood vessels.

As with muscle and joint pain, with ME/CFS the response to simple over-the-counter painkillers is often far from satisfactory. It should also be noted that constant frequent use of ordinary painkillers may actually worsen the very symptom for which they are being used (reference: *British Medical Journal*, 1995, 310, 479–480). This review concluded that *'Large daily doses of analgesics may aggravate headaches'* and *'. . . mixed analgesic compounds containing aspirin or paracetamol in combination* [with other painkillers] *are probably the strongest inducers of chronic analgesic headache'.*

Stronger analgesics are best avoided altogether, unless really necessary, and then only for very short periods of time.

In America, some doctors who treat ME/CFS patients prescribe a drug called Diamox, something which is normally only used to decrease pressure inside the eye in glaucoma. Diamox is not usually used in the UK for treating headaches and it has a number of side-effects (drowsiness, depression, paraesthesiae, blood disorders) which seem to make it a rather unsuitable choice in ME/CFS.

I personally find that the occasional use of a simple painkiller combined with local heat (in the form of a hot water bottle or facecloth) is the best solution. A soak in a warm bath can also be helpful if there is tension in the neck muscles.

The general use of painkillers in ME/CFS is described in more detail on pages 194–8.

For headaches that take on a more migrainous character (i.e. one-sided, and associated with nausea and visual disturbances) there are specific and effective drugs available both over-the-counter (e.g.

Migraleve) and on prescription. Imigran (sumatriptan) affects blood flow to the brain by acting on 5HT receptors and may be worth trying. It's also a good idea to try cutting out foods such as cheese and chocolate, as well as red wine and coffee for a while.

For details of self-help groups dealing with migraine see Useful Addresses, page 424.

# How ME/CFS Affects Other Parts of the Nervous System

The human nervous system consists of millions of individual nerve cells, which store and pass on information and instructions rather like a computer. Various control centres for all this nervous activity are situated in different parts of the brain. From here, messages pass down the spinal cord and then out via numerous tiny nerves to muscles, blood vessels and body organs which are under nervous control. One particularly important part of the nervous system affected by ME/CFS is the autonomic nerves and the results of a number of different research studies looking at this aspect have now been published (see pages 144–5).

## The autonomic nervous system

This consists of two complementary sets of nerves, known as sympathetic and parasympathetic fibres, which both pass to the part of the body they are controlling, but have opposing functions. For example, sympathetic nerves to the heart will speed up its rate, whereas parasympathetic fibres will slow down the rate. These nerves are controlled by 'higher centres' in the brain, particularly in the brain stem. The nerves are called autonomic, because unlike nerves which control muscle movements, we don't have much voluntary control over their actions. If we become worried about something, this will trigger activity in the sympathetic nerves and speed up the pulse rate, but there's no way we can cancel out this automatic overactivity.

The autonomic nerves try to maintain a 'status quo' by exerting control over a wide range of body functions. They pass to the heart, intestines and bladder, where they control emptying functions. They also have a very important role in body temperature control.

## Temperature control and night sweats

One particularly important autonomic control centre in the brain is known as the hypothalamus and it's from here that the body is programmed to maintain its constant internal temperature.

People with ME/CFS frequently have difficulties with the control of body temperature, in particular being abnormally sensitive to any extreme of temperature, be it a hot bath or climatic heat or cold. This is also quite a common finding in multiple sclerosis where marked fatigue follows a hot bath.

People with ME/CFS often feel cold and shivery and may even want to wrap up when the external temperature is quite warm. It's not unusual to record body temperatures which are constantly a degree or so below normal. One strange aspect of this, which I personally experience, is that whenever I succumb to an infection I rarely have a raised temperature, but just feel cold and shivery.

One of the normal body mechanisms for losing heat is to sweat, and profuse night sweats (just like those some women experience during their menopause) are quite a common feature. Sheets and bedclothes may have to be frequently changed as a result. Sometimes the sweating episodes occur night after night for a while and if the body temperature is taken at the time with a thermometer, it may be lower than normal. Sweating attacks can also occur when people try to 'push on' – mentally or physically – beyond their limitations.

Night sweats are a prominent feature of a lymph node cancer known as Hodgkin's disease. Here the trigger factor is thought to be increased production of an immune chemical known as interleukin–1. This can induce an abrupt increase in the manufacture of a substance called prostaglandin E2 within the hypothalamus, which then affects the body's thermostatic control. It is possible that similar mechanisms could be involved in temperature control defects related to ME/CFS.

Unfortunately, there's no effective medical therapy for problems with temperature regulation apart from avoiding, wherever possible, situations where they might occur. This is particularly appropriate if you go on holiday to hot climates.

## The heart and blood vessels

ME/CFS, through dysfunction of the nervous system, may affect the heart and small blood vessels. Overactivity in the sympathetic nervous system can cause a sudden increase in the pulse rate (a tachycardia) and this may be accompanied by the frightening sensation of actually feeling the heart beating inside the chest – palpitations. These palpitations will be exacerbated if you're also feeling anxious. If you experience either rapid pulse rates or palpitations, it's important to avoid anything else which will overstimulate these nerves, including coffee, alcohol and even the contents of some cold cures and nasal sprays. If in doubt do ask your pharmacist.

There are drugs available, known as beta-blockers, which can dampen down this overactivity and help to control symptoms. When palpitations are particularly bothersome, such treatment may be worth trying. Before using these drugs, your doctor may wish to check the heart rhythm using an electrocardiogram (ECG), just to make sure that there's no other problem with the heart itself. One disadvantage of using beta-blockers is that they have side-effects, some of which can be similar to the symptoms already caused by ME/CFS (see also pages 185-6).

The sympathetic nerves also control the size of tiny blood vessels which supply blood to the hands and feet. The ghastly facial pallor which is noticed in some people may be part of this malfunction, if blood supply to the skin is reduced. Cold hands and feet are a common accompaniment to ME/CFS, and are often brought on by cold weather, when these tiny blood vessels seem to be unduly sensitive and clamp down. Inhalation of cigarette smoke and the use of beta-blocking drugs will exacerbate this problem.

The most effective way of dealing with cold hands and feet is by the following simple practical advice:

- In the house, try to make sure that at least one room is as draught free as possible; to save on heating bills in winter keep at least one area of the house constantly warm.
- At night, have a warm drink before going to bed. Take a hot drink in a flask upstairs in case you feel cold in the night. A nightcap, bed-socks, gloves and pyjamas should all help to keep you warm, along with an electric blanket or covered hot water bottle if necessary.
- Lack of physical exercise isn't very good for the circulation, so try to avoid sitting still for long periods of time. If you are going through a relapse and are very inactive, it's worth carrying out some passive exercises in bed.
- Never warm up cold hands or feet by putting them straight on to a radiator or under hot running water – they *must* be warmed up gradually.
- It's vital to keep the trunk warm; this is best done by wearing several layers of thin clothing rather than one very thick layer. Air becomes trapped between the various layers and helps to insulate the body.
- Before going outside in winter always wear a hat (a considerable amount of heat is lost from the scalp and face), a scarf and thermal clothing if it's really cold.
- Hands and feet must always be adequately covered. Woollen tights, leg warmers and thick woollen socks are all ideal. Footwear can be insulated by lining it with aluminium foil or thermal 'space age' inner soles.
- Don't forget that the body needs plenty of warm 'fuel' on cold winter days. A bowl of hot porridge is an ideal way to start; then try to have regular small meals throughout the day to maintain energy levels.

- Avoid touching cold surfaces and objects; don't go into the fridge or freezer without wearing insulated gloves.
- Don't smoke cigarettes (nicotine constricts the tiny blood vessels even further); avoid other people's smoke wherever possible.
- Try using a Mycoal Warm Park which acts as a portable body warmer. These come as sachets, which when exposed to the air will generate heat from 50° to 70°F. They can then be used to insulate gloves, shoes, etc. Hand and Foot Warmers last up to six hours, Body Warmers up to 20 hours. If cold hands and feet are causing a lot of difficulties, especially outdoors in winter, it may be worth taking more radical measures, and purchasing some battery-heated shoes and gloves. The Reynaud's Association Trust (see Useful Addresses, page 429) deals specifically with this condition, and can give further practical advice.

Although many people experience palpitations and rapid pulse rates from time to time, this doesn't mean that the heart has become affected by ME/CFS. The most likely reason is overactivity of the sympathetic nerves which are telling it to beat faster.

However, there are a few people with ME/CFS who have associated heart disease, because, as mentioned earlier, enteroviruses can affect both the heart muscle (the myocardium = myocarditis) or the heart lining (the pericardium = pericarditis). In these cases the person is often quite seriously ill at the beginning, due to effects on the heart, and may have to be admitted to hospital. This heart involvement may then start to gradually improve, but in some instances the problems continue.

I must stress that direct involvement of the heart is very unusual. If you are having persistent chest pains and palpitations, your doctor will probably want to do some tests (e.g. an electrocardiogram to trace the heart rhythm), just to be sure there's nothing more serious going wrong. For more information on the way in which ME/CFS can affect the heart see pages 157–8.

## Feeling faint or fainting

One further important function of the autonomic nerves is that of controlling blood pressure by their effect on the size of larger blood vessels. If these vessels are too dilated, then the pressure in the system falls, not enough blood reaches the brain, and you either feel faint or actually faint. When you move from lying or sitting to a standing position, these vessels should contract to keep blood flowing to the brain, but some people with ME/CFS feel faint on suddenly standing up. This is what doctors call postural hypotension – a fall in blood pressure on standing.

Postural hypotension probably isn't the only reason why you may feel faint at times. In some of the earlier outbreaks of ME/CFS, patients were found to have very low blood sugar levels (hypoglycaemia) and were even admitted to hospital because of this. Another factor may be related to drugs being taken. Antidepressants can lower blood pressure as a side-effect, as can alcohol and excessive heat. Lastly, there's a special type of fainting attack, known as micturition syncope, which tends to affect men when they get up in the middle of the night to pass urine. It seems that the combination of postural hypotension and the autonomic nerve activity involved in bladder emptying combine to cause a faint.

If feeling faint is a particular problem, it's worth asking your doctor to check your blood pressure, to see if it does fall significantly when you change from lying to standing.

Whatever the cause, there are measures *you* can take:

- Drink plenty of fluids throughout the day.
- Consider increasing the amount of salt in your diet (but only after discussion with your doctor).
- Try to remain upright as much as possible during the day, but avoid standing still for long periods.
- Avoid standing in a hot shower.
- Blood pressure tends to fall after eating a large meal, so stick to smaller, more frequent meals as well as taking a short rest afterwards.
- Hot weather makes dizziness and fainting symptoms even worse – you may need to increase your fluid and salt intake at such times.
- Consider wearing elastic support stockings, especially when you have to stand up for a long period.
- Straining on the toilet or when lifting a heavy object will also cause a drop in blood pressure. If micturition syncope is a problem, make sure you sit on the toilet when passing urine.
- If postural hypotension is a problem, be careful how you move from lying down to standing up. Sit on the bed for a few minutes and learn to exercise your stomach muscles by pulling them in several times before changing position – this will help to raise the blood pressure.
- If you do start feeling dizzy or faint whilst standing up, lie down or sit on a chair with your feet well elevated. Simply raising both arms up in the air is also said to be helpful.

If feeling faint becomes very troublesome, you should ask your doctor to check that there is nothing wrong with your blood cortisol level. American researchers are currently looking at the problems of low blood pressure in ME/CFS. Their findings and the possible implications for drug treatments are discussed on pages 144–5.

## Problems with balance

The almost constant feeling of unsteadiness experienced by many people with ME/CFS is probably caused by a disturbance in the way that both the inner ear and parts of the central nervous system help to maintain balance. This disturbance in equilibrium is often reported as being very similar to feeling 'drunk all the time' or even 'walking on rubber'. However, most people don't experience the typical spinning sensation that doctors associate with the term vertigo.

For a significant minority, especially where the illness started with a viral labyrinthitis (an infection involving the inner ear), problems with balance can become far more disabling. Tripping over in the dark is a common consequence, and the result can be a serious fall.

These problems with balance are often dismissed by doctors as being due to anxiety or hyperventilation (overbreathing), particularly when tests for balance all turn out to be relatively normal. The doctor's examination is likely to include asking you to stand up with your eyes closed (the Romberg test), and you may well be referred to the ear, nose and throat clinic for more complicated hospital tests.

In my own case, it was only after being referred to the special balance unit at the National Hospital for Nervous Diseases in London that I was finally able to convince my doctors that I did have a genuine problem with balance – the tests showed evidence of viral damage to a part of the brain, the cerebellum, which is involved in maintaining normal body equilibrium.

The only published research on balance problems comes from America (reference 59). This study involved 11 patients with ME/CFS who all had severe problems with balance. The research group looked in particular at the way in which a part of the central nervous system control of balance – the vestibular system – was functioning. This is an area which forms part of the brain stem – where some interesting abnormalities in blood flow have already been reported in ME/CFS using SPECT scans – and receives information from three main sources. These are the inner ears, eyes, and messages from the skin, joints, muscles and neck. All these sources of information help the body to maintain a normal steady balance. If any of this information feeding into the vestibular system is faulty or unco-ordinated then all is not well; the result is some form of disturbance in balance control.

Almost every ME/CFS patient in this particular study had abnormal test results, but not all of them had the same abnormalities. The overall conclusion was that abnormalities in balance were suggestive of what is called 'central vestibular dysfunction'. They were clearly *not* psychological in origin.

Simple testing of the vestibular apparatus at a doctor's surgery can be carried out by using what is known as the Fukada test. With both eyes shut and arms fully outstretched the patient marches on the spot for 30 seconds. If the vestibular apparatus is functioning normally the subject should still be facing in the same direction as at the start of the test. Rotation of more than 30° to one side indicates impaired vestibular function on the side to which the rotation has occurred.

Having carried out this test on several ME/CFS patients, my own findings confirm that vestibular problems may be quite common in those who complain of persisting dizziness, unsteadiness or vertigo (actual spinning around). Unfortunately, confirming that a vestibular problem exists isn't necessarily helpful when it comes to drug treatment of balance disorders, but it may indicate the need for referral to an ENT specialist for further assessment.

As far as management of unsteadiness is concerned, I have not found any prescription drugs used in the treatment of vertigo to be particularly beneficial. Drugs such as prochlorperazine (Stemetil) may be helpful in an acute or severe attack, but they must *not be used continually* because they can cause additional neurological problems as a side-effect. A newer drug called cinnarizine (Stugeron) does appear to be safe and can be purchased in the pharmacy without a prescription. Again, it's unlikely to help with persistent unsteadiness, but it can be useful for preventing motion sickness on car journeys or sea crossings.

Neurologists interested in the practical difficulties associated with vertigo have devised a series of exercises (Cooksey-Cawthorne); on a personal level I haven't found them to be helpful.

## Problems with bladder control

Some of the autonomic nerves help to contract muscles of the bladder wall and cause emptying, whereas others keep the bladder exit sphincter closed till the body wishes to pass urine.

Symptoms such as frequently wanting to pass urine, getting up in the night to pass urine or the feeling of having an 'irritable bladder' seem fairly common in both men and women with ME/CFS.

Poor muscle control may be the reason why some men have a poor urinary stream and dribble at the end, but there is also a small group around the age of 40 who develop definite symptoms of prostate gland enlargement and inflammation (e.g. perineal pain and various difficulties in passing urine). This may be due to the fact that enteroviral infection is persisting within the prostate gland tissues and causing chronic inflammation. This is an extremely difficult complication of ME/CFS when it comes to treatment. I know of several men who have had prolonged courses of various antibiotics and prostate gland massage, all to no avail. In the end, the only solution has been to have a prostate operation, but again the results have often been far from satisfactory

In women, there may be weakness of the pelvic floor muscles which produces what is known as 'stress incontinence'. Here, sudden abdominal pressure from coughing, straining or exercise can suddenly produce an embarrassing leak of urine, as the pelvic muscles fail to contract properly around the urethra. If this is happening, a properly taught course of pelvic floor exercises will probably help. A recently researched method is now being taught which involves inserting cones of varying sizes into the vagina for short periods each day; the effort of keeping the cones in place specifically strengthens the weak pelvic muscles.

If you do want to pass urine frequently, your doctor will need to exclude infection by sending a specimen to the laboratory. If no infection is present, then the reason may well be to do with the nervous control of bladder function. The doctor may decide to carry out a full investigation of the whole urinary tract from kidneys to bladder, by doing an IVP test (intravenous pyelogram) or ultrasound examination.

More sophisticated techniques are now available in specialised urological units to accurately assess the nerve-muscle control of bladder function, and it would be interesting to examine a group of ME/CFS patients who have bladder problems using these methods.

If bladder symptoms such as frequency are becoming very incapacitating, there are drugs which may be of help, but these would only be prescribed after careful consideration.

## Disturbances involving sensory nerves

One last part of the nervous system which can be affected are the sensory nerves. These carry information on sensation, pain, pressure and temperature change back to the brain. If there are problems here, symptoms such as numbness (hypoaesthesiae), 'pins and needles' (paraesthesiae) or an increased awareness of sensation (hyperaesthesiae) can occur.

I'd had ME/CFS for about five years before ever experiencing any of these changes. Then one very cold November day I'd been out walking my dog, and on returning home I noticed that my right foot had started to feel cold and numb. Over the following few days I also started to develop pins and needles in my fingers. These symptoms continued intermittently all through the winter till spring arrived and now they return each year, in varying degrees of severity according to how cold the weather is.

Other people notice that these sensory changes tend to come and go, and particularly affect the hands and feet, but are not necessarily related to the cold. A few also notice altered sensations on their tongues and inside their mouths.

There are no obvious medical solutions to these abnormal sensations. They can have several other causes, some of them treatable. It's important, if such symptoms come on after ME/CFS has been present for some time, to exclude other possible explanations. These include:

- Diabetes (increased thirst, weight loss, calf pains and skin infections)
- Pernicious anaemia (sore tongue, anaemic symptoms, previous stomach surgery)
- Multiple sclerosis (balance and speech problems, eye pain and visual disturbances)
- Porphyria (stomach pains and mental disturbances)
- Dysparaproteinaemia.

Vitamin B supplements and injections are often prescribed by doctors for these sensory symptoms, but their value in ME/CFS is very doubtful because no specific deficiencies or problems with absorption have, as yet, been demonstrated.

**Appendix:** Symptoms and signs in 420 patients with ME/CFS

| Commonly found (> 50%) | No | % |
|---|---|---|
| Muscle fatigue | 420 | 100 |
| Emotional lability+ | 411 | 98 |
| Myalgia++ | 336 | 80 |
| Cognitive disturbance+++ | 323 | 77 |
| Headache | 310 | 74 |
| Giddiness, disequilibrium | 302 | 72 |
| Autonomic dysfunction++++ | 289 | 69 |
| Auditory disturbances* | 289 | 69 |
| Reversal of sleep rhythm | 268 | 64 |
| Visual disturbances** | 260 | 62 |
| Paraesthesia, hypo & hyperaesthesia | 256 | 61 |
| Intercostal myalgia/weakness | 247 | 59 |
| Fasciculation, spasm, myoclonus | 239 | 57 |
| Clumsiness*** | 235 | 56 |

+ Includes frustration, elation, depression;
++ characteristically affects limbs, shoulder girdle, spinal muscles;
+++ memory, concentration, anomia, dyslexia;
++++ especially circulation and thermoregulation;
* hyperacusis, deafness, tinnitus;
** mainly loss of accommodation, photophobia, nystagmus;
*** usually due to impaired spatial discrimination.

| Less commonly found (< 50%) | No. | % |
|---|---|---|
| Gastrointestinal symptoms**** | 205 | 49 |
| Disturbance of micturition | 160 | 38 |
| Recurrent lymphadenopathy | 152 | 36 |
| Arthralgia | 118 | 28 |
| Orthostatic tachycardia | 88 | 21 |
| Recurrent abacterial conjunctivitis | 68 | 16 |
| Orchitis/prostatism in young males | 15/113 | 13 |
| Seronegative polyarthritis | 42 | 10 |
| Vasculitic skin lesions | 42 | 10 |
| Myo/pericarditis | 34 | 8 |
| Positive Romberg sign | 25 | 6 |
| Thyroiditis in female patients | 15/307 | 5 |
| Mesenteric adenitis | 5 | 1 |
| Paresis and muscle wasting | 3 | 1 |

**** nausea/disturbance of intestinal motility; frequency incontinence, retention; enlargement, recurrent after prodrome; surgical intervention for abdominal pain.

From E. G. Dowsett *et al*. 'Myalgic Encephalomyelitis – a persistent enteroviral infection'. *Postgraduate Medical Journal*, 1990, 66, 526–30.
*Reproduced by kind permission of the* Journal.

# Secondary Problems

The cardinal features of ME/CFS, already discussed in the previous chapter, are later joined in many instances by a range of other symptoms affecting different parts of the body.

Although you may have successfully cleared the first hurdle and persuaded your doctor that ME/CFS really does exist – causing muscle fatigue and brain malfunction – you may once again be facing an uphill struggle when it comes to having other seemingly unrelated problems being accepted as part of the illness. However, doctors and patients both need to remember that it's unwise to simply blame the development of any new symptom on this illness – the real cause could be a completely unrelated medical condition or even co-existent depression.

## The Ears and Hearing Problems

People with ME/CFS frequently remark on three particular problems connected with hearing:

- The presence of abnormal noises in the ear – tinnitus. These sounds can be high-pitched whistling or hissing noises. They tend to occur at times of stress or undue fatigue.
- Being unable to cope with constant chatter in a room full of people, or a lot of loud noise (hyperacusis). This latter symptom may alternate with periods of deafness or normal hearing.
- Pain in or around the ear.

Sound is normally transmitted in waves through various components of the outer and middle ear to a structure called the cochlea. This is a fluid-filled chamber with thousands of tiny hair cells lining its walls. Sound vibrations pass through it, moving the tiny hairs, and the message is transformed into a nerve impulse, which passes along the auditory nerve (or nerve of hearing) to the brain, where it is decoded. It seems that in ME/CFS, the ability of the auditory nerve to conduct sound waves suffers from interference – rather like a faulty telephone wire.

Tinnitus can be an extremely distressing complaint, and makes any form of concentration even more difficult. There is no effective drug treatment, although some doctors prescribe tranquillisers where stress is a factor, but these are not a long-term solution. Fortunately, in many cases, tinnitus is intermittent, and in my personal experience it can disappear altogether for quite long periods of time.

If tinnitus is persistent and troublesome, then it is well worth trying what is known as a 'masking device'. This acts rather like a hearing aid, and masks the unpleasant noise with a pleasant background sound. An alternative do-it-yourself method for masking tinnitus is using a personal stereo to play soothing music. The Tinnitus Association (see Useful Addresses, page 432) provides useful information and practical advice.

## Eyes and Visual Disturbances

ME/CFS is capable of causing several visual disturbances:

- **Blurring of vision (defective accommodation)** This is very common, especially after prolonged periods of watching television, reading print in a newspaper or book, or when having to switch from near to far vision. The printed words become increasingly difficult to focus on and may start to appear double (double vision = diplopia). The cause is probably related to the fact that correct focusing of the eye is controlled by tiny muscles – ciliary muscles – and just like other muscle groups, they are prone to fatigue after prolonged use.

  Some people make repeated visits to the optician to try and get the problem sorted out. The optician, not surprisingly, finds nothing wrong. So, try not to visit your optician on an 'off day', when you are feeling tired and your vision worse than usual.
- **Photophobia** – dislike of bright lights – is also quite common, and this may stem from increased sensitivity to light in the brain. If you cannot avoid shops, working areas, etc, where there are very bright lights, then try wearing dark glasses when necessary.
- **Pain** in and around the eyes can be quite severe, and become localised behind one eye (retro-orbital pain). The doctor may query a diagnosis of migraine, but the pain is not usually associated with sickness or visual disturbances seen in migraine. This type of eye pain doesn't tend to respond very well to analgesics. Often all you can do is rest quietly until it goes away.
- **Nystagmus**, an involuntary rolling movement of the eyeball, is an occasional complication that is picked up during a neurological examination. There is no specific treatment.
- The problem of **blepharospasm** (involuntary spasm and flickering of the eyelids) is discussed on pages 44–5, and **dry eyes** on pages 102–3. Further information on eye symptoms can be found in references 61 and 62.

# Irritable Bowel

## *Symptomatology*

People with ME/CFS often have problems with their digestion and bowels. Some become unduly worried about such symptoms, which is only likely to make them worse. So, if you have gastric problems, do discuss them with your doctor, and get any tests done that seem appropriate to rule out other causes such as coeliac disease, Crohn's disease, and giardia infection (see also Chapter 6: Other Causes of Chronic Fatigue).

In a few people, food sensitivity or allergy may be a problem, but please don't embark on drastic dietary restrictions without expert supervision.

Among the wide variety of fluctuating or persisting digestive symptoms are nausea, vague colicky pains in the stomach, bloating or feeling abnormally full after a meal, and alterations in bowel habit, which can veer towards diarrhoea or constipation. Vomiting, progressive weight loss or blood in the motions should *not* be ascribed to ME/CFS, and a search must be made for an alternative explanation.

Trying to establish the reason for these symptoms so that treatment can be devised isn't always easy, but a number of explanations have been put forward. The whole gastrointestinal tract consists of a long hosepipe-like tube which starts at the oesophagus. From here, food enters the stomach, where digestion takes place, then it continues its journey through many feet of intestines where nutrients are absorbed and waste products excreted. The lining of the intestine is made up of cells which form a membrane called the mucosa. Surrounding the mucosa are layers of muscle fibres, whose function is to rhythmically contract in a wave-like manner to propel food and waste products along. Like any other muscle, this is under nervous control, and may therefore be affected in ME/CFS.

Where there is a combination of colicky stomach pain, bloating or wind, and alteration in normal bowel habit, the explanation may be what doctors term the 'irritable bowel syndrome'. This seems to be a common problem in ME/CFS, but it has also been estimated that about 15 per cent of all adults suffer from irritable bowel.

One suggested cause for irritable bowel is overactivity of the nerves controlling propulsive movements of the muscle in the bowel wall, and as these movements become unco-ordinated, muscle spasm and pain result. It has been shown in experiments that if a balloon is introduced into the intestine, and the pressure inside is increased, the characteristic colicky pain can be reproduced. As a result of this abnormal or increased propulsion of bowel contents, there may also be diarrhoea. Gastric infections such as giardia sometimes initiate the development of irritable bowel, and it is not unknown for this condition to develop after a nasty stomach upset caught abroad on holiday.

## Treatment

Whatever causes irritable bowel in the first place, symptoms will inevitably be exacerbated by any associated anxiety about the condition, so it is worth emphasising that it has no serious consequences, cannot lead to cancer and frequently resolves or improves in the course of time. The way the medical profession treats irritable bowel is by trying to alleviate individual symptoms. Colicky pain can be helped by drugs that have a direct relaxing effect on the muscle. Colofac, taken 20 minutes before meals, is one such drug, but it requires a prescription from your doctor. A course of capsules containing peppermint oil (Colpermin, available over-the-counter with one or two capsules being taken half an hour before meals) is an alternative that may be worth trying. This also relaxes the intestinal muscles to help with colic and bloating, though some people find it causes gastric irritation and heartburn.

The most popular method of managing irritable bowel symptoms is increasing dietary fibre. This means ensuring that the diet is rich in fruit, vegetables and wholemeal bread, or even adding bran directly on to food, such as the morning breakfast cereal. This sort of dietary change has to be introduced *gradually* (especially if you are going to try added bran), as a drastic change in diet may exacerbate symptoms, and increased fibre does not suit everyone. In a few people, where nerve-muscle control seems to be at fault, increasing fibre can lead to more pain and bloating. In this case one of the now unfashionable stimulant laxatives (e.g. Senna) may be helpful.

However, many doctors are now seriously questioning whether a high-fibre diet really is the best way to manage the symptoms of irritable bowel syndrome. There is growing evidence that food intolerance may be a significant factor in up to half of all cases. The main provocative foods appear to be dairy produce (particularly milk in people with a defect in an enzyme called lactase which helps to break up milk and aid its absorption), corn, wheat (unfortunately, the main constituent of a high-fibre diet), fried foods, chocolate, caffeine (which acts as a laxative) and citrus fruits. It can be worth experimenting with an exclusion diet and completely cutting out *all* these foods for a period of two to three weeks to see if any improvement occurs. Groups of foods are then re-introduced one by one to see if any obvious reaction occurs. If it does, the 'culprit' food(s) should be totally excluded from the diet. This sort of dietary manipulation should only be carried out with careful thought and with the help of an interested doctor or dietician – after all, people with ME/CFS have quite enough restrictions imposed on their lives without having to cut out all their favourite foods as well!

Wind, bloating and flatulence can often be helped by a preparation containing dimethicone, which helps to make the wind bubbles in the stomach coalesce. Alternatively, it may be worth trying one of the preparations containing charcoal.

When constipation is the predominant symptom, it can help to use a laxative that increases the bulk contents of the stools, such as Fybogel or Isogel. These drugs help the stool to retain water, so expanding the size, and thus increasing the motility.

If diarrhoea accompanies the pain, then management is rather different. The diarrhoea of irritable bowel isn't usually like that of true infective diarrhoea – it has the consistency of toothpaste, and may alternate with normal stools or constipated pellet-like motions. In a phase of diarrhoea, a prescribed anti-diarrhoeal drug such as codeine phosphate or loperamide (Imodium) may be useful. If you have persisting watery diarrhoea, a stool sample should be sent to the local laboratory to check for infection with giardia (see page 90).

Your doctor may also wish to arrange further hospital investigations including a sigmoidoscopy (a look inside the lower bowel using a long flexible tube) or barium examination, just to make sure there is nothing more serious going on.

Blood in the motions is *not* part of irritable bowel or ME/CFS; if this occurs you *must* go to your doctor – it may simply be piles, but it could indicate something more serious.

A couple of new approaches to the management of irritable bowel include hypnotherapy and anti-allergy drugs. Self-hypnosis centres on the idea that spasm inside the intestines can be overcome by producing a mental picture of 'knotted muscles' in the gut. Then, with hands on the stomach, soothing massage movements and concentration are used to reduce the knot.

Researchers from Italy have reported some success in severe cases of food intolerance by using a drug called sodium cromoglycate, which seems to make the gut lining less sensitive to various foods.

If you are having problems with any of these irritable bowel symptoms and your own general practitioner is finding it difficult to know what to do next, you could ask to be referred to a gastroenterology specialist.

Research into the link between ME/CFS and irritable bowel syndrome is described in reference 64.

## Weight Changes in ME/CFS

Some people, especially children, lose a significant amount of weight in the very early stages of the illness, and then experience considerable difficulty in putting it back on again, no matter how hard they try. Unfortunately, a few also go on to develop a true anorexic state (see reference 71). It should be noted that significant or progressive weight loss is *not a normal feature of ME/CFS*, and when it occurs alternative explanations (e.g. an overactive thyroid gland) should always be excluded. For advice on how to increase weight see pages 212–3.

Other people experience quite the opposite problem and find that their weight is gradually increasing. A relatively inactive lifestyle imposed by the illness obviously decreases energy requirements quite substantially, so it may be necessary to cut down on calorie intake. This should be done by reducing sugar and fat content in the diet, *not* by any dramatic starvation-type diets involving a very low calorie intake.

Weight gain can occasionally be associated with a hormonal problem, such as an underactive thyroid gland (see pages 87–8) or Cushing's syndrome (see page 871). Weight gain also occurs as a side-effect when taking some of the tricyclic antidepressant drugs.

Some women find that they have a marked cyclical weight gain around the mid point of the menstrual cycle. This is known as cyclical ideopathic oedema, and several patients studied in Professor Behan's unit in Glasgow have been found to put on an extra 10–12 lbs over this period. This type of menstrual weight gain may be related to a disturbance in the hormonal control of fluid retention (see page 108).

# Nausea

Intermittent feelings of nausea affect a minority of people with ME/CFS, but aren't usually associated with vomiting. Why this should be isn't certain – there is an area in the brain which, if disturbed, can cause a feeling of sickness; nausea can also be associated with anxiety. If necessary, there is a variety of drugs that can help, including metoclopramide (Maxalon) and a phenothiazine like Stemetil, which is probably more helpful in acute attacks. This latter drug should *not be used continuously* over long periods of time because of its side-effects on the nervous system. There are also some new anti-sickness drugs being developed which are proving to be particularly useful in cases associated with cancer treatment, where nausea can be severe and continuous. These drugs act on chemical transmitters in the brain (5HT/5 hydroxytryptamine), and may turn out to be useful in other illnesses associated with nausea. They are, however, very expensive. Two natural solutions reported as being effective are root ginger and acupressure. Acupressure is similar to acupuncture but involves pressure to a precise point on the wrist (the Neiguan point). This is achieved by an elasticated wrist band and stud which press on this acupressure site, about three fingers above the first wrist crease.

## Oesophageal Spasm

Spasms in the oesophagus (gullet) tend to come and go, and may cause difficulty with swallowing. Such spasms may be related to those elsewhere in the gut which cause irritable bowel. Any continual difficulty with swallowing is a symptom you must see the doctor about, as it will require further investigation. If oesophageal spasm becomes persistent, then there are drugs that can help, but you must take advice from a gastroenterologist.

## Proctalgia Fugax

This is the name given to a severe cramp-like pain in the rectum. It often comes on suddenly, but may then last for up to half an hour or so before gradually starting to subside. Limited relief may be obtained by going to the toilet or having a warm bath. Otherwise, there is no effective treatment. Tranquillisers should be avoided if possible.

## Hypoglycaemia

It is widely assumed that episodes of hypoglycaemia (abnormally low blood sugar) are a problem in ME/CFS. However, apart from one or two isolated reports, there is very little objective evidence to back up these claims. In fact, when Dr David McCluskey and his colleagues in Belfast measured blood sugar levels in a group of ME/CFS patients during exercise, the results turned out to be no different from the control group of people with irritable bowel syndrome (reference 248). What I suspect may be happening is that people with ME/CFS, just like many women with premenstrual syndrome, become *more sensitive* to lower levels of blood sugar, and this is why they develop hypoglycaemic symptoms (e.g. sweating, light-headedness, headaches and tremor). Once again, if this particular problem becomes severe, it is worth being referred to a diabetic specialist who can rule out any other possible causes of low blood sugar.

Advice on how to prevent these types of hypoglycaemic symptoms occurring is contained on page 211.

## Pre-Menstrual Tension (PMT)

If you're unlucky enough to have both ME/CFS and symptoms of premenstrual tension, both conditions will inevitably interact and make each other worse. PMT symptoms characteristically start towards the latter part of the cycle from the time of ovulation and then rapidly improve within a day or so of starting the period. There is a long list of symptoms, both mental and physical, associated with PMT, but among the commonest are irritability, depression, stomach bloating, breast enlargement or pain (mastalgia) and fluid retention. Although there are a large number of treatments being advocated for PMT, very few have been scientifically proven to be of value. The most popular ones include:

- Vitamin B6 (pyridoxine). This can be taken at a dose of up to 50mg per day. *Do not exceed this level* as large doses of this vitamin can damage the sensory nerves (see pages 276–7).
- Vitamin E and magnesium supplements are widely promoted by health magazines but are of doubtful value.
- Efamol (evening primrose oil) can be taken at a dose of eight x 500 mg capsules per day from day 15 till the onset of menstruation. Regular use can become very costly as this supplement is not yet available on the NHS. It can, however, be prescribed as Efamast for cyclical breast pain (mastalgia).
- Diuretics (water-losing tablets) in small doses may help when bloating or fluid retention is a particular problem.
- Relaxation techniques can be extremely useful – see Relaxation for Living in Useful Addresses, page 430.
- Dietary changes advocated include the reduction of refined sugars, salt and fat. It may also be beneficial to cut out coffee, cola drinks and chocolate. Taking a regular snack of a complex carbohydrate (even just a Ryvita biscuit) sometimes seems to help prevent rapid swings in blood sugar and resulting hypoglycaemic-type symptoms.
- Hormonal treatments are sometimes necessary when symptoms become more severe. These include the use of oestrogen skin patches and implants which prevent ovulation – now regarded by some gynaecologists as the most effective way of dealing with PMT. It also seems that the contraceptive pill is not very effective in alleviating this condition. More potent types of hormonal drugs such as Danol can be effective, but they are invariably accompanied by unpleasant side-effects (e.g. sickness, dizziness, more fluid retention and headaches), making them a far less suitable choice in ME/CFS. Some gynaecologists recommend the use of natural progesterone hormones given by vaginal or rectal suppository, but there is no universal agreement on this particular approach.

There is no simple solution to PMT; what suits one woman may not help another, so trying several different treatments may be necessary before relief is obtained. Further help and advice are available from the Premenstrual Society (see Useful Addresses, page 429).

## The Menopause and Osteoporosis

The menopause is the time of life when the ovaries start to decrease their production of the hormone oestrogen. The first sign may be an increasing irregularity in the pattern and blood loss of periods – though this should not automatically be ascribed to the menopause. Some women start to experience menopausal symptoms as early as 40, whereas others may be over 50 before anything changes. Many women go through the menopause with no problems at all, but in others, falling levels of oestrogen produce definite symptoms such as hot flushes, sweats and aching joints. Vague emotional symptoms may also occur, including irritability and depression – just as with PMT.

The problem for women with ME/CFS who are approaching the menopause is that many of the symptoms overlap, particularly vasomotor instability (hot flushes, night sweats, palpitations), which is probably due to problems with overactivity of the autonomic nervous system. Consequently, the two conditions will interact to exacerbate one another.

If there is any doubt as to whether vasomotor symptoms are due to ME/CFS or the menopause, the latter is more likely if there are associated changes in period pattern, with vaginal dryness and a rise in the hormone FSH, which can be measured by your doctor. Vaginal dryness may cause pain during sexual intercourse and this can be helped by increasing the lubrication with KY Jelly (from the pharmacy) or a locally applied oestrogen cream available on prescription.

Another problem related to the menopause is osteoporosis – loss of calcium and consequent thinning of bones – a natural ageing process, but one that accelerates in women going through the menopause because of the dramatic fall of oestrogen levels. Osteoporotic bones, especially in the wrist, hip and spine, become fragile and susceptible to fracture.

People with ME/CFS – both male and female – who are already thin and inactive (which also increases calcium loss), and who do not go outside in the sunlight to absorb vitamin D, are increasing their chances of developing osteoporosis, especially if they are also on a diet excluding milk and other dairy products – foods rich in calcium. Cigarette smoking is another contributory factor.

The only clinical trial into the incidence of osteoporosis in people with ME/CFS has been carried out at the Royal North Shore Hospital in Sydney, Australia (reference 67). This study compared bone density measurements, calcium intake and exercise levels in 37 women with ME/CFS and 20 healthy controls. Those with ME/CFS had a decreased level of bone density (a sign of osteoporosis) and a significant reduction in dietary intake of calcium – probably due to intolerance of dairy produce. The researchers concluded that *women with ME/CFS are at high risk of developing osteoporosis, especially around the menopause.*

To try and minimise the risk of developing osteoporosis, anyone with ME/CFS who is not taking sufficient calcium in their diet should be taking some form of calcium supplement (e.g. Sandocal tablets, which can be made into a fizzy drink, or ordinary calcium tablets from the pharmacy), but *do not exceed the recommended doses*, as excess calcium can be harmful (see also page 212).

Hormone replacement therapy (HRT) involves using a low dose of oestrogen which is available in pill form, as skin patches, or as implants which are inserted surgically (a very minor operation) under the skin. This is something to be seriously considered by any female with ME/CFS who is entering the menopause, as it not only helps the vasomotor symptoms, but also slows down calcium loss caused by falling oestrogen levels. In addition, HRT is believed to give increased protection against heart disease. HRT should be discussed with your doctor and may be a viable option provided there are no medical contra-indications – e.g. heart disease, previous cancer of the uterus or family history of breast cancer.

If you require further information about menopausal symptoms and the various treatments available, contact the Amarant Trust (see Useful Addresses, page 409). The Osteoporosis Society (see Useful Addresses, page 428) provides information on this particular menopausal complication. Additional information on the use of oestrogen and progesterone supplements is contained on page 189.

## Thrush

Candida albicans, or thrush, is probably the commonest cause of vaginal discharge in women. For some, though, it's not just an occasional 'one-off' problem, but a recurring nuisance which never seems to go away.

The yeast candida lives quite happily in our bodies without causing any problems. Then, from time to time, it goes out of control and multiplies to start causing symptoms. In the vagina, there is a creamy discharge along with external soreness and irritation, but other parts of the body, particularly the skin and nails, can also be affected.

A variety of explanations have been put forward as to what 'tips the balance' and allows the yeast to start multiplying. These include antibiotics, diabetes and immune-deficiency. Many gynaecologists now doubt that there is any link between thrush and taking the oral contraceptive pill. The fact that candida is a latent organism prone to periodic reactivation has led some doctors to link its presence to ME/CFS, but my personal experience is that *the incidence of thrush is no higher among people with ME/CFS than is found in the normal population*. I am dealing with the subject here for the benefit of those who believe that such a link exists. Treatment of an acute episode of thrush is usually very effective; it is preventing recurrence that causes the problem. Pessaries are the commonest prescribed treatment – these used to have to be inserted for a week or more, but now there are new types which are equally effective in a few days, or can even be taken in one 'megadose'. Some women prefer anti-fungal creams, which can be prescribed along with an applicator. Your male partner may also have the infection on his penis, without any symptoms, so it is usually a good idea to ask him to use some cream twice daily as well.

Self-help measures can significantly reduce the chances of a recurrence:

- Avoid tight-fitting jeans, nylon pants and tights – in fact any clothing that helps to create a warm, moist environment in which the yeast thrives.
- Wipe your bottom away from your vagina as reinfection can come from the bowels.
- Do not 'traumatise' the vagina by using chemicals like bubble baths or vaginal douches; if you are dry during intercourse use KY Jelly.

If attacks of thrush keep recurring, your doctor may be willing to give you a further supply of medication, or a prescription, so you can start treatment as soon as any symptoms recur.

If none of these measures help, then a prolonged course of anti-fungal treatment may be necessary.

## Pain in the Joints (Arthralgia)

In addition to muscle pain (myalgia) which may accompany fatigue in ME/CFS, some people experience a variety of joint and bone pains. This kind of pain – arthralgia – is not usually as severe as muscle pain, and is not associated with any permanent disruption to the joint, which can occur in pure rheumatic diseases.

If the joints are carefully examined by a doctor, it is unusual to find any restriction in their range of movement. There are no changes seen with X-rays. For these reasons the cause may well be due to involvement of the supporting structures – muscles and tendons – which surround the joint. However, it is now recognised that a variety of viral infections can cause a temporary arthritis, with rubella being particularly common (other causes are described on page 41). Lowered levels of cortisol are another possible explanation.

If you are experiencing joint pains, particularly if there is any associated swelling, your doctor should carry out tests to exclude a number of specific rheumatic diseases before ascribing these symptoms to ME/CFS. Conditions such as Sjögren's syndrome and systemic lupus erythematosus (SLE), which are occasionally misdiagnosed as ME/CFS, are described in more detail on pages 102–3. The combination of bone pain in the back and muscle weakness which causes particular difficulty when moving from sitting to standing raises the possibility of osteomalacia being present.

Treatment of arthralgia is normally with one of the anti-inflammatory drugs, whichever seems to suit the individual best. Aspirin, taken four to six hourly, is still a very effective drug as long as it doesn't upset your stomach. If this is unsuitable, one of the new anti-inflammatory drugs (NSAIDs) can be purchased (e.g. Brufen) or prescribed, but they don't suit everyone. Paracetamol is not a very effective drug for arthritic pain. Steroids should *definitely* be avoided in most cases.

One useful alternative approach is evening primrose oil (Efamol), which has been shown in controlled trials to be as effective as conventional drugs in the treatment of mild arthritic pain. It is free from side-effects (see pages 186–7).

Another 'natural' product which has been shown to have similar anti-inflammatory effects to evening primrose oil is a daily dose of olive oil.

## Respiratory Problems

Although a small number of people, generally those who are more severely affected by ME/CFS, find that they develop breathing difficulties, there has been very little research into this aspect of the illness.

The only published study (reference 70) assessed lung function using tests (e.g. FEV1, FVC and PEF) which are very similar to those carried out in diagnosing asthma. Results indicated a *'significant reduction in all lung function parameters'*. In conclusion, the authors of this study reported that in their group of ME/CFS patients, *'There is a moderate respiratory muscle dysfunction resulting in abnormal lung function tests.'*

## Sore Throats and Enlarged Glands

These two symptoms form a common initial presentation of the illness, and in some instances go on to become a recurring problem, possibly due to reactivation of a glandular fever-type virus (Epstein-Barr) or an oversensitivity of the immune system to any 'new' infection that affects the throat.

Throat swabs taken by a doctor seldom reveal any organisms which are sensitive to antibiotics. These drugs are best avoided, and should only be used where a specific bacterium has been grown by the pathology laboratory, or where there is a marked general illness with fever and noticeably enlarged glands in the neck.

Antiseptic mouth washes, gargles and throat pastilles are probably of limited value. A soothing warm drink made from glycerine, honey and lemon, or sucking a boiled sweet are much cheaper alternatives, and probably more soothing. Recurrent sore throats are *not* an indication to have your tonsils removed, although this will be considered if there are several attacks of genuine tonsillitis throughout the year.

## Skin Problems

Quite a few of my ME/CFS patients report on how they seem to bruise more easily, but there is no evidence of any associated blood or skin disorder present which could explain this problem. A more likely cause, which I suspect is commoner than realised, is that clumsiness and lack of co-ordination make people more prone to injuries which, in turn, result in bruising.

Immune system disturbances could account for the fact that cold sores, caused by recurrent herpes infection, become a problem for some adults. Cold sores are extremely common in the normal adult population, but it's interesting to note that reactivation of other types of herpes virus infection have been linked to ME/CFS. If cold sores become severe or persistent, then there are some highly effective antiviral drugs available from your doctor.

## Disordered Sleep

Normal adults vary widely in their nightly sleep requirements. Some are bright and alert after only five or six hours, whereas others must have their statutory eight hours or more of good solid sleep.

A common occurrence in nearly everyone with ME/CFS is increased sleep requirements (hypersomnia). This is especially so in the very early stages of the illness, when sleeping for 14 or 16 hours a day is not unusual. Those who are recovering seldom seem able to cope with being up and about for a full 12-hour day without some form of rest period, unless they're going through an extremely good patch. Even after a full night's sleep, someone with ME/CFS will still wake up feeling unrefreshed.

It's important to remember that the commonest sleep problem – that of requiring too much sleep – isn't necessarily something to fight against. This is your body's way of instructing you to slow down. It's also a very important healing mechanism, which allows the body to repair damaged tissues and aid recovery. Don't feel guilty about going to bed early if you feel the need to. If your body says 'sleep', then this is what you probably ought to do.

Normal human sleep is divided into two quite distinct components, each occurring in alternate periods throughout the night. Dream sleep occupies about a quarter of the total time asleep, coming on in bouts of gradually increasing length. This type of sleep is technically known as rapid eye movement (REM) sleep.

The other type of sleep – orthodox or non-REM sleep – occurs in rather longer periods between each block of dream sleep. During these periods you gradually pass from light sleep into deep sleep and then re-enter a period of dream sleep.

As far as benefits of sleep are concerned, it's the first four or five hours of deep sleep that are really important. Any interruption in these first few vital hours has been shown to significantly affect mental functioning and the ability to learn new tasks the following day. The final few hours of sleep are far less important.

Control of sleep is thought to centre in parts of the brain known as the brain stem and hypothalamus. As I discuss in Chapter 8: Current Research, both of these areas may turn out to be key parts of the nervous system that are involved in ME/CFS. Whether people with ME/CFS have significant changes in the ratio of dream sleep to non-dream sleep is an area that warrants further research in sleep laboratories.

Another possible explanation for these sleep disturbances has been put forward by one of the world's leading authorities on sleep, Professor Harvey Moldofsky. He has suggested that some of the immune system abnormalities (e.g. increased production of cytokines); which are triggered by viral infections, may be affecting sleep control centres in the brain. For more information on research into sleep disturbances see page 156 and references 303–311.

Besides the generally increased requirement for sleep there are several other disturbances in sleep patterns which commonly occur. Some people with ME/CFS find themselves falling asleep at inappropriate times of the day, and in children it is not unusual to find a complete reversal of the normal pattern, with sleeping during the day and being awake at night. However, the three commonest types of disturbed sleep are:

**(1) Difficulty getting off to sleep** This often coincides with a rise in mental activity after retiring to bed. Thoughts of unachieved plans for that day, coming events or a range of unsolvable anxieties may all start to surface and prevent the initiation of sleep.

**(2) Waking up once asleep** Here the cause can be associated with distressing physical symptoms which disturb normal sleep, e.g. sweating, muscle aches and cramps, needing to pass urine, restless legs or jerking movements. These sort of problems may continually interrupt sleep throughout the night, and this difficulty in maintaining good-quality sleep is now thought to be the most common type of disturbance found in ME/CFS.

**Night cramps** in the calf muscles can affect anyone, and if massage or local heat won't provide relief, a simple stretching exercise can often be very effective in relieving the pain.

Stand and face the bedroom wall, with your feet about three feet away from the skirting-board. Then lean forward, using hands and arms to act as support against the wall, and make sure that your heels don't move off the ground. This will stretch the calf muscles. Keep them stretched for about 10 seconds, then relax for a while and repeat the exercise.

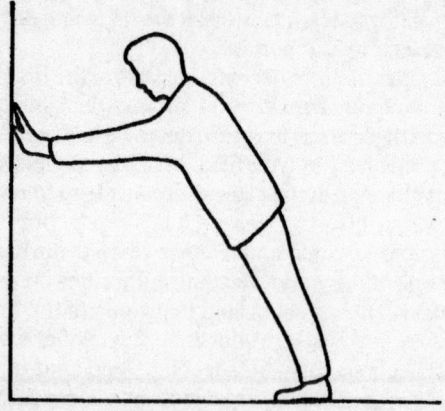

If cramp is occurring regularly, try repeating these exercises three times a day as well.

A wide range of drugs have been tried for treating night cramps. Quinine sulphate is the one that is most frequently prescribed, but it does have disturbing side-effects, including eye damage, tinnitus, confusion and blood disorders. Consequently, *it shouldn't generally be used for more than two or three weeks.*

**Restless legs** are another cause of disturbed sleep, whereby people complain of a variety of strange sensations, which seem to be more in the muscle than the skin. (Doctors sometimes refer to this condition as Ekbom's syndrome.) Tickling, pricking, burning or crawling feelings are frequently mentioned, as well as jerking movements in the legs. This strange activity is usually confined to the lower parts of the leg; the thigh and ankle areas are not usually affected. Symptoms tend to gradually increase in intensity, till the only way of obtaining relief is to get out of bed and walk around the room. Unfortunately, this may have to be repeated several times in one night.

Doctors don't know what causes 'restless legs'; it's certainly not confined to ME/CFS, and has also been linked to rheumatoid arthritis, iron deficiency anaemia and an excessive intake of caffeine – so it's worth trying decaffeinated coffee. Sometimes warming (or cooling) the affected leg may help; other sufferers try exercises before going to sleep, but there doesn't seem to be an effective treatment which suits everyone.

As with night cramps, a variety of drugs have been tried, but the results are not impressive. Fortunately, for many people awoken by this strange phenomenon, it's a transient problem which seems to come and go.

**Vivid dreams**, or even nightmares are reported by some people with ME/CFS. Dreams are often described as being in vivid colours and involving various 'pressures' which seem to be causing anxiety, e.g. getting back to work again, or the frustrations of trying to achieve some other impossible task.

**(3) Early morning wakening** This is when you wake up at, say, 4 or 5 a.m., and then have great difficulty in getting back to sleep again. This type of sleep disturbance is very characteristic of clinical depression, which would obviously require specific drug treatment.

## Helping yourself to a better night's sleep

Here are some useful tips which should help to promote a better night's sleep, without having to resort to sleeping tablets.

### General advice

- Spending excessively long periods of time in bed during the day can result in fragmented and shallow sleep at night. People with ME/CFS often have increased sleep requirements early on in the illness, but as time goes by, spending too much time in bed during the day can have very adverse effects on normal patterns of sleep at night.
- Try to establish a regular waking time each morning. This will help to promote a more normal sleep rhythm on a day-to-day basis. It should also make it easier to go to sleep at a more regular time in the evening.

- Don't forget the importance of sleeping in a room which has fresh air coming in. A comfortable bed with a good firm mattress could be a sound investment!

## During the evening

- Try not to involve yourself in stimulating mental activity or watching exciting television programmes in the hour or so before you normally go to bed. Reading a small amount from a good book is a much better way of 'switching off'.
- If you don't feel fully relaxed at night, try the relaxation technique I describe on pages 247–8, especially if you have any painful 'trouble spots'. An audio cassette tape (e.g. *Sleep Well!* from Lifeskills, see Useful Addresses, page 431) can be helpful as well. You could also try learning some creative visualisation techniques to quieten the mind, e.g. thinking about leaves floating down a river.
- Don't embark on heavy meals, alcohol or caffeine-containing drinks late in the evening. A glass of warm milk or herbal tea such as camomile or lime blossom is a much better alternative.
- Inhaling an aromatic oil, such as ylang-ylang, or orange blossom added to a warm bath are both soothing and relaxing – see aromatherapy in Chapter 13: Alternative and Complementary Approaches. Homoeopaths often recommend arnica for those who feel over-tired and restless, or coffea for those who are wide awake and dwelling on the next day's problems.

## At bedtime

- Let yourself relax and remember that sleep will come when it's ready to do so.
- Don't try to fall asleep. If you try to 'switch on' sleep in this way, all you end up doing is 'switching it off'.
- Make sure that the bed isn't too warm and not too cold.
- If you're still not feeling tired, don't forget that sex is a good way of sending people off to sleep!
- A warm bath can also be very sleep-inducing.

## If you have problems during the night

- When pain is waking you in the night or preventing you falling asleep, try taking a mild painkiller before retiring.
- If you're still awake half an hour later, it's probably better to get out of bed and go to another room for a while or have a cup of tea.

## How can a doctor help?

Unfortunately, all too often going to ask a doctor for help with sleep disorders simply leads to a prescription for 'sleeping pills'. These may well help to break a vicious circle, but are not a long-term solution. If used, this type of medication should *only be taken for a short period* (preferably no longer than a couple of weeks) or intermittently – say every third day over a slightly longer period.

**Antidepressants** A low dose of a sedating tricyclic antidepressant such as amitriptyline (10–25mg given mid-evening) is probably a far better choice when sleep problems become persistent. Side-effects aren't usually troublesome at this dose level and treatment can be continued for a longer period than with a benzodiazepine.

**Antihistamines** These drugs are normally used to treat allergic reactions or skin irritation. They also cause sedation as a side-effect, which is why some people use them for insomnia. Mixtures such as Medinex and Nytol can be purchased over-the-counter, but the main problem with using antihistamines in this way is that they inevitably cause daytime drowsiness. For this reason, I feel *they are generally unsuitable for treating sleep disturbance in ME/CFS.*

**Barbiturates** Although still available on prescription, these potentially dangerous drugs should only be used in very exceptional circumstances for severe intractable insomnia. *They have no place in the management of ME/CFS.*

**Benzodiazepines** These commonly prescribed drugs are chemically very similar to tranquillisers such as Valium (diazepam). They all carry the same serious risk of dependence and side-effects, including headaches, drowsiness, light-headedness, confusion and dizziness the following day.

Benzodiazepines are divided into two main groups. Shorter-acting ones last for about 6 to 10 hours but may cause some degree of drowsiness and confusion the following day. Examples include Loprazolam, Lormetazepam, Normison (temazepam), Rohypnol (flunitrazepam) and temazepam.

The longer-acting benzodiazepines all produce sedating effects which can persist well into the following day. After repeated use they also start to accumulate in the body, especially in the elderly, where they may lead to serious confusion. *I would not recommend their use in ME/CFS.* Examples include Dalmane (flurazepam), Mogadon (nitrazepam) and Nitrazepam.

When benzodiazepines have been taken for a long period of time (several weeks or more), it becomes increasingly difficult to stop taking them, even though they may be having little effect on normalising sleep patterns. The withdrawal symptoms are very similar to those experienced by people coming off tranquillisers used to treat anxiety (see pages 246–7).

**Heminevrin (chlormethiazole)** The use of this drug tends to be restricted to more elderly people with sleep problems. Side-effects include nasal irritation and congestion, gastric upsets, headaches and confusion. *I do not believe that Heminevrin is a good choice for anyone with ME/CFS.*

**Melatonin** This is the body's natural sleep hormone, which is produced by a small part of the brain known as the pineal gland. Levels of melatonin gradually start to decline as we grow older and this decrease in production has been linked to all kinds of human health problems, particularly disturbed patterns of sleep. Melatonin also acts in other parts of the body to affect mood, digestion, reproductive cycles and the immune system.

Research studies involving the use of melatonin have shown that it can improve the quality of sleep as well as helping people who are going to sleep at inappropriate times of the day or night.

Commercially available preparations have rapid but transient sleep-inducing properties. And by manipulating the body's internal clock, they've been found to be extremely useful in reducing the adverse effects of jet lag.

A number of doctors, including myself, believe that melatonin (in a dose of 2–5mg taken at night) can be of significant help to some people with ME/CFS, especially those whose normal sleep/wake cycle has become severely distorted in the course of their illness. I've also found melatonin to be occasionally useful in children who are sleeping during the day and are then awake at night.

Melatonin isn't habit-forming, but around 6 per cent of users report side-effects, including vivid dreams, nightmares and daytime drowsiness. No serious long-term side-effects have as yet been reported. However, this lack of reliable information on safety resulted in the UK Medicines Control Agency deciding to classify melatonin supplements as medicines, so severely restricting their over-the-counter availability. It may be possible to obtain melatonin in the UK on a private prescription from your GP (on a named patient basis), but not all GPs are willing to take the risk of co-operating in this way. Melatonin is still readily available outside the UK, but do take care if you decide to purchase it from a foreign source as some companies have been using pineal glands from cows' brains (risk of BSE) to obtain their supplies.

The use of melatonin in sleep disturbances associated with ME/CFS deserves further assessment as raised levels have now been reported in some patients (see reference 530).

In the UK, pharmacists can obtain supplies of melatonin from PharmaNord Ltd (tel: 0800 591756). You will need to present the pharmacist with a prescription (NHS or private) written out by your GP for melatonin.

**Stilnoct (zolpidem)** This is a new type of drug which is claimed to be as effective as the benzodiazepines, yet has fewer adverse effects on mental performance the following day. Stilnoct has a fairly rapid onset of action, so it can be particularly helpful for those who have difficulty in getting off to sleep at night. Side-effects include gastric upsets, headaches, memory disturbances, lack of co-ordination, nightmares and depression. Some users report daytime drowsiness. Stilnoct is thought to produce fewer withdrawal problems than benzodiazepines.

**Zimovane (zopiclone)** Another new drug which is not in the benzodiazepine group, and like Stilnoct has a fairly rapid onset of action. Zimovane lasts for about six to eight hours and is claimed to have a low incidence of side-effects. However, it can produce gastric upsets, a bitter or metallic taste in the mouth, a dry mouth, irritability, lack of co-ordination, headaches, dizziness and confusion. Zimovane needs to be used with care as some doctors believe that continued use can lead to problems with dependence.

Amitriptyline (in a low dose), Stilnoct and Zimovane are probably the three best drugs to choose from when it comes to the treatment of sleep problems associated with ME/CFS. They are all likely to be effective in the short-term, but are not the long-term solution.

When researchers finally unravel the workings of the biological clock that regulates normal sleep, it seems highly likely that safe and more effective drugs will become available.

Lastly, I'd like to briefly consider two important sleep disturbances – sleep apnoea syndrome and narcolepsy – which are both associated with severe daytime fatigue and are occasionally misdiagnosed as ME/CFS.

## Sleep apnoea

Although not strictly related to ME/CFS, this condition is worth including because it is yet another cause of chronic fatigue that is often overlooked. I know of several patients with suspected ME/CFS for whom this turned out to be the main reason for their ill-health.

Sleep apnoea is a condition of disordered breathing which occurs during the night. The result is a very low level of oxygen reaching the brain. Common causes include obesity (a collar size of more than 17½" is said to be an important clue!) and large tonsils or adenoids. These obstructions to the airway in the throat cause it to collapse during the night, and sleep is constantly disturbed by a series of 'attacks' where abortive breaths are followed by loud snorts and near-wakening. In the morning the bed looks like a battlefield and the constant lack of satisfactory sleep produces severe daytime drowsiness.

Serious sleep disorders like this are best diagnosed in hospitals that have established sleep laboratories. Well-known ones include the City Hospital in Edinburgh, the John Radcliffe Hospital in Oxford, Leicester Infirmary and one at the department of psychiatry, St George's Hospital, London.

## Narcolepsy

This is a rare inherited sleep disorder which almost always starts before the age of 30. Disturbances in sleep control mechanisms within the brain result in periodic and embarrassing attacks of suddenly going off to sleep during the day, each one lasting for about 15 minutes. Attacks commonly occur after meals, while travelling or at times of boredom. Some people with narcolepsy have up to 20 such attacks during the course of a single day. Narcolepsy is sometimes associated with terrifying hallucinations and sleep paralysis. For more information contact the Narcolepsy Association (see Useful Addresses, page 428).

Periods of excessive sleep can also occur in another rare condition known as the Kleine-Levin Syndrome which predominantly affects young men. These may last for days or even weeks. On recovery, there is a phase of abnormal eating.

# Other Causes of Chronic Fatigue

In the previous thee chapters I've described the way in which ME/CFS is commonly triggered by either an infection, vaccination or exposure to some form of chemical toxin, as well as explaining the wide range of symptoms which can occur as the illness enters a more chronic phase.

One of the major problems in making a diagnosis of ME/CFS is that this still has to be done on the basis of your symptoms. Although abnormalities in brain chemistry and body hormones may eventually be used to form a diagnostic blood test, this isn't likely to occur in the near future. Without such an aid to diagnosis, it's vital to make sure that all other forms of chronic fatigue are thoroughly ruled out.

My own personal experience of having seen well over 800 ME/CFS patients is that around 5 to 10 per cent have some other medical or psychiatric explanation – which may be responsive to drug treatment – for their persisting ill health. The medical journals are also starting to report on disturbing cases where ME/CFS has been misdiagnosed by either a doctor, an alternative practitioner or sufferers themselves, and serious conditions such as multiple sclerosis, brain tumours and lead poisoning were the true problem.

To diagnose ME/CFS, extensive and elaborate investigations are seldom required in addition to the baseline blood tests I describe on pages 163–4. However, when a particular symptom – say, joint pain or enlarged lymph glands – predominates, then a careful search must be taken to exclude other possible causes.

It's also worth noting that when an ME/CFS-like illness occurs in someone who works with animals, there are several unusual infections which may need to be ruled out (e.g. brucellosis, leptospirosis and yersinia). The same reasoning applies to anyone who may have picked up an infection whilst travelling abroad, or who works with toxic chemicals or pesticides.

I will now describe a number of important conditions which can produce chronic fatigue as either the presenting or predominant symptom.

## Table 5 Other Possible Causes of Chronic Fatigue

**Blood disorders**
anaemia
haemochromatosis

**Drugs**

**Gastrointestinal disorders**
coeliac disease
Crohn's disease
food allergy/intolerance
irritable bowel syndrome

**Heart conditions**
intermittent claudication
low blood pressure

**Hormonal imbalance**
Addison's disease
Cushings syndrome
pituitary tumours
hyper and hypothyroidism

**Infections**
brucellosis
campylobacter
clostridium botulinum
cytomegalovirus
giardia
hepatitis
HIV
leptospirosis hardjo
Lyme disease
mycoplasma
parvovirus B19
Q fever
toxocara
toxoplasmosis
yersinia pseudotuberculosis

**Liver disease**
primary biliary cirrhosis
Gilbert's disease

**Malignancy**
Hodgkin's disease

**Muscle disorders**
myasthenia gravis
polymyalgia rheumatica
polymyositis

**Neurological disorders**
multiple sclerosis
Parkinson's disease

**Poisoning**
carbon monoxide
lead

**Psychiatric disorders**
anxiety
depression
hyperventilation syndrome
post-traumatic stress disorder
seasonal affective disorder (SAD)
somatisation
stress and overwork

**Respiratory disorders**
sarcoidosis
tuberculosis

**Rheumatic diseases**
Sjögren's syndrome
systematic lupus erythematosus

**Other conditions**
alcohol abuse
raised blood calcium
osteomalacia
sick building syndrome
sleep apnoea and narcolepsy

**Overlapping disorders**
athletic overtraining
ciguatera poisoning
fibromyalgia
fluid retention syndrome
Gulf War Syndrome
organophosphate poisoning
post-polio syndrome

# Blood Disorders

## Anaemia

Symptoms which are common to both ME/CFS and anaemia include palpitations, headaches and dizziness. However, ME/CFS doesn't usually cause marked pallor of the nailbeds and tongue, ankle swelling or shortness of breath.

Everyone suspected of having ME/CFS *must* have a routine blood test to check for the presence of anaemia (see pages 165–6). *ME/CFS does not cause anaemia*, and if this is detected, a thorough assessment needs to be made by your doctor to find the true cause. Common explanations for anaemia include a poor dietary intake of nutrients, malabsorption, and blood loss from the bowels or from heavy periods. It's also worth noting that several other important causes of chronic fatigue can cause anaemia. These include brucellosis, coeliac disease, hypothyroidism and lupus (SLE).

Anyone who experiences recurrent soreness of the tongue, along with tingling sensations (paraesthesiae) and/or numbness in the arms or legs should be checked for pernicious (vitamin B12 deficiency) anaemia.

## Haemochromatosis

Although most people have never even heard of haemochromatosis, it's one of the most common inherited disorders. A genetic fault causes increased absorption of iron, which then starts to accumulate in various body tissues.

Early on, there may be fatigue, weakness, headaches, joint pains (particularly in the knuckles of the first and second fingers), stomach pains and loss of sex drive. Later on, haemochromatosis can cause diabetes, a tanned appearance to the skin, decreased amounts of body hair and mood swings.

If the diagnosis is suspected, then various blood tests (to check for increased levels of serum ferritin and a transferrin saturation of greater than 50 per cent) will need to be arranged.

# Drugs

Fatigue is one of the most frequently reported side-effects to be associated with both prescription-only and over-the-counter medications. Among the more common examples are drugs for treating allergies (e.g. antihistamines), anxiety (tranquillisers such as Valium), depression (sedating tricyclic preparations) and heart conditions (beta-blockers). There shouldn't usually be any confusion with ME/CFS. However, the use of these, and a number of other drugs, can obviously cause a further increase in fatigue, and so they need to be used with caution by anyone who has ME/CFS.

# Gastrointestinal Disorders

If you have fatigue plus a number of stomach and/or bowel symptoms, then it may be advisable to exclude some of the conditions listed below, along with infections such as giardia.

## Coeliac disease

Many doctors still regard coeliac disease (sensitivity to gluten in wheat products) as a disease of childhood. In fact, one in every 300 adults is thought to be affected.

The commonest presenting symptoms are fatigue, weight loss, stomach pains and diarrhoea – symptoms which are easily confused with a diagnosis of ME/CFS plus an 'irritable bowel'. Other less common features of coeliac disease which should *not* be confused with ME/CFS include anaemia (due to iron or folic acid deficiency), recurrent mouth ulcers, arthritis (which can be a presenting feature), hair loss and low blood pressure.

I now know of several adults who were initially diagnosed as having ME/CFS, but then experienced a dramatic improvement in general health once they had tried removing wheat products from their diet. Hospital investigations – including the removal of a minute piece of small bowel tissue (a biopsy) for examination under the microscope – should confirm the diagnosis.

Interestingly, carnitine deficiency has been reported in both coeliac disease and ME/CFS (see page 140), and antigliadin antibodies (a blood marker of untreated coeliac disease) appear to be quite common in people with neurological illness of unknown cause (reference 81).

## Crohn's disease

This is a chronic form of inflammation that can affect any part of the bowel lining from the small intestine right down to the anus. Common symptoms include diarrhoea, rectal bleeding, stomach pain and weight loss. Episodes of fever may accompany exacerbations of Crohn's disease.

As with coeliac disease, Crohn's disease is occasionally misdiagnosed as being ME/CFS plus an 'irritable bowel'. However, ME/CFS *does not cause* progressive weight loss or rectal bleeding.

Blood tests in Crohn's disease may reveal anaemia (due to low iron or folic acid levels), a raised ESR (erythrocyte sedimentation rate, see page 255–60) and a low level of potassium. The diagnosis is confirmed by hospital investigations (e.g. a biopsy of the lining mucosa and X-rays).

## Food allergy/intolerance

Besides producing 'irritable bowel'-type symptoms, genuine food allergy/intolerance can cause chronic fatigue, migraine attacks, aching joints and depression. Some of the most commonly eaten foods are the main culprits, with 60 per cent of patients with food allergy being affected by wheat, 44 per cent by milk or corn, 39 per cent by cheese, 33 per cent by coffee and 24 per cent by citrus fruits.

If you suspect that food allergy or intolerance could be the underlying cause for your symptoms, I strongly recommend that you see an NHS specialist who is competent in this controversial area of medicine. Further details on allergy diagnosis and treatment are contained on pages 255–60.

## Irritable bowel syndrome (IBS)

Varying degrees of IBS affect around 20 per cent of all adults, with a significant female predominance. Besides the common symptoms of stomach pain, distension, diarrhoea (often described as a frequent urge to pass loose or pellet-like stools with an 'early morning rush' to the toilet), IBS quite often co-exists with ME/CFS (reference 64). IBS can also produce gynaecological symptoms (urgency to pass urine and pain on intercourse) and joint pains. It *does not cause* weight loss or rectal bleeding. The management of IBS is described on pages 63–4.

# Heart Conditions

## Intermittent claudication

Muscle pain in the arms or legs can sometimes be quite severe in ME/CFS, and when this occurs it may be necessary to rule out other possible muscle disorders (see later in this chapter).

One important cause of severe muscle pain in the legs is intermittent claudication – a condition caused by narrowing of the arterial blood supply. This type of muscle pain is almost always *brought on by exercise and quickly relieved by rest*. Later on, though, it may occur at night. The pain is usually described as being 'cramp like', and mainly involves the calf or thigh muscles. It's often worse in one leg and may cause a limp.

If your muscle pain feels more like intermittent claudication, especially if you have any other heart problems, then ask your GP to check the state of the pulses in your leg. If necessary, you can be referred to hospital for further investigations on the blood supply to the legs.

## Low blood pressure (hypotension)

Most people who are found to have a low blood pressure (defined as being below 110/60) don't usually have any signs of ill health. However, research suggests that low blood pressure can be associated with symptoms such as fatigue, dizziness and depression (reference: *British Medical Journal*, 1992, 304, 75–8). It also appears that a subgroup of ME/CFS patients have low blood pressure as part of this illness (see pages 144–5).

If low blood pressure is found during a medical examination, then it is important to rule out a number of conditions (e.g. Addison's disease, Parkinson's disease and diabetes) which could be the cause. Drugs such as antidepressants can sometimes be responsible as well.

In contrast to several other European countries, doctors in the UK are reluctant to treat low blood pressure, but research from America suggests that drug treatment can sometimes be helpful when it is associated with ME/CFS (reference 143).

# Hormones

## Addison's disease

This a rare but potentially fatal hormonal disorder which shares a number of common symptoms (e.g. fatigue, muscle weakness, dizziness, low blood pressure, stomach pains and headaches) with ME/CFS. It is caused by the destruction of the outer layer of the adrenal gland – usually due to infection or an immunological problem – and so produces a dramatic fall in the output of cortisol. Interestingly, cortisol is a hormone which also appears to be deficient in ME/CFS (see pages 149–50).

Symptoms of Addison's disease which *do not occur* in ME/CFS include vomiting, weight loss, increased pigmentation (brown skin) in the mouth, scars, pressure areas and palmar creases, and loss of body hair.

Routine blood tests often reveal:

- a low level of cortisol (0900 sample)
- increased urea and potassium
- low sodium
- low thyroxine (T4) and increased thyroid stimulating hormone (TSH)

If a diagnosis of Addison's disease seems at all possible, you need *urgent referral* to a hospital specialist for further investigations and treatment with steroids.

## Cushing's syndrome

This refers to a combination of symptoms which are caused by a persistently raised level of cortisol – a finding which is *not* characteristic of ME/CFS. Symptoms include weight gain (particularly around the trunk and abdomen), muscle weakness, skin problems (easy bruising, acne, fungal infections and red or purple lines/striae on the abdomen), raised blood pressure and depression. A 48-hour low-dose dexamethasone suppression test is a simple and reliable way of making the diagnosis.

## Pituitary tumours

One of the most disturbing reports involving misdiagnosis of ME/CFS concerned a 65-year-old man with a four-year history of chronic fatigue and weight loss who had been treated by a herbalist (reference 82). When he was finally referred to hospital it emerged that he was suffering from a pituitary gland tumour in the brain. This was successfully removed and, with the help of hormone replacement therapy, he was able to resume a normal lifestyle. Sadly, this was not the only instance I know of where a brain tumour has been misdiagnosed as ME/CFS.

Although this type of brain tumour isn't usually cancerous, it can lead to serious problems if left untreated. Characteristic symptoms of a pituitary tumour include headaches (dull in nature, often at the front of the head and made worse by coughing or sneezing), disturbances in temperature control (as with ME/CFS), abnormal eating patterns and general fatigue. GP blood tests may reveal disturbances in hormone levels (e.g. prolactin, thyroid and cortisol), but the diagnosis needs to be confirmed by special radiological investigations in hospital.

## Thyroid gland disorders

Underactivity (hypothyroidism or myxoedema) and overactivity (hyperthyroidism or thyrotoxicosis) of the thyroid gland are two important hormonal disorders which *must* be ruled out in anyone who is suspected of having ME/CFS.

*Hypothyroidism* This doesn't usually occur in the under 45s but thereafter starts to appear with increasing frequency. It can cause a wide range of symptoms affecting almost any part of the body. General complaints include fatigue, increasing weight, depression and intolerance to the cold. As with ME/CFS, hypothyroidism can cause muscle pain and problems with normal mental activity. Symptoms which are *not seen in ME/CFS* include progressive hoarseness, dry puffy skin, hair loss (especially the outer third of the eyebrows) and a low pulse rate. Hypothyroidism sometimes produces an obvious enlargement of the thyroid gland at the front of the neck (a goitre).

Abnormal blood test results quickly confirm the diagnosis. These include:

- decreased levels of free and total thyroxine (T4) and increased levels of thyroid stimulating hormone (TSH)
- increased levels of TSH and a normal T4 – often seen early on or in mild cases
- decreased free and total T4 and normal or slightly decreased TSH, indicating that the problem is due to lack of stimulation on the thyroid gland by either the hypothalamus or the pituitary gland.

At present, there is no scientific evidence to suggest that people with ME/CFS have low levels of thyroid hormones, but studies are in progress to investigate this possibility (see page 167).

*Thyrotoxicosis* commonly causes fatigue, muscle weakness, sweating, heat intolerance and palpitations – all common symptoms of both ME/CFS and anxiety. In addition, thyrotoxicosis produces weight loss, tremor, puffiness or a gritty feeling in the eyes, and hand tremor – symptoms which are *not* seen in ME/CFS.

Blood tests will show an increased level of free and total T4 along with a reduced level of TSH.

## Infections

### Brucellosis

This is an infection which can be transmitted from various animal sources, including cattle (from unpasteurised milk), dogs, goats (from cheese) and sheep. Although nowhere near as common as it used to be, brucellosis can still be picked up during foreign travel, particularly in the Gulf States and Saudi Arabia.

After an incubation period lasting one to three weeks, the onset is usually 'flu-like with fever, chills, malaise, joint pains, loss of appetite, headaches and profuse sweating.

Brucellosis sometimes produces a slow-onset illness with ME/CFS-like features such as fatigue, excessive sleep requirements, low-grade fever, sweating episodes, depression and joint pains (particularly in the lower back). There can also be a significant loss of weight and recurrent chest infections.

Blood test abnormalities include a low white blood cell count (a leucopenia) and minor elevations in liver enzymes. A raised level of antibody IgG indicates active or recent infection with brucellosis. Further confirmation of the diagnosis can sometimes be obtained by culture of the organism from a blood sample. Treatment with a combination of antibiotics may then be necessary.

Brucellosis certainly needs to be considered in anyone with chronic fatigue who has been in the Middle East or works closely with farm animals, especially if there is associated weight loss, back pains or fever.

## Campylobacter

This produces attacks of gastroenteritis, particularly during the warm summer months. Sources of infection include undercooked food (chicken and pork) and contaminated milk or water (even bathing water in lakes).

After an incubation period of three to five days, early symptoms consist of severe cramp-like stomach pains and loose watery stools, which are frequently blood-stained.

A small minority of people fail to recover from the acute attack and continue to complain of fatigue, sometimes accompanied by joint pains and persisting loose motions.

Diagnosis can normally be confirmed by sending a stool specimen to the hospital laboratory. Antibiotic treatment with erythromycin may be recommended if symptoms persist.

## Clostridium botulinum (botulism)

Infection with this bacterium results in the production of a powerful chemical toxin (neurotoxin) which causes life-threatening muscle paralysis. The best-known clostridium infection is tetanus, but the infection that is of most interest in relation to ME/CFS is *Clostridium botulinum*.

An outbreak of this infection – which is usually contracted by eating contaminated tinned food – occurred in north-west England and Wales during June 1989. It was reported in *The Lancet* (reference 77) by Dr E. M. Critchley, the neurologist who looked after the patients. A follow-up study revealed a high incidence of ME/CFS-like symptoms three years later (reference 78) – further evidence to support the idea that triggering infections could be causing the production of toxins that affect various aspects of brain and muscle function (see also ciguatera poisoning and Gulf War syndrome later in this chapter).

## Cytomegalovirus

I know of a small number of cases where this herpes virus appears to have triggered a particularly severe ME/CFS-like illness, often with a marked degree of ongoing glandular fever-type symptoms, and sometimes other complications which are associated with this infection. As with glandular fever, various antibody tests can help in making a diagnosis. Treatment with ganciclovir may be worth considering (see page 185 and reference 390).

## Giardia

This is a gut parasite which can cause an extremely unpleasant attack of gastroenteritis with watery diarrhoea. Most cases seem to occur in both adults and children who have been travelling abroad, especially in countries where standards of hygiene are poor. However, giardia can also be picked up in the UK.

Chronic infection may produce persistent loose stools or diarrhoea, malabsorption of nutrients, fatigue and weight loss.

The best way to check for the presence of giardia is to have a series of stool samples examined by the hospital laboratory. If the result is positive, treatment with the antibiotic metronidazole will probably be recommended. If your ME/CFS started with an attack of gastroenteritis and some of these symptoms have persisted, then chronic giardia infection ought to be ruled out.

## Hepatitis

There are several different viruses which can cause an attack of hepatitis (inflammation of the liver):

- **Hepatitis A** is often picked up as a result of visiting a country where hygiene conditions are poor or by eating seafood which has been contaminated with human sewage.
- **Hepatitis B** is usually transmitted through direct contact with infected body fluids. Those at particular risk include drug users who share contaminated needles, homosexuals and anyone who has had a blood transfusion in a part of the world that doesn't routinely test for this virus.
- **Hepatitis C** is largely passed on through infected blood. Unfortunately, there were no effective testing procedures in place in the UK prior to September 1991 and it is now estimated that up to 1 in 500 of the adult population could be carrying this virus without even realising it.
- **Hepatitis D and E** are 'new' viruses which are becoming increasingly common.

The importance of hepatitis in relation to ME/CFS is two-fold. First, it has long been recognised that infection with hepatitis A can result in a prolonged period of fatigue. This has now been confirmed in a research study which followed the recovery pattern of 40 patients with hepatitis A or B who had been admitted to an infectious disease unit in London (reference 74). The patients with prolonged fatigue also had several other typical features of ME/CFS, including alcohol intolerance.

Second, a considerable number of people who carry the hepatitis B or C virus do so for quite some time without ever feeling unwell and with no clear recollection of a previous attack of hepatitis (it could in fact, have just been a simple 'flu-like illness). The first sign of anything being wrong may be general ill health plus fatigue, which can easily be diagnosed as ME/CFS. So, if you fall into one of the 'at risk' groups for catching hepatitis, it is important to have this possibility excluded by the appropriate blood tests.

For further information on hepatitis contact The British Liver Trust (see Useful Addresses, page 423).

## HIV

Also known as 'the AIDS virus', this infection obviously needs to be considered if your lifestyle may have placed you at increased risk of catching HIV.

The infection usually produces little or nothing in the way of symptoms during the very early stages. There can, however, be enlargement of lymph glands in the neck, under the arm and in the groin. Skin diseases such as seborrhoeic eczema, boils or shingles may appear for the first time.

As the white blood cell (CD4) count starts to fall, more generalised symptoms appear, some of which can easily be confused with ME/CFS. These include fatigue, muscle pain, concentration problems, intermittent diarrhoea and sweating. Chest infections and candida in the mouth or vagina may become troublesome at this stage. More severe complications of HIV tend to occur rather later on. By then the diagnosis should be obvious.

If you feel that you may have put yourself at risk of catching HIV, this should be discussed with your GP. Alternatively, you could visit a sexually transmitted disease clinic (NHS or private) for *confidential advice and HIV testing.*

## Leptospirosis hardjo

For anyone in regular contact with farm animals, this is another infection, besides brucellosis and yersinia, which may need to be excluded.

*Leptospirosis hardjo* is an organism which infects cattle and can then be passed on to farm workers and vets who come in contact with contaminated urine. The infection can easily enter the human body when urine is splashed on to skin or even via the lining membrane covering the eye.

An acute infection will cause a 'flu-like illness, often with severe headache, fever, muscle pain and mental confusion. Chronic infection with

*Leptospirosis hardjo* may produce an ongoing 'flu-like illness with *severe malaise*.

In the UK, public health laboratories offer a diagnostic service for blood samples. The Leptospirosis Reference Laboratory at Hereford County Hospital accepts samples where the diagnosis is in doubt. Treatment is with an antibiotic called amoxycillin.

## Lyme disease

This is a recently recognised infection due to an organism called *Borrelia burgdorferi*. Lyme disease is transmitted by bites from ticks which live on sheep and deer. The infection is becoming increasingly common in woodland and heathland areas of Europe (particularly the New Forest in the UK) and North America (where there are now over 4,000 cases per year being reported).

Lyme disease frequently commences with a highly characteristic circular skin rash (*erythema migrans*), which appears between two and 30 days following the tick bite. The circular rash has a pronounced margin and gradually spreads outwards. The lymph glands may also become enlarged.

The second stage to Lyme disease involves a vague 'flu-like illness with muscle pain and joint pain which tends to affect the small hand joints and the knee (which may become quite swollen). In addition, there may be further skin rashes, neurological signs (e.g. a facial paralysis) and heart problems.

The diagnosis can be confirmed by using blood tests which identify specific antibodies directed against the infection. Unfortunately, these tests are not entirely accurate because a variety of other illnesses (e.g. glandular fever) produce false-positive results. If there is any doubt about the results from blood testing, ask for another opinion from a specialist screening laboratory.

A considerable number of people have been misdiagnosed as having ME/CFS when they really have Lyme disease. This is one diagnosis which really shouldn't be missed, as early treatment with a long course of antibiotics can be effective. Later on, antibiotic treatment is far less reliable, and a minority of chronic sufferers go on to develop severe ill health and disability.

An interesting account of the current controversies surrounding the misdiagnosis and mismanagement of Lyme disease has been published in the *Archives of Internal Medicine* (ref. 1996, 156, 1493–1500).

## Mycoplasma

This infection usually causes a 'flu-like illness which is followed by chest symptoms (cough and sputum production), and sometimes even pneumonia. Malaise and fatigue quite often persist for a considerable period of time after the acute episode is over, but I have now seen several patients who have gone on to develop ME/CFS as a result.

The diagnosis can be confirmed by looking for specific antibodies in the blood. Mycoplasma can be successfully treated with a course of antibiotics.

## Parvovirus B19

Children between the ages of four and ten quite frequently catch this viral infection and then develop nothing more than a transient mild illness with fever, headache, malaise and a red 'slapped cheek' rash on the face.

Adults who catch parvovirus infection may again develop nothing more than a 'flu-like episode and a lace-like rash on the limbs. A few, though, have a more prolonged illness involving fatigue, joint pain (mainly affecting the knees, wrists and hands) and anaemia.

The diagnosis can be confirmed by checking the blood for a specific immunoglobulin called anti-B19 IgM. Unfortunately, there is no effective antiviral drug treatment yet available for parvovirus infection. If symptoms are severe or persistent, then treatment should be discussed with an infectious disease specialist.

A research study is currently underway in the UK to look at the possible relationship between parvovirus infection and ME/CFS. See also reference 83, which describes the case of an 18-year-old woman with persistent parvovirus infection who was treated with intravenous immunoglobulin.

## Q fever

This is one of those unusual infections which is seldom even referred to in the medical journals. With only about 100 cases being reported each year, many doctors never even see a patient with Q fever during their working lifetime. Not surprisingly, it's a diagnosis which isn't always made when it should be.

The infection is caused by an organism called *Coxiella burnetii* (a close relative of the Rickettsiae group of infections), and usually affects cattle, sheep, goats and Australian marsupials (where it was first recognised in the 1930s). Although Q fever is usually passed on to humans via infected milk, it can also be acquired by inhalation. High risk occupations include farmers, abattoir workers and vets.

In most cases there are chest and 'flu-like symptoms – predominantly headaches, bodyache and weight loss – which last for about seven to ten days. A small minority of sufferers go on to develop more chronic problems including fatigue and problems with the liver, heart or bones. Q fever is diagnosed by finding raised levels of antibodies in the blood. Treatment involves painkillers and tetracycline antibiotics.

I have now seen several patients with suspected ME/CFS – all with farming connections – who have turned out to be suffering from Q fever. Two reports in *The Lancet* suggest that the incidence of prolonged ME/CFS-like symptoms following Q fever may be much more common than realised.

The first report, from doctors in Adelaide, Australia (reference 84) gave details on a group of agricultural workers who originally had Q fever but then continued to remain unwell with either 'chronic Q fever' or 'recurrent Q fever'. Ongoing symptoms included incapacitating fatigue, muscle pains, nausea, headaches, night sweats, joint pains, alcohol intolerance, sleep disturbances and enlarged lymph glands. A considerable number of this group met CDC criteria for CFS, and the authors speculated that '*a persistence of* Coxiella burnetii *or its antigens may cause dysregulation of the macrophage/T lymphocyte axis with aberrant monokine and cytokine [both immune chemicals] production which in turn mediates the symptoms* – a theory which has also been applied to ME/CFS.

The second report, from doctors at Birmingham's Heartlands Hospital, described their follow-up study on an outbreak of Q fever, which affected 147 people in 1989 (references 72 and 73). Although no specific source of this unusual outbreak was ever identified, the authors suggested that windborne spread of infection from smallholdings with sheep was one distinct possibility. Six years on, 83 of this group were then questioned about the persistence of ME/CFS-like symptoms. There was a high incidence of fatigue (66%), joint aches (69%), sleep disturbance (65%) and sweating (53%). These findings add weight to the idea that a chronic Q fever syndrome exists with remarkable similarity to ME/CFS.

Further research into the possible link between Q fever and ME/CFS is now under way in Australia to look at the possibility that the symptoms may be related to an abnormal immunological response involving cytokines (reference 213).

## *Toxocara*

This is a worm infection found in dogs, especially puppies and those which are not regularly wormed. The eggs are passed out in faeces and these can then remain in the soil as potential sources of infection for up to two years.

Young children who pick up worms on their fingers and then swallow them can develop an illness which commonly includes fever, chest symptoms and abnormal blood tests for liver function. Toxocara also produces a number of more chronic symptoms which are similar to those found in children with ME/CFS. These include stomach pain and nausea, fatigue, sleep disturbance, headaches and behaviour changes, so this is a diagnosis which may need to be ruled out in children with suspected ME/CFS.

The diagnosis can be confirmed by looking for evidence of specific antibodies in the blood. Children with toxocara frequently have raised levels of eosinophils (a special type of white blood cell) and immunoglobulin E (IgE) – two findings which should raise suspicions about this potentially serious infection.

## Toxoplasmosis

Anyone who comes into frequent contact with cats, or has been eating raw/undercooked meat, should consider the possibility of infection with toxoplasmosis.

Around 30 per cent of all adults have antibodies to toxoplasmosis and so have probably had a mild infection at some stage in their life. The acute illness is 'flu-like with fever, headaches and joint pains. Sometimes, though, these symptoms persist, along with enlarged lymph glands in the neck. There is also a risk of severe complications affecting the eye.

Blood tests are of limited value in making a diagnosis of toxoplasmosis. You may need to be referred to a specialist laboratory if this infection is seriously suspected.

If the diagnosis is confirmed, then specific antiparasitic treatment will need to be discussed with an expert in infectious diseases.

## Tropical infections

There are a number of more unusual tropical infections which are capable of precipitating an ME/CFS-like illness. If this is a possibility you should ask to be referred to a specialist hospital unit that deals with tropical diseases (there are several such hospitals in the UK). This is because some of these tropical infections, once correctly identified, may need to be treated with antibiotics or other drugs.

## Yersinia pseudotuberculosis

The case of a 25-year-old veterinary nurse with a six-year history of chronic fatigue, arthritis and irritable bowel symptomatology (reference 80) illustrates how important it is to exclude more unusual infections in anyone whose job brings them into close contact with animals. The cause turned out to be infection with yersinia. Following treatment with a course of tetracycline antibiotics she went on to make a substantial degree of recovery.

Yersinia infection is normally found in rodents and birds. It can then be spread by eating contaminated food or handling an affected animal. Early symptoms include gastroenteritis, arthritis (especially in the lower back) and 'flu-like symptoms. Chronic low-grade infection with yersinia can cause a combination of fatigue, arthritic pains and ongoing stomach or bowel symptoms. Blood tests for antibodies should help to confirm the diagnosis.

# Liver Diseases

## *Primary biliary cirrhosis*

This is a fairly rare liver disease that tends to affect middle-aged females. During the early stages it can produce severe and debilitating fatigue, but this is usually combined with skin irritation. Other symptoms associated with this type of cirrhosis include increased pigmentation on the arms and trunk, dry eyes/mouth, thyroid disease and problems with absorption of fat-soluble vitamins.

Abnormal blood test results include:

- increased levels of alkaline phosphatase and gamma glutamyl transpeptidase – both liver enzymes
- increased levels of aminotransferases and bilirubin
- increased levels of IgG and IgM immunoglobulins
- the presence of antimitochondrial antibodies (AMAs)

Primary biliary cirrhosis can progress to cause severe liver damage, so it's a diagnosis which must be excluded, particularly in females who have severe fatigue and skin irritation.

## *Gilbert's disease*

Most liver experts believe that this rather unusual liver problem causes no real harm apart from an occasional attack of mild jaundice. However, when Gilbert and colleagues first described the illness in 1907, they also reported on an association with neurasthenia (an historical equivalent of chronic fatigue) and blood disorders. Other reports in the medical literature since then have noted associations with chronic fatigue, nausea and stomach pains over the area of the liver.

Two reports in *The Lancet* have indicated that Gilbert's disease seems to be more common in people with ME/CFS, particularly men. The first study (reference 76) noted that 16 per cent of a small group of ME/CFS patients had the same liver abnormality – a raised level of bilirubin, the jaundice-producing pigment – compared to between 2 and 5 per cent of the normal population. A second report (reference 88) noted an incidence of 11 per cent.

Research into Gilbert's disease has found that it is a genetic disorder which affects an enzyme that controls the way the liver removes bilirubin.

Apart from this abnormality, there are no serious indications of liver damage and other liver function tests are usually normal. No specific treatment is necessary.

Why there should be an increase in the incidence of Gilbert's disease in people with ME/CFS remains a mystery. One possibility is that the presence of the genetic defect increases the susceptibility to developing ME/CFS when the right trigger (e.g. an infection) appears. Even so, the vast majority of adults with Gilbert's disease appear to have no health problems whatsoever.

# Malignancy

A number of common forms of cancer can present with fatigue as the main symptom, so this is something which may need to be considered if there are other symptoms (e.g. weight loss or unusual stomach pains) which cannot be linked to ME/CFS.

## Hodgkin's disease

This is a type of lymph-node cancer that is mainly seen in young adults. It causes a painless enlargement of the lymph glands (particularly in the neck), anaemia, weight loss, itching of the skin, night sweats and fatigue. This diagnosis should always be queried in anyone with ME/CFS who also has significantly enlarged glands and night sweats.

# Muscle Disorders

Although fatigue, pain, weakness and twitching in the muscles are all common symptoms in ME/CFS, there are muscle diseases which may need to be excluded if there are no other typical symptoms present, or where actual muscle wasting is occurring (this is not usually present unless there has been a prolonged period of immobility). Unfortunately, there are very few muscle specialists in the UK and you may need to travel to London or Scotland if an expert opinion is required.

## Myasthenia gravis

Although this serious muscle disease can affect all age groups, the onset is most common during the early 20s. Weakness is often first noticed in the eye muscles, sometimes resulting in double vision. Exercise-induced fatigue then occurs in the limb muscles – something which is exacerbated by stress or infection. Sufferers frequently report having difficulties in getting out of chairs, climbing stairs or hanging out washing. Problems with facial muscles can lead to speech difficulties (which may become slurred when tired), chewing and swallowing. In severe

cases, or where the diagnosis has been missed, respiratory muscle problems may lead to shortness of breath.

Various blood tests can help to confirm the diagnosis. These include
the presence of harmful antibodies (anti-AchR and anti-striated muscle
antibodies) and an EMG investigation (which records how the muscles
respond to nerve impulses). Treatment involves the use of drugs which
help to reverse the chemical defect in muscle–nerve co-ordination.

## Muscle pain

As already described earlier in this chapter, a number of infections cause
quite severe muscle pain, but this can also occur in other diseases and
as a side-effect of drugs.

Medical conditions causing muscle pain include *polymyalgia
rheumatica* (widespread pain and stiffness, particularly in the mornings,
often accompanied by headache and eye problems in a more elderly age
group); *polymyositis* (pain and tenderness, especially in the neck
muscles, joint pains, skin rash, cold hands/feet); and *biochemical disorders of muscle* (where pain is often made worse during exercise).

A large number of drugs can produce muscle pain and/or weakness
as a side-effect. These include cimetidine (for stomach ulcers),
isotretinoin (for acne), propranolol (for heart conditions), salbutamol
(for asthma) and statins (for lowering cholesterol).

# Neurological Disorders

## Multiple sclerosis (MS)

Professor Charles Poser, one of the world's leading authorities on multiple sclerosis, has reported that in a review of 336 patients, all of whom
were referred to him for a second opinion, only 236 actually had MS
(reference 87). Out of 130 with a misdiagnosis of MS, 28 were suffering
from ME/CFS.

These findings are not that surprising because a number of symptoms are common to both conditions and MS isn't always easy to diagnose in the very early stages. Two of the most interesting similarities are
the way in which people with MS and ME/CFS both have problems with
fatigue and normal mental (cognitive) functioning, and that many of
their symptoms are made much worse in hot weather. Paraesthesiae
(patches of abnormal sensation in the skin), difficulties with balance and
co-ordination, and pain also occur quite commonly in both conditions.
Key features of MS which are not seen in ME/CFS are attacks of severe
pain and loss of vision in one eye (optic neuritis).

If there is any doubt about a diagnosis of MS, then I suggest you ask to be referred to a neurologist who knows about ME/CFS as well. There are various neurological investigations which should help to differentiate between the two. These include abnormal visually evoked potentials, changes in proteins in the cerebrospinal fluid (i.e. increased oligoclonal IgG), and characteristic lesions in the brain shown by magnetic resonance imaging (MRI) scans.

Incidentally, the drug amantadine has also been used in MS as a possible treatment for fatigue with some reports of success (see pages 184–5).

### Parkinson's disease

Early Parkinson's disease should always be considered in someone over the age of 50, especially where there is a gradual deterioration in health. In this disorder there is a progressive slowing down of all body movements (often first noticed by changes in facial expression) followed by increasing muscular rigidity, fatigue and tremor (most noticeable in the hands when resting). People with Parkinson's disease, as with ME/CFS, have difficulties with balance, co-ordination and normal mental functioning. An unusual symptom, which is quite characteristic early on, is loss of sense of smell (anosmia). It's important to recognise Parkinson's disease as soon as possible because effective drug treatments are now available.

## Poisoning

A number of poisonous substances, especially when low levels are being taken into the body over prolonged periods of time, are capable of causing general ill health that can be mistaken for ME/CFS.

### Carbon monoxide poisoning

This is normally due to a small leak from a faulty home gas appliance. It can lead to headaches, dizziness, diarrhoea, muzziness in the head, fatigue and 'flu-like feelings. Around 100 people in the UK die each year from carbon monoxide poisoning and several disturbing cases have appeared in the press involving people who have been misdiagnosed as having ME/CFS. Carbon monoxide poisoning should certainly be suspected where more than one member of a family develops an ME/CFS-like illness at around the same time with no obvious precipitating event. The diagnosis can be confirmed by a blood sample estimation.

### Lead poisoning

A report in *The Lancet* (reference 86) described the case of a 47-year-old woman with a 10-year history of debility, weight loss, constipation and

YEOVIL COLLEGE
LIBRARY

difficulty with concentration, which had been confidently diagnosed as being due to ME/CFS. The presence of anaemia on a routine blood test fortunately led to her hospital doctors carrying out some further investigations, which included the discovery of a high level of lead. This lady's lead poisoning had been caused by contamination of the domestic water supply from lead in the hot water cylinder. The case illustrates how important it is to properly follow up any abnormalities which are found on routine blood tests, as well as the dangers of including a symptom such as weight loss as being due to ME/CFS (which it is not).

# Psychiatric Disorders

Chronic fatigue, problems with normal mental functioning and sleep disturbances all occur quite commonly in anxiety, depression, somatisation and chronic hyperventilation (overbreathing). These four conditions, and their possible associations with ME/CFS, are discussed in more detail in Chapter 12: Mind and Body, but there are two other psychiatric disorders which can produce ME/CFS-like symptoms.

## Post-traumatic stress disorder

This is a newly recognised condition which has to follow some form of extremely traumatic event such as a serious accident, witnessing the violent death of someone, or being the victim of terrorism or torture. Symptoms include a wide variety of emotional and psychiatric reactions commonly seen in stress. These include irritability, loss of interest, limited feelings, detachment from other people, poor concentration and difficulty falling asleep. There will also be recurring thoughts about the incident which triggered this reaction.

Although there shouldn't be any difficulty in differentiating the condition from ME/CFS, it is interesting to note that a small minority of people develop ME/CFS after a major stressful event, and research into post-traumatic stress disorder suggests that similar disturbances in the hypothalamic control of hormones such as cortisol may be present.

## Seasonal affective disorder (SAD)

This is a special type of depression where symptoms tend to occur during October or November each year and then persist right through until the following spring. Most sufferers are aged between 20 and 40. The vast majority are female.

Besides symptoms normally associated with depression (e.g. hopelessness, apathy, fatigue, mood swings), people with SAD complain of sleep disturbances (usually increased sleep requirements), weight gain (due to cravings for carbohydrate foods) and loss of interest in sex.

Even though the cause of SAD isn't yet fully understood, it's possible that decreased amounts of winter sunshine are interfering with hypothalamic function and brain chemical transmitters such as serotonin (as can also occur in ME/CFS).

One form of extremely effective treatment for SAD is the use of light boxes which emit high-intensity light. SSRI drugs such as Lustral can also be helpful.

For more information contact the SAD Association (see Useful Addresses, page 431).

## Somatisation disorder

This is a psychiatric condition which consists of numerous physical symptoms (e.g. abdominal pain, headaches, chest pain, dizziness, allergies, fatigue) for which no obvious physical cause can be found. It is frequently accompanied by depression or anxiety and results in a severe degree of disability.

There is currently a great deal of debate amongst psychiatrists as to whether those people with ME/CFS who have a large number of physical symptoms are more likely to be suffering from somatisation. A number of research studies on this possible association have now been published (references 427, 430, 432–5 and 446) but the results are not always consistent. Some studies have indicated that up to 10 per cent of patients seen in specialist ME/CFS clinics may be suffering from somatisation. Other studies put the figure much lower.

True somatisation disorder is most effectively treated using cognitive behaviour therapy. There are no specific drug treatments which appear to be effective. Unfortunately, many people with this disorder remain in a state of chronic ill health.

## Stress and overwork

In Chapter 2, I described how chronic stress can have a powerful effect on the production of hormones such as cortisol and so possibly predispose people towards the development of illnesses like ME/CFS. Chronic stress can also lead to a significant decrease in the efficiency of the body's normal immune defence mechanisms.

One of the major sources of chronic stress is in the workplace – a situation which has not been helped by the way in which both the length and intensity of many people's working hours have steadily increased over the past 20 years.

A combination of chronic stress and overwork can easily result in a condition which has popularly become known as 'burnout'. Common symptoms include fatigue, problems with mental functioning, headaches, increased sweating, decreased appetite and dizziness.

It's important that this type of reaction to stress is recognised for what it is and not misdiagnosed as ME/CFS. Otherwise, the chances are that the correct approach to management will not be initiated and recovery is unlikely to follow.

# Respiratory Conditions

## *Sarcoidosis*

This is a mysterious disease which can affect almost any part of the body. It most commonly occurs in females in the 20–40 year age group.

The onset can be acute with fever, malaise, skin rash (tender red nodules on the shins) and joint pain (ankles and knees). Around 5 per cent of people with an acute attack of sarcoid go on to develop an illness which includes chronic fatigue (reference: *Sarcoidosis*, 1993, 10, 1–3).

A less common presentation is a more gradual onset with chest symptoms (cough and shortness of breath), increasing fatigue, mild fever and eye problems – a combination which can be mistaken for ME/CFS.

Various investigations will help to confirm a diagnosis of sarcoid. These include blood tests (an increased level of calcium may be present) and skin tests. Interestingly, there may be an elevation of an enzyme called serum angiotensin-converting enzyme (ACE) – a finding which has also been reported in ME/CFS (reference 361).

## *Tuberculosis*

During the past 10 years there has been a steady increase in the incidence of tuberculosis in both the UK and America. Although this serious infection usually produces quite obvious chest symptoms, it can sometimes present with rather more vague general ill health and a number of ME/CFS-like symptoms (e.g. fever, sweats, fatigue, enlarged lymph glands), especially in children. It is a diagnosis which ought to be considered if you've been travelling abroad in an at-risk area or are suffering from weight loss.

# Rheumatic Diseases

## *Sjögren's syndrome*

An unusual condition which should always be excluded when chronic fatigue is accompanied by joint pains and dryness in the mouth and/or eyes.

Sjögren's syndrome is a serious immune system disorder which causes widespread inflammation in various body tissues, particularly the joints and glands that produce secretions. Constant dryness in the mouth can lead to dental decay; dryness in the eye makes them feel 'gritty and sore'. Loss of glandular secretions elsewhere causes vaginal dryness. Other common symptoms include skin rashes on the legs and cold hands or feet.

Characteristic blood test abnormalities found in this disease include:

- a raised ESR
- a low white blood count
- the presence of antinuclear antibodies
- raised amounts of IgG, IgA and IgM immunoglobulins

Dryness in the eyes should be assessed by a Shirmer test, where a strip of filter paper is hooked on to the lower lid to test the output of tears.

Similarities between ME/CFS and Sjögren's syndrome are discussed in medical reference 75.

For further information contact the Sjögren's Syndrome Association (see Useful Addresses, page 431).

## Systemic lupus erythematosus (SLE)

Rheumatologists who see patients with this fairly unusual condition are all aware of a minority of cases, mainly women, who have initially been misdiagnosed as having ME/CFS. This is probably because both conditions have a considerable number of symptoms in common. These include fatigue (which can be quite disabling in SLE), muscle pain, enlarged glands, painful tender joints with morning stiffness, depression, headaches, problems with normal mental functioning and cold hands or feet. Symptoms of SLE which are *not* usually seen in ME/CFS are hair loss, chest pain, skin that becomes extremely sensitive to the sun and a highly characteristic 'butterfly rash' on the cheeks.

Another interesting similarity between the two conditions is that both may involve an overactive response by the body's immune system. In SLE, this results in the production of harmful autoantibodies – something which can occasionally occur in ME/CFS.

A number of investigations are helpful in confirming or refuting the possibility of SLE. These include:

- anaemia
- a raised ESR
- a low white blood count
- the presence of antinuclear autoantibodies in 95 per cent of cases

For more information on SLE contact Lupus UK (see Useful Addresses, page 423).

# Other Conditions

A complete list of all the remaining medical and psychiatric disorders which can produce chronic fatigue or an ME/CFS-like illness would be endless. However, there are a number which continue to cause confusion and are worth a brief mention.

## Alcohol abuse

This is obviously something which few people would admit to, and very seldom occurs in association with ME/CFS, as excess alcohol inevitably makes the condition worse. Alcoholics can end up with serious damage to almost any organ in the body. Not surprisingly, they often complain of general ill health, weakness and problems with mental functioning. If you have abnormal liver function tests, then your doctor may well query if excess alcohol consumption could be the explanation, but as I explain on page 166, there are several other causes for this finding in ME/CFS.

## Calcium

A raised level of blood calcium can cause a gradual loss of appetite, sickness, constipation, excessive thirst, muscle weakness and depression. These symptoms tend to come on gradually, so a blood test for calcium should always be arranged if this is how your ME/CFS started. Further hospital investigations will be required if your calcium level is raised in order to find out the true cause (see also page 164).

## Osteomalacia

This is a fairly rare bone disease caused by vitamin D deficiency which, in turn, results in a lack of absorption of calcium and phosphate from the diet. The three principal symptoms are fatigue, muscle weakness (particularly when trying to stand up) and bone pain. Blood tests will usually reveal low levels of calcium and phosphate along with a raised level of alkaline phosphatase.

## Sick building syndrome

The idea that buildings and working environments can make people ill isn't something that all doctors accept. Despite this fact, there do appear to be genuine instances where more people than normal start to suffer from a range of symptoms, including itchy, watery eyes and noses, sore throats, headaches, fatigue, difficulty concentrating and irritability, for no obvious reason. And it's quite common to find that these symptoms often disappear at weekends or when time is spent away from the 'sick' building. Possible explanations include hot dry atmospheres inside many modern buildings, coupled with irritating chemicals and working with VDUs for long periods of time.

Various types of *sleep disturbance*, including sleep apnoea and narcolepsy, which can cause chronic fatigue, are discussed on pages 79–80.

# Conditions Which Overlap with ME/CFS

Now that ME/CFS has finally become accepted as a genuine medical illness, it is becoming clear that there are a number of other newly recognised conditions which have very similar symptoms and abnormal research findings. Once a further understanding of these conditions starts to emerge, it seems likely that this information will assist in our understanding of ME/CFS. Some of the more important overlapping conditions are described below.

## *Athletic overtraining syndrome (OTS)*

There are frequent reports in the newspapers of athletes and sportsmen suffering from either ME/CFS or a condition known as overtraining syndrome (OTS), which has a number of overlapping features in common with ME/CFS.

The precise cause of OTS is unknown, but some athletes seem to catch minor infections – which could be an important precipitating factor – every time they increase their level of training. Research into OTS suggests that a combination of factors (many of which also appear to play a role in perpetuating ME/CFS), including disturbances in brain chemical transmitters and hormones, immunological function and reductions in the amino acid glutamine, could be involved. Such similarities with ME/CFS have resulted in research now being carried out in parallel into both conditions.

OTS is characterised by prolonged fatigue and underperformance being associated with periods of intensive training. A period of high-intensity exercise with little time for rest is another precipitating factor, so OTS is less likely to be seen in sprinters, who manage to train with longer periods of rest. OTS can also occur when an athlete changes from low-intensity winter training to high-intensity summer training.

The main symptoms of OTS are fatigue, a 'heavy' feeling in the muscles, significant underperformance and depression. Sleep disturbances are extremely common, along with the familiar ME/CFS complaint of continually 'waking up feeling unrefreshed'. Other symptoms include emotional lability, irritability, excessive sweating, a raised pulse rate, loss of appetite and loss of weight.

Early detection of OTS is obviously important for competitive athletes, and there are several early warning signs to indicate that all is not well. These include a rise in the early morning pulse rate, a steady decline in normal performance and changes in mood.

Recovery rates from OTS seem to be far better than seen in ME/CFS. The general advice to any athlete suffering from OTS is to start off by having a five-week period of rest. Time spent on aerobic exercise then needs to be resumed at a very low level, which may only mean light training for a few minutes each day. This can be gradually increased over the following 12 weeks. Apart from treating any co-existent sleep disturbance or depression, drugs seem to be of little value in the management of OTS.

For a more detailed review of OTS see reference 89.

## Chronic ciguatera poisoning

This rather unusual cause of an ME/CFS-like illness has been reported by Professor John Pearn, from the Royal Children's Hospital in Brisbane, Australia (reference 93).

Ciguatoxin is an extremely potent chemical toxin that affects the nervous system. It is passed on to humans who are unlucky enough to eat 'gourmet' fish (such as coral trout and various species of mackerel) which have been caught in tropical and sub-tropical regions of the Atlantic, Pacific or Indian Oceans.

An acute attack produces a diverse range of symptoms affecting the nervous system (problems with temperature control, abnormal skin sensations), heart (fall in blood pressure), gastrointestinal system (diarrhoea and vomiting) and skin (allergic type rash).

In most cases, these symptoms gradually start to resolve over a period of days or weeks. However, around 20 per cent of victims have persisting ill health, and about 2 per cent develop a serious ME/CFS-like illness. It's also quite common for anyone who has been affected to experience an exacerbation of symptoms after eating pork or chicken which have been obtained from animals fed with fish meal.

An interesting fact to emerge from research into ciguatera poisoning is that the toxin affects the way in which sodium molecules pass across cell membranes in nerve and muscle tissue – something which could be relevant to our understanding of what is going wrong in more typical cases of ME/CFS (see also page 157–8).

## Fibromyalgia

This is a diagnostic label which is used with increasing frequency by rheumatology specialists when they see patients with quite severe muscle aches and pains for which no obvious muscle or arthritic condition seems to be responsible.

The three principal symptoms of fibromyalgia are:

- **Pain**, mainly in the muscles of the back and neck, which is often made worse by stress, cold weather or physical activity. Generalised early morning stiffness frequently accompanies the pain.
- **Sleep disturbance**, which is usually described as leaving the person concerned feeling 'completely unrefreshed' the following morning.
- **Fatigue**, often severe and disabling, which is exacerbated by minimal amounts of physical exertion.

Other symptoms, which may or may not be present, include hands/feet which feel intermittently swollen, pins and needles sensations (paraesthesiae) in the skin, poor memory and concentration, irritability or mood swings, frequently passing urine, irritable bowel symptomatology.

As you can see there is a considerable degree of overlap between many of the symptoms of ME/CFS and fibromyalgia, and many people who are diagnosed by rheumatologists as having fibromyalgia would also receive a diagnosis of ME/CFS if they were to visit another type of specialist instead! However, people with fibromyalgia don't usually have an acute onset associated with infection, although a stressful or traumatic event (e.g. a road traffic accident) can sometimes act as a trigger for fibromyalgia. For a diagnosis of fibromyalgia to be confirmed, there must be a number of well-defined tender spots present in various muscles and ligaments.

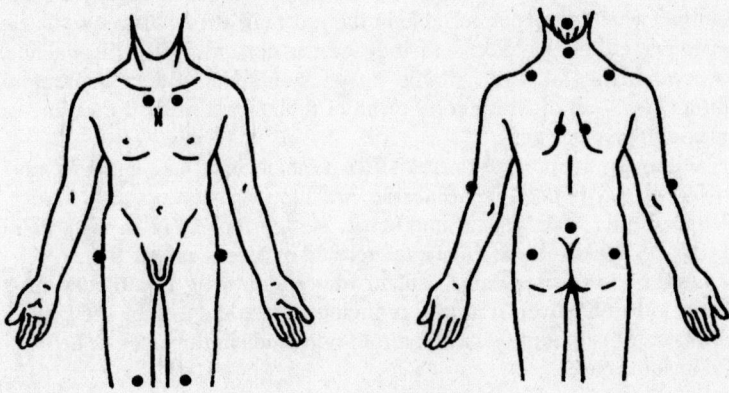

**Sites of tender spots which indicate a diagnosis of fibromyalgia**

At present, nobody is quite certain about what causes fibromyalgia, but some form of major sleep disturbance which interferes with the normal nightly episodes of deep sleep or 'restorative' sleep seems quite likely. In fact, fibromyalgia symptoms can easily be reproduced in perfectly healthy volunteers by simply depriving them of a normal night's sleep on a regular basis. There is also some interesting research in progress which suggests that people with both fibromyalgia and ME/CFS have similar abnormalities in the control of growth hormone.

As far as treatment is concerned, the main aim is to try and reduce muscle pain and improve the quality of sleep. This is why a low dose of a sedating tricyclic antidepressant such as amitriptyline is usually recommended along with a course of exercise (e.g. swimming), which helps to improve aerobic (oxygen-carrying) fitness. Other treatments which may be advised include steroid injections (into particularly tender areas), yoga and relaxation techniques (where stress is playing a major role). Normal types of analgesics don't seem to be very helpful in relieving the pain associated with this condition. (For more detailed information on fibromyalgia see medical references 90–1 and 524.)

## Fluid retention syndrome (FRS)

Also known as 'idiopathic cyclical oedema', this is a condition which often overlaps with the normal symptoms associated with pre-menstrual tension. Abnormal accumulation of fluid, which can sometimes result in a weight gain of 10 pounds at this time of the month, causes a feeling of swelling in the face, arms and abdomen. Some women with FRS notice that their weight steadily increases during the course of the day, so that clothes which were comfortable in the morning are no longer so in the evening. Other symptoms include depression, sweating, headaches, overwhelming fatigue, irritable bowel symptoms and concentration difficulties – all of which tend to be at their worst around the time of maximum weight gain.

Although the precise cause of FRS remains uncertain, it may involve a disturbance in both hypothalamic function (reference: *British Medical Journal*, 1983, 286, 1691–3) and female sex hormones. As in the case of ME/CFS, it also seems to be exaggerated by stress or infection.

Apart from water-losing tablets (diuretics), drug treatments don't seem to be effective. Gradually reducing any excess weight and cutting down on the amount of carbohydrate-rich foods in the diet can be helpful in some cases.

## Gulf War Syndrome (Gulf War illnesses)

Perhaps the most controversial and mysterious illness to emerge during the 1990s is the Gulf War Syndrome (GWS). As with ME/CFS, the condition has been frequently dismissed as 'all in the mind', and sufferers ridiculed by both doctors and the popular press. Soldiers affected by GWS have also had to endure a long frustrating struggle with both government and the medical establishment to have their chronic ill health taken seriously and properly investigated.

Among the various symptoms reported by members of the UK and US armed forces who served in the August 1990 to March 1991 Gulf War are chronic fatigue, muscle and joint pains, problems with normal mental (cognitive) functioning, depression, anxiety and sleep disturbances. Others have reported unusual skin lesions, allergies, chest complaints such as asthma or bronchitis, and symptoms (e.g. paraesthesiae) suggesting nerve damage. There are anecdotal claims that there is a higher incidence of birth defects amongst children born to mothers/fathers who served in the Gulf War.

Although some of these personnel are clearly affected by an illness which is very similar to ME/CFS, others have a range of symptoms which are *not* consistent with this diagnosis. Consequently, the term 'GWS', which implies a single illness, should probably be replaced with the umbrella term 'Gulf War illnesses'.

The fact that an ME/CFS-like illness is frequently reported has prompted researchers to look at how service in the Gulf War could have resulted in exposure to factors which are already known to be involved in the development of ME/CFS.

First is the very late acknowledgement by the UK Ministry of Defence that some soldiers were exposed to organophosphate (OP) pesticides – a fact which was repeatedly denied in early ministerial statements to Parliament. OPs used in sheep-dipping, etc, are now being accepted as a recognised trigger for ME/CFS (see later in this chapter), and there is a further possibility that these troops were exposed to other types of toxic nerve chemicals including DEET (an insect repellent) and the nerve gas sarin.

Second is the use of multiple vaccinations – including those which were given to protect against whooping cough, plague, anthrax, typhoid, tetanus and cholera – which were only administered to the troops once they were in the war zone, when they would have been under a considerable amount of stress. Vaccinations can also trigger ME/CFS in some circumstances (see pages 35–7), and researchers from University College, London, have put forward a hypothesis in *The Lancet* (reference 99) that these vaccinations could have produced a significant and harmful shift in the type of cytokines being produced by the immune system (see pages 135–6).

Third is the fact that these soldiers were undoubtedly under a considerable amount of physical and mental stress throughout their time in the Gulf. It may well be that this allowed the protective barrier – the blood–brain barrier – that normally isolates brain tissues from toxic agents and infections to become defective – yet another explanation that has been suggested in the case of ME/CFS (see page 31).

The true cause of Gulf War illnesses remains a matter of intense medical and political debate, but some of these troops do appear to have developed an ME/CFS-like illness as a result of service in the Gulf, and exposure to multiple vaccinations and/or OPs may well have played a crucial role.

In both the UK and the USA, a considerable amount of money is now being devoted to Gulf War illness research. One such study, from Dr Goran Jamal at the Institute for Neurological Sciences in Glasgow, has already found evidence of nerve damage (reference 97). Other results are awaited with interest by patients, lawyers and politicians.

Further references to research into Gulf War illnesses are on pages 447–8.

## Organophosphate (OP) pesticides

These powerful nerve poisons were originally developed back in the 1930s for possible use as weapons in chemical warfare. However, it soon became obvious that OPs were extremely effective at killing all kinds of pests and insects. This discovery led to their widespread use on the farm as crop sprays and sheep-dips, in the garden for general pest control, and in the house for killing pet fleas. OPs have also become a standard form of treatment for head-lice in small children.

Although there's no doubt that high doses of OPs can cause serious damage to the nervous system – even paralysis and death – it is only recently that concern has been expressed about the dangers of chronic low level exposure and possible links with ME/CFS.

During the late 1980s, a number of doctors, including myself, became aware of farmers who were developing an ME/CFS-like illness which was jokingly being referred to as "farmers' 'flu" (reference 110). Many of these farmers had all the typical symptoms of ME/CFS, but others experienced a much greater degree of depression, suicidal intentions and mood swings than is normally the case in ME/CFS.

A considerable number of these farmers were regularly being exposed to OPs through sheep-dipping (during which they hadn't always used an effective range of protective clothing), and in some instances an acute onset to the illness could be clearly dated back to a specific episode of dipping.

Research into a possible link between ME/CFS and OPs has been followed up by Professor Peter Behan at the Institute of Neurological Sciences in Glasgow. His first results, published in 1996 (reference 103), indicate that the farmers had very similar abnormalities to those found in ME/CFS when tests were carried out to assess the activity of various brain hormones and chemical transmitters which are under the control of the hypothalamus (see pages 146–50).

The farming patients also had an increase in sensitivity to a brain chemical transmitter called acetylcholine similar to that found in some cases of ME/CFS. This finding was hardly surprising given the fact that OPs disrupt the nervous system by inhibiting the action of an enzyme called cholinesterase, whose normal function is to break down acetylcholine (and so increase its activity).

It is also disturbing to note that two of the farmers in this group went on to develop a tumour known as non-Hodgkin's lymphoma. This finding may be more than coincidence because OPs are known to (a) adversely affect the body's immune system (by depressing the function of natural killer cells), (b) allow the reactivation of latent viral infections (such as herpes and Epstein-Barr) which have been implicated in the development of this tumour and (c) damage genetic material (reference 108).

Dr Bob Davies, a psychiatrist from Taunton, has been investigating the type of psychiatric problems and dangers of suicide which appear to be associated with low level exposure to OPs in other groups of agricultural workers. These findings have also been published (see reference 105).

Despite the fact that the government and manufacturers of OPs still maintain that there is no proven link between low level exposure and adverse effects on the nervous system, evidence is clearly mounting to support the view that these pesticides are involved in various neurological, cardiological (heart) and psychiatric illnesses, including ME/CFS. Consequently, anyone who already has ME/CFS needs to be extremely cautious about coming into direct contact with *even small amounts* of OPs in either the house or garden. The use of suitable alternative pet flea remedies and head-lice products should be used whenever possible.

Not surprisingly, the case against OPs is now being tested in the courts. In 1997, the Supreme Court of New South Wales, Australia, awarded A$71,000 to three sheep-shearers who had suffered OP-toxicity. In the UK, a Peterborough farmhand who developed an ME/CFS-like illness following exposure to a grain store insecticide, won a limited victory in the High Court in the same year in which it was accepted that *'exposure to organophosphate probably can and does cause persistent neuropsychological and neurobehavioural effects'* (reference: *The Lancet*, 1997, 350, 1457).

For further medical references on OP toxicity see page 448. Advice and information on OPs can be obtained from the OP Information

Network (see Useful Addresses, page 419).

## Post-polio syndrome (PPS)

Thanks to a highly effective vaccine, polio infection has almost been eradicated from most developed countries. However, there appear to be a growing number of people who succumbed to an acute attack of paralytic polio 15, 20 or even 30 years ago, who are now developing (sometimes after full recovery from polio) a group of symptoms which have been named the post-polio syndrome (PPS). This unusual long-term complication of polio has a number of important similarities with ME/CFS and a better understanding of PPS could well improve our knowledge of what is going wrong in ME/CFS.

The first similarity is that polio viruses belong to a group known as enteroviruses (see pages 32–4), which have long been thought to act as triggering infections in the case of ME/CFS. The possibility of a much stronger link with polio viruses themselves occurred in many of the early outbreaks of ME/CFS described in Chapter 1.

The second similarity is that many of the symptoms of PPS are exactly the same as those found in ME/CFS. Among the most common PPS symptoms are incapacitating fatigue; weakness, pain and twitching (fasciculations) in the limb muscles; problems with memory, concentration, word-finding; and joint pain. Other symptoms of PPS, which occur less frequently, include difficulty with swallowing and breathing. In some cases, these symptoms appear in a fairly gradual manner. In others, as with ME/CFS, there is a sudden onset precipitated by an infection.

The third important similarity with ME/CFS concerns research into PPS, which has largely been carried out by Dr Richard Bruno and his colleagues at the Post-Polio Rehabilitation and Research Service – part of the Kessler Institute for Rehabilitation, New Jersey, USA. It appears that people with both ME/CFS and PPS have abnormalities in the production of hormones relating to the hypothalamus gland in the brain, particularly growth hormone and CRH release (see pages 146–50), along with similar problems with normal mental (cognitive) functioning (reference 114).

In the case of PPS, it has also been possible to obtain samples of brain tissue from patients who have died. These results demonstrate the presence of polio lesions in key parts of the brain, including the brain stem, hypothalamus and reticular activating system – three sites which have also been implicated in ME/CFS (reference 113).

Although symptoms of the two conditions are often very similar, there are a number of investigations – including muscle biopsies, electrophysiological studies and examination of the spinal fluid – which should help in the confirmation of PPS.

At present, there is no generally agreed treatment for PPS, although trials are being carried out in America to assess the value of drugs such as bromocriptine and edrophonium, a drug which helps to improve nerve–muscle co-ordination, see reference 118). Otherwise, management of PPS is very similar to that recommended for people with ME/CFS.

Unfortunately, there are very few physicians in the UK who are either interested or knowledgeable about PPS and the only specialist unit which treats polio is the Lane Fox Unit at Saint Thomas's Hospital in London.

You can obtain further information on polio from the British Polio Fellowship (see Useful Addresses, page 429). Other medical references relating to PPS are listed on page 448–9.

# Quality of Life, Disability Assessment and Recovery from ME/CFS

## Quality of Life with ME/CFS

Although many doctors are now becoming aware of and interested in the diverse range of symptoms associated with ME/CFS, very little attention has been paid to the way in which a combination of chronic ill health and resulting disability affects relationships and the ability to work and participate in social activities, along with various other aspects of normal daily living. And in what often appears to be a preoccupation by researchers into looking for a cause of ME/CFS, one of the most crucial parts of the illness for sufferers – namely their quality of life – has been badly ignored.

We all know what quality of life is, but measuring it objectively isn't that easy to do. In medical jargon it's often referred to by terms such as 'health status' or 'life satisfaction'. In fact, there is no general agreement as to how it can or should be measured in something like ME/CFS, even though sufferers clearly all agree that their quality of life has been dramatically reduced since the onset of this illness. Perhaps the most useful way to try and assess the impact of ME/CFS on quality of life is to look at three separate aspects which can be measured with some degree of accuracy: physical ability, mental health and social functioning. This is what several different research groups have now done in considerable detail.

### Australian research

This was carried out by Robert Schweitzer and his colleagues in Queensland (reference 121). Their study involved 47 ME/CFS patients using what is known as a Sickness Impact Profile assessment – a 136-item questionnaire covering 12 main areas of daily living activity, including mobility, mental health, recreational activity and employment. Their results confirmed that ME/CFS produces a very significant impact on all areas of normal daily living, and the scores indicate a far more severe reduction in quality of life than in conditions such as renal failure, heart disease or a comparable group with multiple sclerosis. Only those suffering from terminal cancer or stroke had a worse quality of life using this particular method of assessment.

Not surprisingly, the main areas of daily living to be affected in ME/CFS turned out to be work-related activities, household tasks, sporting or recreational pastimes and social contacts. Almost everyone who was interviewed had been prevented from participating in physical activities because of the inevitable exacerbation of symptoms. Problems with home management meant that everyday tasks such as shopping, cleaning and repairs were either being left unattended or cancelled. For those still in work, having ME/CFS often resulted in far less attention being given to the accuracy of whatever duties were being carried out. Social contacts were severely reduced, and in many cases were now restricted to immediate family and a few remaining close friends and relatives. Rather more variable was the impact on physical capabilities and mental health (e.g. mobility, sleep patterns and emotions), but there was no doubt that physical symptoms still placed many restrictions on what the whole group could do.

## American studies

Two research studies on what is termed 'functional status' were published in the *American Journal of Medicine* in 1996 (references 119 and 120).

Dr Dedra Buchwald and colleagues in Seattle looked at 185 ME/CFS patients using the Medical Outcomes Study Short-Form General Health Survey (SF-36). They compared the results to those obtained from 111 patients with acute glandular fever (infectious mononucleosis) and 25 with major depression. Those with ME/CFS were found to be 'strikingly disabled', particularly in areas of social functioning and general vitality. In fact, Dr Buchwald's group concluded that people with ME/CFS *'demonstrated greater impairment across all functional domains than previously observed for any medical or psychiatric disorder'* and that *'a constellation of symptoms, reminiscent of an infectious illness, are responsible for a substantial proportion of disability experienced by CFS patients'*.

Professor Tony Komaroff and colleagues in Boston once again used an SF-36 assessment to compare 223 ME/CFS patients with others suffering from congestive heart failure, diabetes, heart attacks, multiple sclerosis and depression.

They found that ME/CFS was having a significantly greater impact on social functioning and ability to work than on physical abilities or mental health symptoms. Even so, the scale of impairment across all types of activity was more severe than in any of the other conditions being assessed. Interestingly, the ME/CFS patients had a very different pattern of results from those of people suffering from depression.

Professor Komaroff and his colleagues concluded that : *'Several of the key symptoms of CFS – particularly fevers, pharyngitis [sore throat], muscle weakness, post exertional malaise, and difficulty thinking – or an underlying pathophysiological process associated with them – produce much of the functional impairment seen in CFS; and most of the symptoms of CFS are unlikely to represent expression of an underlying depressive disorder.'*

None of these findings are likely to come as a surprise to anyone who actually suffers from ME/CFS, but they do vividly illustrate and confirm the way in which this illness results in a severe reduction in quality of life. Social isolation and the inability to carry out a meaningful role in the home, community or workplace can combine to severely deflate your self-esteem and confidence. Work, in particular, provides people with social contacts, status, financial security and a structured way of life. Pulling the plug on this aspect of daily living can sometimes be the most devastating consequence of having ME/CFS. The combination of numerous restrictions being placed on normal daily life, along with distressing physical symptoms, could also help to explain why some sufferers then go on to develop depression or other psychiatric problems.

Finally, it's worth noting that the above research findings might be of considerable assistance should you become involved in a dispute with an employer or benefit/pension provider over the level of disability this illness can cause.

## Assessing your Own Level of Disability

The type of detailed questionnaires I've just described are fine for research purposes, but are of limited value when it comes to any form of regular personal assessment of disability levels. To help with this I've modified a well-used disability scale (see table). You should find that one of the percentage figures in the left-hand column corresponds to your usual state of health. There will also be one or two percentages above and below this figure to where you fluctuate during good and bad periods of health.

It may be helpful to use a disability scale like this to monitor your own progress from time to time. Alternatively, the scale could be useful when you're trying to explain to a doctor, employer or benefit/pension provider how ME/CFS is affecting your ability to carry on with activities associated with normal daily living in both the home and workplace.

**Table 6: ME/CFS Disability Scale**

0%   Fit and well for at least the past three months. No symptoms at rest or following activity. Capable of full-time employment.

10%  Generally well. No symptoms at rest. Occasional mild symptoms may follow activity. Capable of most forms of full-time employment.

20%  Occasional mild symptoms at rest. More noticeable symptoms following activity. Some restriction of capabilities which require physical exertion. Able to work full-time but difficulty with work that requires physical exertion.

30%  Mild symptoms at rest. Limited ability to carry out some tasks which require physical exertion. May be able to work full-time.

40%  Mild or moderate symptoms at rest. Variable ability to carry out tasks associated with normal daily living. Unable to work part-time in a job involving frequent physical exertion. May be able to work part-time in other types of employment.

50%  Mild to moderate symptoms at rest. Moderate to more severe exacerbation of symptoms following physical and/or mental exertion. Unable to carry out any strenuous physical tasks. Able to perform light duties or desk work for several hours a day, provided adequate rest periods are provided.

60%  Moderate symptoms at rest. Moderate to severe symptoms following any form of physical or mental exertion. Unable to carry out any strenuous duties. Able to carry out light duties/desk work for one to three hours per day, provided adequate rest periods are available. Generally not confined to the house.

70%  Moderate to severe symptoms at rest. Severe symptoms follow any physical or mental activity. Able to perform desk work or light duties for one or two hours during the day. Often confined to the house and may require wheelchair assistance at times.

80%  Moderate to severe symptoms at rest. May only be able to carry out a very minimal range of physical activities relating to personal care (e.g. washing, bathing). Frequently unable to leave the house and may be confined to wheelchair or bed for much of the day. Unable to concentrate for more than short periods of time.

90%  Severe symptoms at rest. Bedridden and housebound for much of the time. Experiences considerable difficulties with many aspects of personal care. Marked problems with mental functioning (e.g. memory, concentration). Requires a great deal of practical support.

100% Severe symptoms on a continual basis. Bedridden and incapable of living independently. Requires a great deal of practical social support.

# Recovery Rates

'Will I ever get better?' is one of the first questions that anyone with ME/CFS wants an answer to once the diagnosis has been confirmed. Yes, you can recover from this illness; it may take several years, but it is still possible after quite long periods of time. Rest and convalescence in the very early stages, along with appropriate changes in lifestyle, seem to have the most positive effect on outcome – which is why late diagnosis and inaccurate management advice can be so harmful. But until all doctors are able to recognise ME/CFS in its initial phase, and then offer their patients the correct advice, many sufferers will continue to spend months, sometimes years, adhering to management programmes which are either unsuitable or sometimes even harmful.

## *Good and bad prognosis*

The Department of Social Security in Britain has become so concerned about recovery rates in ME/CFS that it decided to set up an expert group of doctors to look at various factors which may influence recovery. The group concluded that there appear to be certain factors which help to determine whether an individual will have a good or bad outcome. These findings have now been published in the *British Medical Journal* (reference 122).

A good prognosis is thought to be indicated by:

- A definite history of viral illness (particularly glandular fever) in the presence of an uncomplicated psychological background.
- A pattern of evolution towards functional recovery.
- An early diagnosis aimed at eliminating associated physical disorders and identifying psychiatric illness and any another complicating psychological or social factors.
- A management regime encompassing physical, psychological and social elements that concentrates on modification of the person's lifestyle, striking a balance between overactivity and the risks of deconditioning and taking a stepwise approach towards achieving functional improvement while addressing factors such as sleep disturbance.

A poor prognosis is thought to be indicated by:

- The onset of symptoms without any clear precipitating factor but set on a complex background of adverse psychological and social factors or occurring after a severe infective illness.
- Severe and unremitting symptoms, particularly if lasting for over four years. The presence of multiple symptoms, especially those suggesting somatisation. (See page 101).

- Delayed diagnosis and especially self-diagnosis, with the patient becoming convinced of a single cause to the exclusion of all others.
- A management regime overemphasising the importance of complete rest or advocating a rapid return to pre-illness levels of physical activity. Failure to recognise the need to treat such features as depressive illness or sleep disturbance.

## Predicting your own outcome

My own view is that anyone who makes steady progress during the first year or two can reasonably expect this to continue into the third or fourth years, although nothing is absolutely certain with ME/CFS. However, the longer the condition remains chronic, without any form of significant progress being achieved, the less likely any recovery is going to occur.

ME/CFS is a very individual condition; some of the symptoms will come and go or vary in severity, whereas others will be there for most of the time. Almost everyone will go through both good and bad periods, which again makes predicting what will happen in the long term extremely difficult to do.

Does having an acute or gradual onset make any difference to the chances of recovering? At present, there are no accurate statistics available, but many doctors believe that those who develop ME/CFS in a more gradual manner, with repeated infections producing a slow deterioration in health, probably don't do so well (a view shared by the DSS expert group).

The majority of people with ME/CFS tend to fit into one of four broad groups when it comes to looking at how the illness progresses. First are those who, after months or years, begin to make a full or significant degree of recovery, and may even return to their normal way of life. Figures from recently published research studies (see later) indicate that the percentage who fit into this category is fairly small.

The second group tend to follow a much more erratic course, with periods of remission and relapse. During periods of remission they may return to relative normality, even going back to work and resuming a normal social life once again. Then the symptoms return – often quite suddenly and precipitated by another infection, or undue stress, or an excessive bout of physical activity. A few just seem to fall back into ill health again for no obvious reason. Periods of remission can sometimes be quite prolonged, and I know people with ME/CFS who have enjoyed reasonably good health for several years before a relapse occurs. For those whose time in remission seems to be increasing, and their relapses less severe, the eventual outlook is probably quite optimistic.

Results from research studies suggest that the majority of people with ME/CFS fall into this second grouping.

The third group are those who develop a chronic and sometimes severe form of ME/CFS. The late Dr Melvin Ramsay described ME/CFS as 'a baffling syndrome with a tragic aftermath'. Follow-up studies of patients involved in the outbreaks described earlier in this book have revealed that very high numbers remains chronically and severely disabled. Some of the nurses involved in the 1934 Los Angeles outbreak were thoroughly reviewed 15 years later and found to be suffering from the same problems with muscle fatigue and brain malfunction. They never managed to return to work. Similarly, over 40 years on from the famous Royal Free Hospital outbreak, many of the medical staff remain unwell. In the survey carried out by Dr Ramsay and Dr Betty Dowsett (reference 124) 31 per cent of patients reported a steady improvement; 20 per cent fluctuating remissions and relapses; 25 per cent a constant level of disability; and 24 per cent had no remissions or actually felt worse.

Sadly, a small but significant minority experience no real improvement and may even start to gradually deteriorate, although this latter course is unusual. The outlook here is poor, and this group requires a great deal of practical, emotional and social support.

## Research studies on outcome/prognosis

More recently, a number of detailed studies have been carried out to assess what happens to people with ME/CFS over a prolonged period of time. The most important findings to be published in medical journals include:

- Sixty-four per cent of all patients in an American study experienced some degree of improvement. Only 2 per cent reported a 'complete resolution' of symptoms and 40 per cent remained unable to work at all (reference 123).
- Nineteen per cent of those referred to a Belfast clinic reported a full degree of recovery. The majority of patients had a fluctuating pattern of illness with relapses and remissions. Around 5 per cent reported deterioration. Younger patients (particularly those under 20) were more likely to show signs of recovery (reference 125).
- Sixty-four per cent of a group of 137 patients followed up for a period of one year at London infectious diseases hospital reported some degree of improvement. Twenty-one per cent remained the same and 15 per cent became worse (reference 127).
- Thirteen per cent of those attending an infectious disease clinic in Oxford considered themselves to be 'fully recovered' two years later.

Sixty-five per cent still had significant problems with many aspects of daily living and 38 per cent had been forced to leave or change their employment/studies as a result of continuing ill health (reference 128).

- Three per cent reported a complete recovery and 17 per cent indicated some degree of improvement in an 18-month follow-up study reported from the Netherlands (reference 129).
- Six per cent of patients taking part in an Australian treatment trial had recovered after three years. Almost half were still unable to work and around a third were unable to carry out physical activities (reference 130).

These results, which do make rather gloomy reading, obviously need to be viewed with caution, as they tend to refer to patients who have been referred to hospital specialist clinics. Consequently, they almost certainly represent a more severely affected group of people with ME/CFS than those who are purely managed by general practitioners.

There is no doubt that many people with ME/CFS have to learn to live with a long-term illness that fluctuates in severity, as well as coping with the sort of difficulties faced by those who have other chronic neurological diseases such as multiple sclerosis. Although some of the symptoms will undoubtedly come and go, and there will be good days to help compensate for many of the bad ones, the cardinal features of muscle fatigue and brain malfunction will be present for much of the time. This means accepting that life for the foreseeable future is going to be governed by a plateau of ill health interspaced with periods of remission and unexpected exacerbations.

Whichever group you seem to fit into, *never give up hope*. In the meantime accept your limitations, listen to what your body is saying, and don't try to fight ME/CFS – it just won't work!

## Death Associated with ME/CFS

Considering the fact that there are probably over 100,000 people with this illness in the UK, deaths associated with ME/CFS remain unusual. However, tragedies do occur, with suicide being the most common cause of death. Many of these suicides are clearly linked to the associated despair and depression which may accompany ME/CFS, but there are often other factors involved as well.

There is no epidemiological evidence to indicate that people with ME/CFS have a decreased life expectancy as a direct result of the illness. Neither is there any evidence to link ME/CFS to other serious medical conditions such as cancer or heart disease, which could shorten life expectancy. The only possible exception to this rule is where a trig-gering infection clearly involved an organ such as the heart or pancreas and produced definite damage at the time. This information may be rel-evant to applications for life insurance policies (see page 179).

Apart from suicide and unrelated causes of death, the only other reasons for premature death in ME/CFS are complications arising from prolonged immobility (thrombosis and osteoporotic fractures are real risks for people who have been confined to bed for long periods) or mis-management (e.g. weird restrictive diets leading to malnourishment and weight loss or complications of drug treatments).

There are very few researchers currently interested in or capable of making use of post-mortem material in order to find out more about the underlying cause(s) of ME/CFS, and the only published report of such an examination is described on page 128. However, this type of exami-nation could prove to be useful in discovering what is going wrong inside the brain in ME/CFS.

# Current Research

In Chapter 3, I discussed how various different factors – genetics, hormones, life stresses, etc – may be involved in *predisposing* someone to develop ME/CFS. Then, when the right 'trigger' comes along – be it an infection, vaccination, pesticide exposure or even some form of major stressful event – the person concerned fails to follow a normal recovery pattern and goes on to develop ME/CFS.

It's this third and final stage – factors which *maintain or perpetuate* ill health and disability in ME/CFS – where most research activity is being concentrated.

The history of good-quality scientific research into this illness really dates back to the early 1980s when Professor Peter Behan, from the University of Glasgow, published his first results in the *Journal of Infection* (reference 131). This study examined the possible role for viral (mainly enteroviral) infection, immunological disturbances, and abnormalities in muscle – three aspects of research which were considered at that time to offer the most likely chance of providing an answer to the question: what is going wrong in ME/CFS?

Since then, well over 400 research papers have been published in the medical literature on all aspects of ME/CFS. Many contain conflicting or inconsistent conclusions about the role of infection, immune system responses, muscle abnormalities and the interrelationship with psychiatric illness. However, there is growing consensus that disturbances in brain function – particularly in relation to hormones, chemical transmitters, blood flow patterns and sleep – do occur in ME/CFS, and that further research studies into these aspects of the illness probably represent the most likely way of finding an effective drug treatment.

I'm now going to try and provide some answers to the most commonly asked questions relating to research findings. I don't have all the answers – and neither do the scientists carrying out this research – but some of the results do now mean that various pieces of the 'ME/CFS jigsaw' are starting to fit into place.

## The Role of Viral Infections

All viruses are made up from two separate components. On the outside is a protective layer of protein (the capsid) which contains unique

# How ME/CFS may be affecting the brain and nervous system

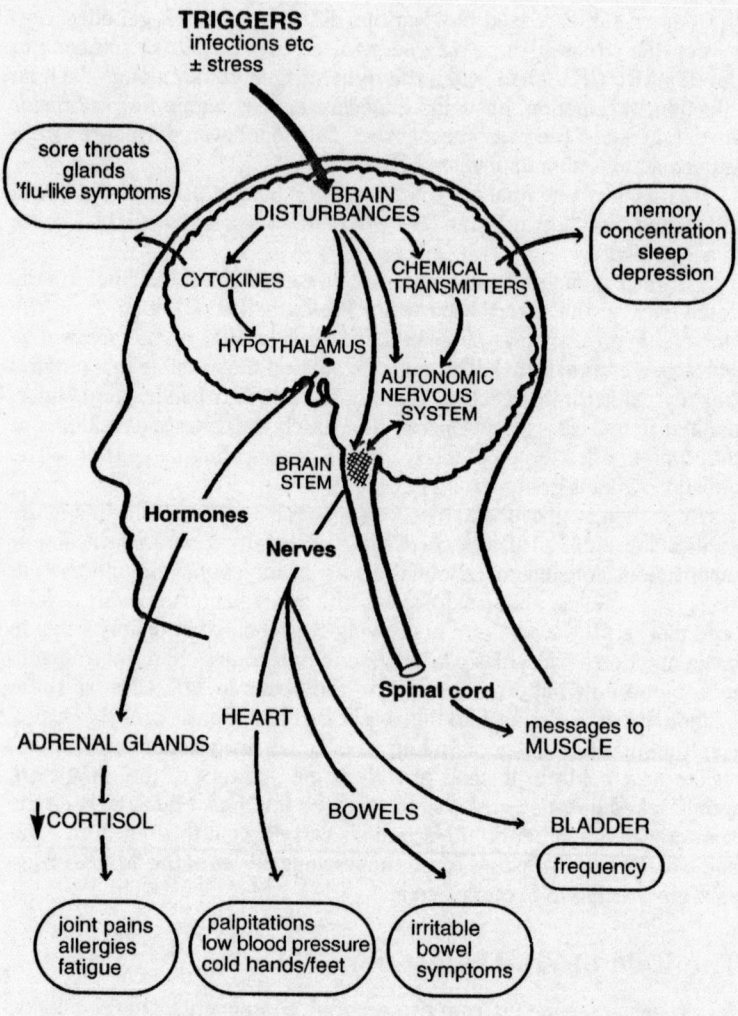

markers against which human antibodies are directed. Inside is a core of nucleic acid (the genome) which contains genetic material known as deoxyribose nucleic acid (DNA), or a close relative, ribose nucleic acid (RNA).

Viruses are classified according to which of the two types of nucleic acid are present. Some, like herpes viruses (Epstein-Barr virus and chicken-pox), contain DNA. Others, like enteroviruses, contain RNA.

## How viruses invade cells and replicate

To make further copies of themselves, viruses have to invade healthy human cells and 'hijack' the chemical machinery which the cells use to carry out their normal everyday functions. This is a process which involves several separate stages:

1. The virus meets the host cell and becomes attached to its outer surface. This is rather like a key fitting into a lock, as the virus has to find specific receptor sites on the cell surface. If viral antibodies are being made, part of their function is to block these receptor sites.
2. The virus then penetrates through the cell wall; this is called viropexis.
3. The capsule or capsid of the virus is stripped off by intracellular enzymes, so allowing its genetic information to be released.
4. The viral nucleic acid then takes over the host's own genetic apparatus, using it to manufacture new viral particles.
5. Once the new viral particles have been assembled and recoated by the host cell, they pass out through the cell membrane.

## The outcome of viral infections

In most cases, the body makes a successful immune response, which removes the virus in question. A normal state of health is gradually resumed.

Sometimes, though, the invading virus may replicate with such voracity that the host cell ends up being permanently damaged or ceases to function and dies. This is what happens when permanent damage follows a serious viral infection such as polio.

Alternatively, the virus may persist and remain dormant inside the cells, without causing any obvious damage or disturbance to normal function, as can be the case when Epstein-Barr virus (glandular fever) occurs during childhood or adolescence.

A further possibility is that the virus remains inside the cell without causing any harm, but the body's immune system continues to react against it, and so causes damage in the process – an autoimmune reaction with the production of autoantibodies. This type of response may be involved with liver damage associated with chronic hepatitis B

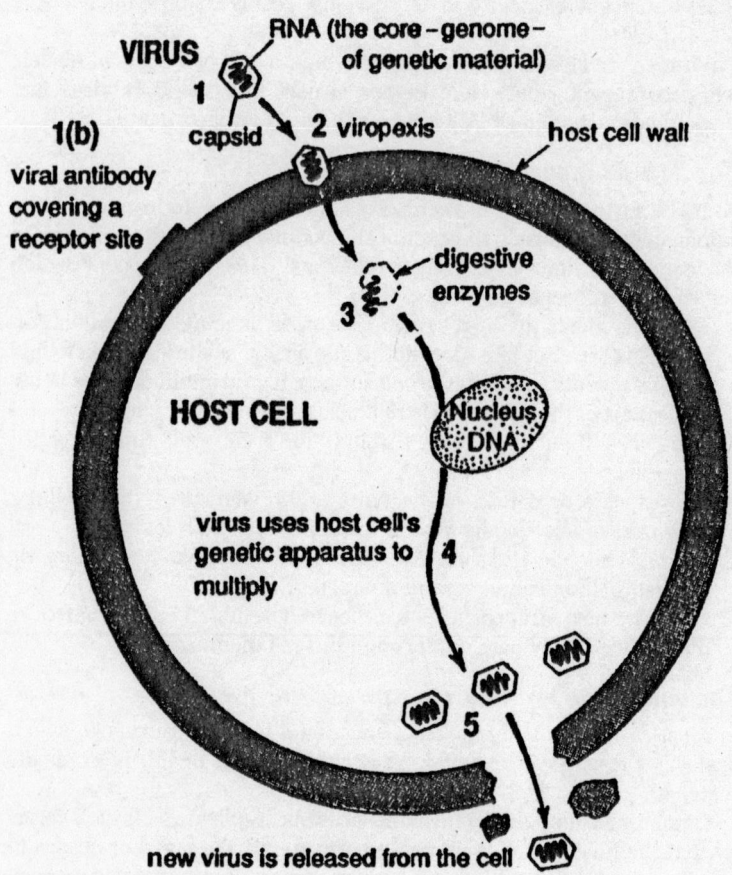

**VIRUS** — RNA (the core –genome– of genetic material)

1

**1(b)**
viral antibody
covering a
receptor site

capsid    2 viropexis    host cell wall

digestive
3    enzymes

**HOST CELL**    Nucleus
DNA

virus uses host cell's
genetic apparatus to    4
multiply

5

new virus is released from the cell

infection. A similar mechanism, also involving autoantibody production, has been suggested in ME/CFS (see page 133).

Finally, it's possible for viruses to remain inside cells without producing any obvious microscopic damage, but instead cause important changes in the way they carry out normal functions (e.g. the manufacture of brain chemical transmitters or hormones), again something which it has been suggested could be happening in ME/CFS.

## Is there any evidence of persisting viral infection in ME/CFS?

Although there is a considerable amount of evidence to show that viral infections (and some non-viral infections) can *trigger* ME/CFS, the evidence for *persisting* viral infection is far less certain.

The most accurate way of obtaining information on the presence of viral infection in the body is to use a procedure called polymerase chain reaction (PCR). This is an enzyme technique which involves taking samples of human blood, muscle, faeces or any other tissue which might contain an infection. Using PCR, it is then possible to magnify the minute amounts of genetic material present and so obtain evidence of the presence of viral particles in the tissue under investigation.

PCR was first used by Professor Behan's group to look for the presence of enteroviral infection in small muscle samples (biopsies) from patients with a post-viral fatigue syndrome. Initial results from Glasgow found evidence of enteroviral RNA in 53 per cent of the samples from ME/CFS patients compared to only 15 per cent in a control group (reference 329). However, when this experiment was repeated in a group of 121 ME/CFS patients and compared to 101 patients suffering from other types of nerve and muscle disease, there was no significant difference between the two – 26 per cent positive in the ME/CFS group and 20 per cent positive in the controls (reference 330). Researchers from the University of Liverpool have also failed to find any evidence of persisting enteroviral infection in muscle biopsies (reference 331), but a research group from Charing Cross and Westminster Medical School in London obtained positive results using a different technique from PCR (references 319, 321 and 325).

PCR has also been used to look for the presence of persisting enteroviral RNA in blood and stool samples from people with ME/CFS. Dr Geoff Clements, from the Regional Virus Laboratory in Glasgow, found positive results in 41 per cent of a patient group compared to only 3 positive results from a group of 126 healthy controls when blood samples were analysed (reference 324). Early research during the late 1980s, carried out by Professor James Mowbray at Saint Mary's Hospital in London, indicated that enteroviral infection could be persisting in both the intestines and blood samples (reference 339), but researchers from the University of Nijmegen in the Netherlands could find no evidence of persisting infection when they examined stool samples from 76 patients and an equal number of controls (reference 337).

The overall conclusion from these studies is that *there is insufficient conclusive evidence to support the view that persisting viral infection is a cause of ME/CFS*. Even so, there remains one crucial part of the body – the brain – where it is extremely difficult to obtain reliable evidence of persisting infection. For obvious ethical reasons, brain biopsies are not generally permitted in medical research and so the only practical way of obtaining brain tissue is from post-mortem material. Interestingly, the only post-mortem so far carried out on someone with ME/CFS who has died, found evidence of enteroviral RNA in the brain stem and hypothalamus as well as in the muscle and heart (reference 332).

It should be noted that raised levels of antibodies to enteroviral infections such as Coxsackie B do *not* indicate that a persisting viral infection is present. Neither can they be used as a diagnostic test for confirming or refuting the presence of ME/CFS (reference 334).

For a more detailed review of the current debate into the role of persisting enteroviral infection see references 333 and 335. Further information on studies into the possibility of persisting enteroviral infection is contained in references 315, 327, 328 and 336. The possible role of *retroviruses* in ME/CFS is discussed on pages 17–8. Information on research into a link with Borna virus disease is contained on page 22.

## Could reactivated viruses play a role?

Although most UK research into viral activity in ME/CFS has tended to concentrate on enteroviral infections, other investigators have examined the possibility that dormant infections such as cytomegalovirus and Epstein-Barr virus could be *reactivated* in the course of this illness.

*Epstein-Barr virus (EBV)* This is the virus which causes glandular fever in teenagers and young adults, and as already discussed on page 34, there is no doubt that glandular fever can be followed by a prolonged illness that is very similar to ME/CFS.

A number of studies have found evidence of raised levels of antibodies to EBV – mainly IgM anti-viral capsid antibodies (VCAs) and early-antigen antibodies (EAs) – in people with ME/CFS. Such antibodies are normally only present in the early stages of glandular fever and then tend to disappear. However, they can sometimes be present in perfectly healthy adults.

A number of explanations have been put forward for these findings. First, they may simply be the result of an immunological disturbance – such as a defect in T cell function – that is present in many cases of ME/CFS. Second, lowered levels of cortisol could be allowing reactivation of a dormant virus because this is a hormone which can also affect immune responses. Whether or not reactivation of EBV is playing a role in symptom development in some cases of ME/CFS remains an unanswered question, but the view of most experts is that it probably isn't.

For more information on research studies into EBV see references 340–53.

*Human herpes virus type 6 (HHV6)* This is a 'new' herpes virus which was first identified in 1982 and has subsequently been linked to a number of different illnesses, including ME/CFS. Once again, a finding of raised levels of antibodies to HHV6 doesn't necessarily mean that this infection caused ME/CFS or that it is still persisting. However, there are reports suggesting that reactivation of HHV6 could be more common in people with ME/CFS (reference 258), something which could turn out to be relevant, as HHV6 is known to infect the nervous system and white blood cells (where it could lead to the release of various immune chemicals/cytokines which have been implicated in ME/CFS).

## *Viral infection in ME/CFS – unanswered questions*

Perhaps the most important unanswered question in the whole debate surrounding the role of viral infections in ME/CFS is what might be happening if viruses do actually go on to persist inside the body.

One intriguing possibility stems from the work of Michael Oldstone and his colleagues in California, USA. They have produced compelling evidence from animal model experiments to show that viral infections can lead to permanent changes in the way that infected cells carry out their normal functions, long after signs of the initial infection have disappeared (references 317 and 318). Using a virus called lymphocytic choriomeningitis, they have shown that this can go on to affect the production of brain chemical transmitters such as acetylcholine as well as hormones produced by the hypothalamus and pituitary glands – abnormalities which have also been reported in ME/CFS.

Of equal interest is the fact that the cells in question show no obvious signs of structural damage, even though a significant and ongoing disruption of their normal functions is clearly occurring.

Whether or not such a process is occurring in ME/CFS remains pure speculation, but it is certainly one avenue of research that is worthy of further exploration.

Results from other types of research (e.g. upregulation of the 2–5A synthetase pathway and one SPECT scan study), which do support a role for persisting viral infection, are described later in this chapter.

# Immunology and ME/CFS

The second strand of research into ME/CFS concerns the way in which the body's immune system responds to whatever event triggers the onset of this illness.

Interest in possible immune system abnormalities initially stemmed from the fact that people with ME/CFS frequently complain of a number of ongoing 'flu-like symptoms (sore throats, enlarged glands, problems with temperature control) which suggest that the immune response hasn't been properly 'switched off' after the triggering event.

## The body's immune response

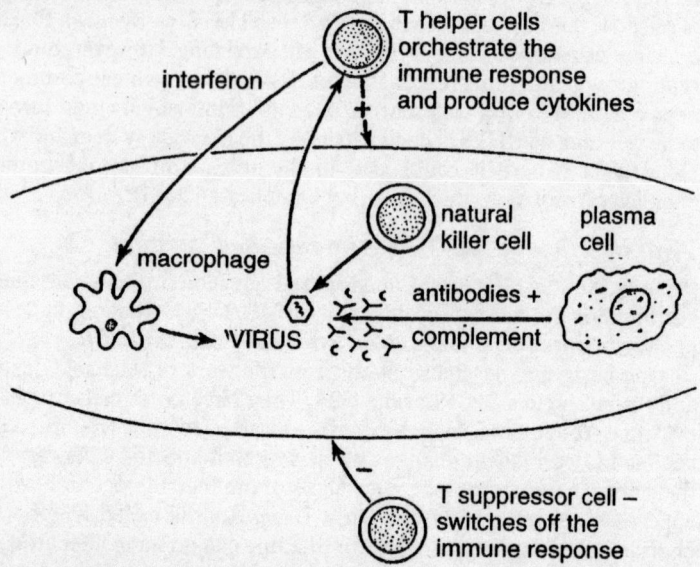

## *How the body's immune system works*

The immune system is made up of numerous different components – antibodies, cytokines and immune chemicals, T cells, etc – which are all 'switched on', rather like a cascade, whenever the body recognises something which is 'foreign'. Then, rather like an orchestra, the various different components should all act in a co-ordinated manner to first neutralise and then remove whatever has triggered the response, be it an infection, allergen or toxin.

As already described in Chapter 3, there may be several important co-factors (age, sex, hormonal status, life stresses) which affect the normal immune response in ME/CFS. And if the immune system fails to respond in an appropriate manner, or continues to function inappropriately, then this could affect activity in the brain, muscles and other parts of the body.

The main players in the immune orchestra are antibodies, immune chemicals known as cytokines and cells called T lymphocytes, all of which have their own specific functions. The immune response is first 'switched on' by white blood cells – the T helper cells – and then 'switched off' again by another group of white cells called T suppressors.

These are the most important components of the immune orchestra in relation to ME/CFS:

**Antibodies** consist of a group of proteins called immunoglobulins, which recognise and lock on to invading organisms. They are produced by plasma cells which originate in the bone marrow where most of the blood cells are produced. This is why bone marrow transplants are sometimes carried out on people whose immune systems have been seriously damaged by leukaemia cells infiltrating the bone marrow. Antibodies make infections more susceptible to attack by cells called macrophages. They also activate an immune chemical called complement (see below).

Following any viral infection, antibody production quickly gathers pace. IgA antibodies are the first line of defence, and act rather like an 'antiseptic paint' to protect the delicate lining membranes of the throat and intestines, and so prevent further spread of virus via the bloodstream. IgA antibodies are produced by the regional lymph glands, which is why those in the neck quickly swell up during a throat infection.

IgG and IgM antibodies are the next to be produced. Their role is to prevent blood spread of virus to tissues like the heart and brain. These type of antibodies often remain long after the initial infection has gone (or after vaccination) and so prevent any further attack by that particular virus.

IgE antibodies are commonly produced during allergic reactions. A raised level of IgE may indicate a co-existent problem with allergies, or even a parasitic infection such as toxocara.

**Autoantibodies** form a special group of antibodies, whereby the body's immune system 'turns on itself' and starts to attack its own tissues. Some researchers have speculated that this could be happening in ME/CFS where autoantibodies are occasionally found.

**Complement** is the name given to a group of about 20 different proteins which circulate in the blood. Along with antibodies, complement helps to neutralise any invading virus.

**Cytokines** are a group of immune chemicals which are mainly produced by the T helper cells. These substances act as messengers within the immune system, and help to co-ordinate the attack on a virus. They also have direct effects on the brain and produce some of the common 'normal' reactions to any type of infection. It now seems that changes in sleep pattern, body temperature control, energy levels and mood, which are associated with most infections, are largely due to changes in the level of cytokines called interleukins acting on a particular part of the brain known as the hypothalamus. Cytokines are also responsible for the general aches and pains in muscles and joints which accompany 'flu-like infections. Interesting new research from America indicates that two specific cytokines – interleukin-6 and interferon alpha – both of which have been implicated in ME/CFS, are responsible for the development of most 'flu-like symptoms (reference: *Journal of Clinical Investigation*, 1998, 101 643–9).

**Immune complexes** are, as the name suggests, combinations of antibody and antigen which also circulate round in the blood. Their presence has been linked to inflammation in the joints, kidneys and skin.

**Lymphocytes** are a vital group of white blood cells which are also made in the bone marrow. One group, the B cells, turn into short-lived plasma cells and produce antibodies. Another group migrates via the blood to a small gland in the neck called the thymus (hence T cells) where they mature into various subgroups, each with a particular number (e.g. T4, T8) according to their specific function. T cells are responsible for general immune surveillance against viruses and bacteria. The T4 (helper) cells have been likened to the conductor of the immune orchestra because of their role in 'switching on' and maintaining the response. These are the cells that become severely depleted in patients with AIDS. The T8 (suppressor) cells send out messages which instruct the immune system to slow down or cease its activities once the infection is under control.

**Macrophages and phagocytic cells** are another important group of cells which act rather like scavengers, and are literally capable of 'mopping up' infected cells and immune complexes. They are one of the first group of cells to recognise an invading organism and envelop it under their membrane. The macrophage then goes on to present the 'captured virus' to the rests of the immune system, but principally to the T4 helper cells and the antibody-producing B cells.

**Natural Killer cells (NK cells)** are part of our primitive immune system. They are always ready to attack anything that the body recognises as 'foreign', and this ranges from infections through to cancerous cells. The way they do this is to produce proteins which damage the outer coating of virus-infected cells. NK cells also help to regulate the production of antibody from B cells.

## Immune system abnormalities in ME/CFS

A large number of subtle immune system abnormalities have been reported by different research groups in the UK, USA and Australia. Unfortunately, these results have often been conflicting and some of the research has not always met high scientific standards. These inconsistencies may well stem from the fact that researchers have been looking at patients who are in different stages of their illness as far as severity and duration are concerned. Equally, age, sex, level of physical activity and degree of co-existent psychiatric problems will all have an effect on immune function tests, as can the time of day when the blood sample is taken. These sort of variables must be taken into account in the design of future immunological research studies if such abnormalities are going to be taken seriously.

Below are some of the more interesting immune system abnormalities to be described so far from nearly 40 different research studies:

*Autoantibodies* occur more frequently in people with ME/CFS than in the normal population. Antinuclear antibodies are found in up to 20 per cent and rheumatoid factor in up to 10 per cent. Levels are usually quite low and occur without any obvious evidence of systemic lupus erythematosus (SLE) or rheumatoid arthritis (see page 103). Autoantibodies against the thyroid gland and some other tissues are also occasionally found (see page 166). One possible explanation for the presence of these autoantibodies is an increased level of activation of the T cells. (See also references 367 and 368.)

**Cytokines and immune chemical** abnormalities have been implicated as a possible cause of symptoms in ME/CFS. Support for this hypothesis first comes from the discovery that a number of ME/CFS-like symptoms (in particular profound fatigue and problems with normal mental functioning) are commonly seen when patients with chronic hepatitis or cancer are treated with an immune chemical called alpha interferon (reference 205). Second, two separate studies in ME/CFS patients have found raised levels of an enzyme known as 2' 5' oligo adenylate synthetase, which is activated when cells are exposed to the presence of interferons (see page 156).

Several studies have reported a diverse range of sometimes rather conflicting results relating to the levels of inflammatory cytokines found in the blood (and sometimes the cerebrospinal fluid) in ME/CFS. However, there are several consistent reports (references 183 and 189) describing raised levels of a specific immune chemical known as transforming growth factor beta (TGF-beta), whose level appears to rise even further during exercise (reference 214). And, in one of the most recent cytokine studies, elevation of TGF-beta was found to be higher than in other conditions where there is a combination of fatigue and immune system disturbances (reference 183).

The fact that very few consistent cytokine abnormalities have so far been identified needs to be viewed with caution because minor changes in blood levels may not be an accurate reflection of what is happening in localised areas within the brain.

Among the more interesting findings from other studies on cytokines are:

- Increased levels of alpha interferon (references 192 and 196).
- Marginally raised levels of alpha interferon in the cerebrospinal fluid (reference 200).
- Normal levels of gamma interferon but increased levels of interleukin 1-alpha (reference 198).
- Normal levels of interleukin-1 (reference 208).
- Abnormal secretion of interleukin-1 beta which may be related to altered sensitivity to oestrogen and progesterone hormones (reference 187).
- Very high levels of interleukin-2 (reference 190).
- Higher levels of interleukin-2 in those who were ill when the sample was taken (reference 204).
- Normal levels of interleukin-2 and undetectable amounts of alpha interferon (reference 217).
- Raised levels of interleukin-6 in febrile patients (reference 184).
- No obvious abnormalities in cytokine production (reference 220).
- Aberrant production of interleukin-6, TNF-alpha and interleukin-10 (reference 191).
- Cytokine dysregulation involving accentuated release of interleukin-6 from mononuclear cells in ME/CFS following Q fever (reference 213).

**Immune complex** abnormalities occasionally occur and one research group found them to be raised in 34 per cent of a patient group compared to only 2 per cent in the controls (reference 367). It doesn't seem that raised levels of immune complexes go on to produce any of the harmful effects that can occur in association with this particular immunological abnormality.

**Immunoglobulin** abnormalities, which are usually fairly minor, are quite frequently reported when this particular aspect of immune function is assessed. Once again, the results from different research groups aren't always consistent.

Most reports of immunoglobulin abnormalities have shown lowered levels than normal, especially with IgA, IgD, IgG or IgM. However, several other studies have reported normal levels of immunoglobulins.

Deficiencies in IgG subclasses, mainly IgG1 or IgG3, have also been reported (references 197, 199, 215 and 224).

**Natural killer** *(NK) cell* abnormalities in both number and function are probably the most consistent immunological finding to date. The majority of research studies have found a *decrease* in the absolute number of NK cells, although there are a few reports of increased amounts.

NK cell abnormalities could be due to an underlying chronic infection, but when this occurs it is usually severe and obvious (as in the case of HIV). Alternatively, they could be secondary to other T cell defects and production of immune chemicals such as gamma interferon and interleukin 2.

It is interesting to note that treatment of ME/CFS patients using the drug lantinan – which results in increased NK cell function – has been reported to be of benefit in a small group of patients (see page 194).

Research references relating to NK cell activity in ME/CFS include numbers 180, 181, 186, 188, 193–5, 207, 218 and 221.

**T cell numbers and function** have been assessed in several studies with, once again, some rather confusing findings.

Measurement of T cell subsets have shown absolute numbers of CD4 (helper/inducer) cells and CD8 (suppressor/cytotoxic) cells to be either *normal or reduced* in number, but one of the more interesting reports comes from Professor Jay Levy and his colleagues at the University of California, USA. They found evidence of what are termed 'activation markers' on the CD8 cells. These findings add further weight to the hypothesis that some form of ongoing immune system activation, possibly involving cytokine abnormalities as well, may be taking place in ME/CFS (reference 195; see also reference 529).

Five controlled studies have demonstrated a deficiency in the ability of T cells to proliferate when they are stimulated by a substance known as phytohaemagglutinin (PHA) – an abnormality in the immune response which is not found in psychiatric disorders.

Allergic skin responses to a range of proteins have been shown to be abnormal in a series of experiments carried out by Professor Andrew Lloyd's team in Australia. This particular test is a useful way of measuring the efficiency of T cells – a process known as cell-mediated immunity. Hypoergy (a significantly reduced level of skin response) was found in up to 50 per cent of ME/CFS patients in this study (reference 201).

## How should we interpret these abnormalities?

Although many of these results raise more questions than answers, there is no doubt that a range of diverse immunological abnormalities can be found in people with ME/CFS. Some of the most important findings support the idea that there is a continued overactivity of the immune system taking place. Some of these results have similarities to those found in psychiatric conditions such as depression, which can undoubtedly affect various aspects of the body's immune response (see page 222). However, such abnormalities are much more characteristic of severely ill hospitalised patients with depression, not those with mild to moderate depression.

None of these immune system abnormalities can yet be used as a basis for a diagnostic test and their relationship to symptoms remains uncertain. However, one recent study (reference 529) has found a definate correlation between abnormal immunological findings and certain specific symptoms, and it is possible that changes in the levels of cytokines could be contributing towards muscle fatigue, brain malfunction and sleep disturbance, as well as upsetting the normal control mechanisms of the hypothalamus gland (see pages 146–50). One intriguing hypothesis relating to immune dysfunction put forward by researchers from University College, London, in *The Lancet* (reference 216) is that both ME/CFS and Gulf War Syndrome (see pages 108–10) may involve a shift in the balance of cytokines from those normally produced by the T helper 1 (Th1) cells to those produced by the T helper 2 (Th2) cells. If this hypothesis is correct, then new types of immunological therapy which are capable of reversing such a disturbance could be of value. The University College researchers are currently investigating the possible use of an experimental drug called SRL 172, which is claimed to be able to push the immune system back into a Th1 mode.

## Muscle Abnormalities

The fact that muscle symptoms – always exercise-induced fatigue, frequently pain and sometimes twitching – are present in ME/CFS has led researchers to use various techniques in order to examine both the structure and function of muscle.

### What causes muscle fatigue and weakness?

Muscle symptoms can have many different causes, depending on which part of the nervous system, or the muscle itself, is at fault.

Messages to move or contract a particular group of muscles originate in a part of the brain called the motor cortex, from where they pass down the spinal cord to peripheral nerves, which then control activity in individual muscles. Between the end of the nerve and the muscle fibre is a gap, known as the neuro-muscular junction. The message to contract a muscle is conducted across this gap by a chemical transmitter known as acetylcholine. When the nervous impulse finally reaches the muscle, large numbers of fibres rapidly contract and so an arm or leg starts to move. Muscle weakness can therefore originate in either the brain, the nervous system, at the neuro-muscular junction or in the muscle itself.

People with spinal cord injuries are obviously unable to pass messages effectively below the site of damage, and so may be completely unable to move their arms or legs. In conditions such as multiple sclerosis – where some sufferers experience a remarkably similar type of fatigue and weakness to that seen in ME/CFS (reference 230) – the problem lies in the nervous system. Even though the weakness here can be quite profound, there is nothing actually wrong with the muscles themselves. In myasthenia gravis, the problem lies with a disorder of chemical transmission involving acetylcholine, and it is interesting to note that abnormal responses involving this chemical transmitter in the brain have now been reported in ME/CFS (see pages 153–4). Diseases in which weakness is purely due to a problem in the muscle are known as myopathies. In children, these are generally the result of inherited genetic defects (like muscular dystrophy), whereas in adults they can be caused by alcohol, drugs, hormonal problems and infections.

The unresolved question as far as ME/CFS research is concerned is whether the muscle symptoms are being caused by a defect in the muscle, the brain (so-called 'central' fatigue), or a combination of both. On a very simple level it's rather like searching for a fault in a car that won't accelerate properly – does the reason lie in the engine (i.e. the muscle) or is it due to the fact that the driver (i.e. the brain) isn't providing clear instructions via the gears and accelerator!

Many doctors involved in the ME/CFS debate remain extremely sceptical about research findings pointing to muscle abnormalities, and the Royal Colleges' report (see page 439–9) concluded that there is *'no convincing evidence of any changes in muscle structure or function other than those secondary to inactivity'* (para 6.1). The real problem, maintain the sceptics, lies centrally in the brain, and this involves a disturbance in the complex co-ordination of messages which pass to and from muscle in order to maintain its power and activity. The fact that people with ME/CFS have normal muscle power when they are examined at rest is not in dispute, but the origin of their fatigue, weakness and pain certainly is.

Those who unreservedly believe that the origin of fatigue in ME/CFS lies wholly in the brain support their position by reference to several research studies which indicate that people with ME/CFS have muscles which are neither weak nor more easily fatigued than in normal healthy controls (references: 231, 234, 238–40, 250–1).

Others, like myself, believe that the results from a number of other research studies – as discussed below – cannot simply be dismissed as being solely due to inactivity.

## Muscle problems and persisting viral infection?

As I've already discussed earlier in this chapter, there is conflicting evidence about the role of persisting viral infection in ME/CFS, with the current position moving away from the idea that virus in muscle is a cause of ongoing symptoms. Even so, the possibility remains that a precipitating viral infection, or the consequent production of inflammatory immune chemicals (cytokines), could be responsible for some muscle symptoms.

## Biopsies and mitochondrial abnormalities

This type of investigation, aimed at looking for structural abnormalities in muscle, involves taking a minute piece of tissue (which can be done almost painlessly using local anaesthetic and a small needle) from the thigh and examining it under a microscope.

Normal muscle is made up of two distinct types of fibre. Type 1 fibres are aerobic (oxygen requiring) and rich in mitochondria. This type of muscle is supposed to be fatigue-resistant, and thus able to withstand prolonged contraction, such as standing up for long periods of time. Type I fibres are also said to be more susceptible to the effects of muscle disuse than the type II variety.

Type II fibres are much more concerned with fine movements, such as performing delicate tasks with the fingers or moving the eyes.

Professor Behan's unit in Glasgow has performed muscle biopsies on several hundred ME/CFS patients. In their most recent series, 50 out of 60 biopsies showed a significant reduction in size (atrophy) of the type II fibres. A research study carried out by Dr Russell Lane and colleagues at Charing Cross Hospital in London (reference 592) has also concluded that changes in muscle fibre ratios are not consistent with inactivity.

Using high-powered electron microscopy, the Glasgow researchers have also been looking at individual structures within muscle known as mitochondria. These are aptly named the 'power house of the cell' because it is here that glycogen is broken down to produce energy. Muscle is extremely rich in mitochondria, but these structures are also present in many other body tissues.

Under the electron microscope, various changes have been noted which appear to be fairly specific to ME/CFS. First, the mitochondria were found to be abnormally situated in the cell, clustering around its outer perimeter. Second, there appeared to be damage to their internal structure. Instead of the normal convoluted pattern there was swelling, vacuole formation and the development of definite compartments (reference 227).

The significance of these changes has still to be evaluated, but it seems doubtful that such mitochondria can be performing their normal tasks in an effective manner. Once again, as with the SF-EMG findings described later, these are abnormalities which can also occur during the acute stages of viral infections. As mitochondria have their own genetic material in the form of DNA, it is possible that one effect of a viral infection is to 'switch off' enzymes concerned with normal energy production. Alternatively, viral infections could be causing mitochondrial damage as a 'hit and run' effect, although the only other research group to study this aspect of muscle failed to agree with these findings (reference 245).

Interestingly, there is one report from Australia of genetic damage to mitochondrial DNA occurring in a patient with ME/CFS (reference 257). Mitochondrial abnormalities could also help to explain the various biochemical changes described later.

One additional test that can be carried out using muscle biopsy material is to stain it for the presence of enzymes which catalyse various functions inside the cell, and several deficiencies have been observed in

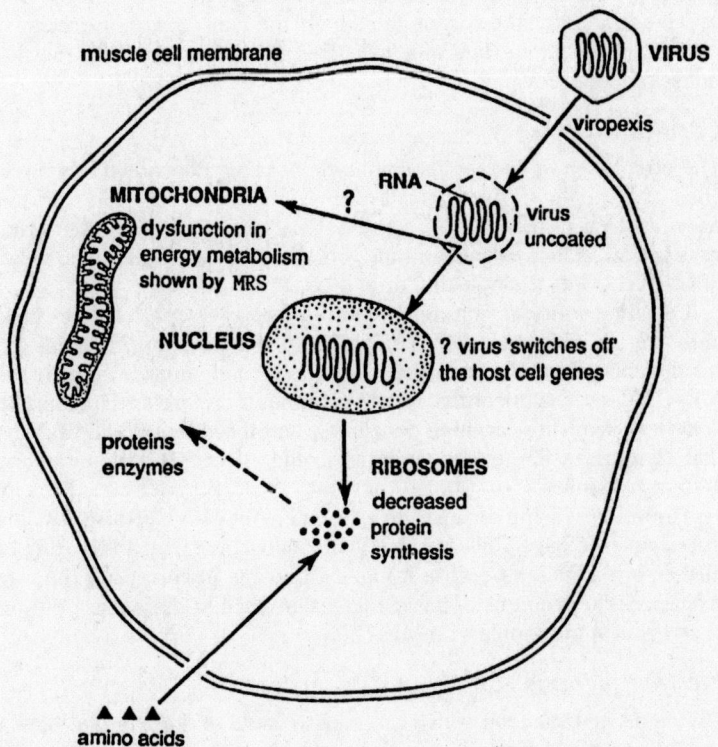

mitochondrial and cell respiration enzymes. Some of these changes are probably the consequence of relative inactivity in the muscle, whereas others (e.g. adenylate deaminase deficiency) do seem to be related to viral infections.

Professor Timothy Peters, from King's College Hospital in London, has been looking at yet another aspect of muscle cell function using biopsy material. He has measured the total content of genetic material (DNA and RNA) and protein in patients' muscles. The results revealed a significant 15 per cent decrease in RNA, most of which is probably in the ribosomes – structures within the cell that manufacture proteins from dietary amino acids (reference 247).

As a follow-up to this work, he has used a radioactively tagged amino acid (leucine C13) to follow its uptake into protein manufacture within both the muscle and the whole body. The preliminary results, both showing decreased protein manufacture, suggest that there may be a similar problem outside the muscle (reference 244).

This is additional evidence to support the view that an intracellular virus may be interfering with selective aspects of the cell's normal housekeeping activities.

## Carnitine deficiency

The production of energy inside muscle not only depends on the presence of glycogen and oxygen. It also requires vitamins, minerals and enzymes to help catalyse the process. One of the most important catalysts is a substance called carnitine, which acts by controlling the influx of fatty acids into the mitochondria.

Carnitine deficiency has now been reported in research studies from both the UK (reference 242) and Japan (reference 235). Although the relationship between carnitine deficiency and muscle fatigue in ME/CFS remains uncertain, it is known that there are specific muscle disorders involving carnitine deficiency, and that there are indications that changes in the level of carnitine could affect the body's immune system responses.

The value of using carnitine as a treatment for ME/CFS also remains uncertain (see page 199), but this is one substance which is worthy of further investigation because it may be of value in correcting the way that excessive amounts of lactic acid accumulate in the muscle during exercise in some people with ME/CFS.

## Electromyograms (EMGs)

This is an investigation which provides reliable information on how a particular muscle group is responding to electrical stimuli which pass down from the brain and nerve fibres in the spinal cord instructing the muscle to contract. EMGs can show up abnormalities in the way the impulse crosses the gap between the nerve and muscle as well as within the actual muscle fibres.

Conventional EMGs are usually quite normal in people with ME/CFS – a fact which has led most neurologists to assume that there is nothing wrong within the muscle. Using a highly sophisticated technique known as single fibre electromyography (SF-EMG), Dr Goran Jamal, a neurophysiologist working with Professor Behan in Glasgow, has shown that about 75 per cent of people with ME/CFS have an abnormality known as 'prolonged jitter' (reference 233).

The unique feature about SF-EMG is that it enables researchers to study how an impulse is transmitted into two separate muscle fibres supplied by the same nerve. So, any abnormality in conduction can be picked up from the point at which the nerve divides, or across the neuromuscular junction, or in the muscle fibre itself. The lack of what is known as impulse blocking indicates that the problem does not lie in the neuromuscular junction (as in myasthenia gravis), the most likely site being, according to Dr Jamal, inside the muscle.

Increased jitter is not a specific finding in ME/CFS (it can also occur in various other nerve and muscle diseases), but in this case it does strongly suggest a definite conduction abnormality in the muscle fibres. It is also a finding that has been reported by Swedish researchers when they looked at the muscles of people during an acute viral infection.

(For further information on EMG studies in ME/CFS see references 229 and 249.)

## Magnetic resonance spectroscopy (MRS)

This is perhaps the most interesting aspect of muscle research, which originally involved the co-operation of Professor George Radda and his team working at the John Radcliffe Hospital in Oxford. In the early 1980s, they started use a new technique called MRS, which enabled them to make accurate assessments of energy production within the muscle by following various chemical changes which were taking place inside the cells. MRS is a painless non-invasive procedure in which the patient is placed inside a giant cylindrical magnet through which chemical changes and muscle acidity during exercise can be followed using a computer.

Dr Melvin Ramsay asked if I could be the first patient with ME/CFS to be investigated by this new technique, to see if there were any identifiable abnormalities in the way my muscles were producing energy.

The results confirmed that there was a unique biochemical defect in the way energy was being produced that was not observed in any of their healthy volunteers.

To understand the significance of this result, it is helpful to know how energy is produced inside the muscle. The initial source is provided by carbohydrates in food, which are first broken down by digestive processes and then stored in the body as glycogen. This is the fuel which is burned up by exercise and, by a process known as glycolysis, converted into energy. For glycolysis to take place, two essential ingredients must be present. These are oxygen, brought to the muscles by the red blood cells, and enzymes, produced on site in the muscle cell, which act as catalysts in the burning process. When oxygen and enzymes are present in the right quantities, glycolysis takes place and energy is produced. This is known as aerobic metabolism. However, when oxygen is lacking, the result is anaerobic metabolism, in which excessive amounts of lactic acid are produced instead of energy.

All normal human beings produce lactic acid during exercise, but the results here showed a rapid and excessive acidity in the muscle, indicating a clear abnormality in the way the mitochondria were breaking down glycogen.

When these results were published in *The Lancet* in 1984 (reference 225) it appeared that, at last, a primary defect in the muscle had been discovered.

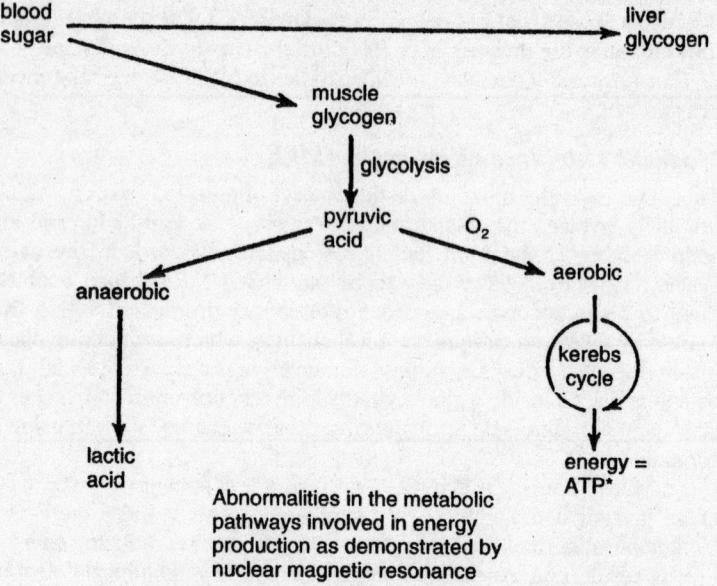

Abnormalities in the metabolic pathways involved in energy production as demonstrated by nuclear magnetic resonance

*ATP (adenosine triphosphate) is a compound which acts as a source of energy storage within a cell

However, a follow-up report by the same research group in 1993 (reference 226) found that this sort of biochemical abnormality was only present in a minority of further ME/CFS patients who had been examined. In fact, out of a total group of 46 extra cases, only six showed an increased acidification of muscle during exercise and another six had a decrease in muscle acidification.

A number of other research groups have also been looking at biochemical changes in muscle during exercise. Some of the more relevant findings include:

- Some ME/CFS patients have impaired muscle energy metabolism (as shown by abnormal amounts of lactic acid produced during exercise). This finding is not readily explained by physical inactivity or a psychiatric disorder (reference 532).
- Oxidative metabolism is reduced in ME/CFS patients compared to sedentary controls (references 243 and 255).
- ME/CFS patients reached exhaustion much more rapidly than normal subjects, at which point they had reduced intracellular concentrations of ATP. This data suggests a defect in oxidative metabolism with an acceleration of glycolysis taking place in the muscle (reference 255).
- Fifteen per cent of cases showed a significant decrease in the maximum rate of mitochondrial ATP production (reference 241).

## Muscle research: what conclusions can be drawn?

Although some doctors still maintain extremely polarised positions as to whether these abnormalities indicate genuine muscle disease or are simply due to immobility and disuse, I believe it is vital to keep an open mind on their relevance. Instinct tells me that there may be a subgroup of people with ME/CFS who have a biochemical problem in their muscle and that further innovative research in this area could even lead to new forms of treatment. Equally, there is good evidence that problems with brain hormones and chemicals are causing the 'central' fatigue that undoubtedly exists in ME/CFS. If we can gain a further understanding of the complex mechanisms involved in the production of fatigue in conditions like multiple sclerosis, this could also end up providing benefits for people with ME/CFS.

# Research into Brain Abnormalities

Research activity into ME/CFS during the 1980s largely concentrated on looking at the possible role of infection, immunological disturbances and abnormalities in muscle. At the same time it was becoming clear that encephalomyelitis (inflammation in the brain and spinal cord) was no longer a tenable explanation for the wide variety of brain symptoms (e.g. clumsiness, poor balance, fainting episodes) and problems with normal mental functioning which are so characteristic of this illness.

The arrival of new and sophisticated investigative techniques means that researchers can now start to look for anatomical (structural) abnormalities in specific parts of the brain, as well how these areas are performing their normal functions.

As a result of using such techniques, some very interesting research findings are starting to emerge, particularly in relation to hormones, chemical transmitters and blood supply to specific parts of the brain.

## The autonomic nervous system – is it involved?

As I've already described on pages 50–54, there are a number of symptoms (e.g. low blood pressure, palpitations, feeling faint, cold hands and feet) which suggest that there may be abnormalities in the co-ordination of nervous messages that are passed from control centres in the brain to the heart and blood vessels via what is known as the autonomic nervous system.

One of the most important studies in this area comes from Professor John Rowe's research group at Johns Hopkins University School of Medicine in Boston, USA. They have examined the relationship between what is known as neurally mediated hypotension (NMH) and ME/CFS. In simple terms, this means that there is abnormal co-ordination of nervous messages passing between the heart and brain. As a result of a fall in blood pressure, people with NMH frequently feel light-headed or faint, particularly after prolonged periods of standing. And because insufficient blood is reaching the brain, there may also be fatigue and problems with normal mental functioning.

To study the possible relationship between NMH and ME/CFS, the American researchers investigated a group of 23 patients using a technique called tilt-table testing (where blood pressure is monitored during changes in posture). An abnormal response was found in 22 of this group and the researchers went on to suggest a treatment regime involving self-help measures (see page 54), carefully increasing the amount of dietary salt intake (which must *only be done with medical supervision*), and the possible use of drugs such as fludrocortisone (see page 189), beta adrenergic blocking agents and disopyramide, either alone or in combination. (For further information on this research see references 143 and 148.)

Other reports of disturbances in the function of the autonomic nervous system include:

- The onset of autonomic symptoms within four weeks of a viral infection in 46 per cent of a group of ME/CFS patients. A positive tilt-table test was found in 25 per cent. Dr Roy Freeman and Professor Tony Komaroff, from Harvard Medical School in Boston, USA, suggested that one possible cause could be a postviral autonomic neuropathy (reference 147).

- Diminished activity involving the vagus nerve (an autonomic nerve which controls heart rate and blood pressure) in both sitting and standing positions. This finding indicates that the parasympathetic part of the autonomic nervous system is not functioning properly at times of increased demand on the heart, which may then result in fatigue which is out of proportion to the physical effort being made (reference 149).

(See also medical references 143–50.)

## EEG and BEAM scans

The long-established method for looking at electrical activity in the brain is known as an electroencephalogram (EEG). Here, electrodes are placed on the scalp and changes in voltage are recorded which correspond to brainwave activity. In the past, EEG measurements have only shown occasional non-specific abnormalities in people with ME/CFS. There are now some highly sophisticated forms of EEG equipment available from America, which can extract more precise information, known as BEAM scans.

One researcher who has been making use of BEAM scans to map out the brain's activity is Dr Marshall Handleman, a neurologist working at the University of Southern California Medical School. He has found that there may be abnormalities in parts of the brain known as the temporal lobes and hippocampus – the latter being an area that plays a key role in the formation of new memories, as well as influencing activity in the hypothalamus.

## Evoked potentials

Dr Leslie Findley and Dr Deepak Prasher at London's National Hospital for Nervous Diseases have investigated what are called cortical evoked potentials – a way of measuring the way the brain reacts to and then processes all kinds of incoming information. Several different tests have been used, and those measuring auditory (hearing), visual and sensory evoked potentials were all found to be normal. (Incidentally, visual evoked potentials are often abnormal in multiple sclerosis, making this a useful test if there is doubt about the diagnosis). The important finding in the ME/CFS group was an absence or delay in what is known as cognitive potential P3 – a finding which could be consistent with the prob-

# Hypothalamus and hormonal control

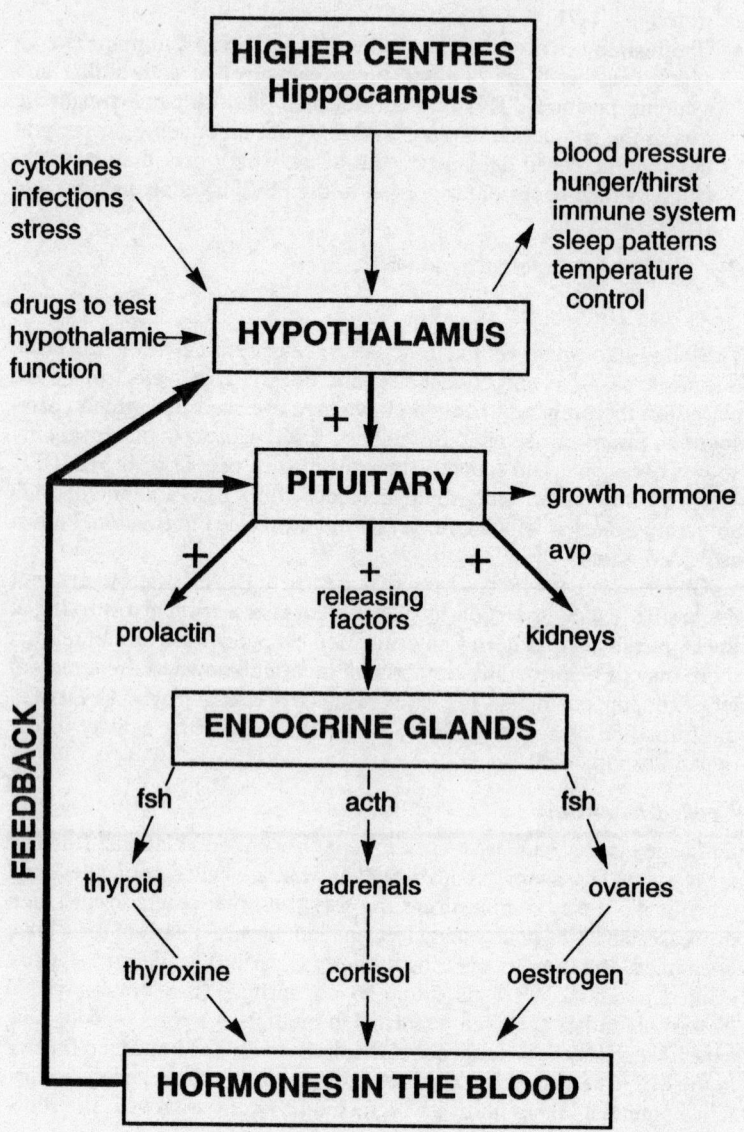

lems of concentration, memory and processing new information. Interestingly, this abnormality was not found in a group of depressed patients, in whom concentration difficulties are also common and often quite severe (reference 154).

## The hypothalamus and hormonal control

The most relevant research findings to date concern the role of the hypothalamus, a small but vital part of the brain which is involved in the regulation of:

- autonomic nerves through what is known as the limbic system
- appetite and food intake
- body temperature control by increasing or decreasing heat loss through sweating or changes in blood supply to the skin
- normal sleep patterns
- numerous body hormones.

Interest in the possibility that there could be a disturbance in hypothalamic function stems from the fact that people with ME/CFS frequently report symptoms which indicate an upset in the normal 'thermostatic' function in this particular part of the brain.

The way in which the hypothalamus finely tunes blood levels of various hormones is best understood by following the diagram on page 146. Firstly, a number of factors including sleep, exercise, and emotions can all influence hypothalamic activity. Of special interest in ME/CFS is the fact that infections and immune chemicals, particularly cytokines such as interleukins 1 and 6, can temporarily upset hypothalamic function, and possibly go on to produce a more permanent disturbance in normal control mechanisms.

As far as body hormones are concerned, their blood levels are constantly being monitored by receptors on the gland; should they rise or fall from normal, then the hypothalamus quickly responds by sending instructions to another hormone-producing gland called the pituitary. It's from here that hormone releasing factors are produced to increase or decrease the levels of other hormones being made by the adrenal glands (cortisol), thyroid gland (thyroxine) or sex glands (oestrogen).

Researchers in both the UK and USA have examined hypothalamic function in ME/CFS by using drugs called agonists which are known to be able to stimulate different aspects of hormone production controlled by the gland. Then, by monitoring the specific levels of hormones such as arginine vasopressin, cortisol, growth hormone and prolactin, it has been possible to demonstrate that normal control mechanisms are clearly malfunctioning.

The precise cause(s) of these disturbances in hypothalamic function remain uncertain. They could be related to infection, cytokines, chemical transmitters such as serotonin, defective stress responses, sleep disturbances (references 163 and 167), or a combination of several of the above.

The main abnormalities in hypothalamic function to be reported concern:

*Arginine vasopressin (AVP)* The function of this hormone is to regulate the amount of water produced by the kidneys and excreted as urine. As described on page 108, some women with ME/CFS seem to have a problem with fluid retention, especially around the mid-point of their menstrual cycle. To study this further, Professor Behan's group in Glasgow carried out tests to see if there were abnormalities in the control of water balance taking place.

One such test involved an overnight fast, which was then followed by the intake of a large quantity of water. Normal healthy people usually remove well over 80 per cent of such a water load within four hours, but the ME/CFS group only managed around 60 per cent. They were also found to have an erratic release of AVP into the blood, and increased amounts of total body water when compared to the control group. The results indicate a definite abnormality in the way that water balance is being regulated by the hypothalamus and pituitary glands (reference 157).

Interestingly, AVP can also help to activate normal stress responses involving the production of cortisol (see pages 30–31).

**Prolactin release** The second hormonal abnormality to be investigated by Professor Behan involved the control of the production of prolactin, a hormone released from the anterior part of the pituitary gland (under hypothalamic control), whose main function is the stimulation of the female breast to produce milk.

Experimentally, prolactin release can be stimulated by using an agonist drug called buspirone (a drug which is normally used for its tranquillising properties). It was originally thought that buspirone stimulated receptors for a brain chemical called serotonin, but it is now realised that it may also act by antagonising the action of another brain chemical called dopamine (whose levels are reduced in Parkinson's disease).

When people with ME/CFS were given buspirone, their output of prolactin far exceeded that of the control group (as well as that of a group with depression). This type of experiment has also been repeated by other researchers, most of whom have reported similar findings (see references 156, 158, 161, 172, 173 and 178).

It has also been suggested that a buspirone challenge could become a useful objective test for monitoring progress in ME/CFS, or even a diagnostic test. Levels of prolactin before administration of buspirone are, incidentally, quite normal in people with ME/CFS. A raised level of resting prolactin may indicate the presence of a pituitary tumour.

*Cortisol* is the third hormone to be assessed in ME/CFS. This is an important stress hormone that is produced by the two adrenal glands, situated immediately above the kidneys. Cortisol has powerful anti-allergy and anti-inflammatory properties through its action on the immune system, and also controls the way in which body proteins and carbohydrates are broken down to produce heat and energy. Levels of cortisol fluctuate throughout the day, being at their highest in the early morning and lowest in the early evening in normal healthy individuals. One of the most important influences on cortisol production is stress and people with more severe forms of depression often have a *marked increase* in their blood levels of cortisol. Dangerously low levels are found in a condition called Addison's disease, which is another cause of chronic fatigue that is sometimes misdiagnosed as ME/CFS (see page 86).

Cortisol production is stimulated from above by an anterior pituitary hormone called adrenocorticotrophic hormone (ACTH), which in turn is influenced by feedback mechanisms, as well as stress, acting on the hypothalamus. The main stimulatory hormone for cortisol, which is produced by the hypothalamus, is called corticotrophin releasing hormone (CRH).

In December 1991, a group of American researchers, including Drs Mark Demitrack and Stephen Straus from the National Institutes of Health, reported their findings of lowered levels of cortisol in 30 ME/CFS patients (reference 162).

This group of patients had a *mild decrease* in cortisol levels, which seemed to be present throughout the day. The results indicated that the adrenal glands themselves were not at fault, although they had become oversensitive to a chronically low level of ACTH. The primary problem was either at the level of the hypothalamus or some other part of the nervous system which influenced its activities. The most likely cause, however, was thought to be a deficit in the production of CRH from a part of the hypothalamus known as the paraventricular nucleus.

The finding of lowered levels of cortisol is currently one of the most exciting research findings to be reported. Besides offering a possible explanation for fatigue, a reduced level of circulating cortisol could be affecting immune function in such a way that it allows an exaggeration of allergic responses (see pages 256–7) and reactivation of dormant infections such as Epstein-Barr virus.

Once again, as with the prolactin experiments, these are completely opposite results to those found in patients with depression. It is also interesting to note that very similar findings were reported in a medical paper back in 1981 (reference 170).

(Details of further research studies – including the use of saliva to test for cortisol levels – see references 171, 174 and 177.)

*Growth hormone* is produced by the anterior part of the pituitary gland and regulates human growth, particularly during childhood. The release of growth hormone is mainly under the control of an inhibitory hypothalamic releasing factor called somatostatin. The relevance of growth hormone release to ME/CFS is that by artificially stimulating its release with a steroid drug called dexamethasone, researchers can gain useful information on the sensitivity of the hypothalamus to circulating levels of steroid hormones in the blood. These experiments, which have been carried out by Professors Ted Dinan and Peter Behan, demonstrated that people with ME/CFS had a blunted (reduced) release of growth hormone when given dexamethasone – results which suggest that there is an abnormality in the way their brains are recognising and responding to naturally produced steroid hormones such as cortisol. Growth hormone levels before stimulation were, incidentally, found to be significantly lower in the ME/CFS patients compared to healthy controls or patients with depression (reference 168), and it is interesting to note that growth hormone deficiency in adults can produce a range of symptoms similar to those found in ME/CFS.

(Details of other research studies looking at hypothalamic function and brain hormone regulation are contained in references 155, 158–61.)

## Neuroimaging: MRI and SPECT scans

**MRI scans** 'MRI' stands for magnetic resonance imaging. Here, the part of the body being examined is placed in a high-powered magnetic field. A perfect picture of the anatomy can then be built up by measuring the amount of electromagnetic radiation being given off from the tissues. In the brain and nervous system, this can give precise information about very small lesions which could never be obtained using conventional X-ray equipment.

Two American research groups, using an even more sensitive MRI scanner, detected small lesions in the white matter of the brain known as unidentified bright objects (UBOs). Dr Sandra Daugherty and colleagues from the University of Nevada School of Medicine reported these findings in a group of 15 patients with severe ME/CFS, some of whom had also started to develop other neurological symptoms. MRI scans revealed small but definite lesions in various parts of the brain, which were not seen in control patients or those with dementia or psychiatric disorders. Along with abnormalities found on psychological testing, the team concluded that these MRI lesions could not be attributed to psychological factors and that they were, in fact, very similar to the disturbances seen in some adults with HIV infection affecting the brain (reference 262).

The results of a much larger MRI study were reported in the *Annals of Internal Medicine* (reference 258). Here, Professor Tony Komaroff's team examined a group of patients who fell ill between 1984 and 1987 – many of whom were involved in the famous Lake Tahoe outbreak that I described in Chapter 2.

These MRI scans revealed numerous pinpoint lesions in the white matter of the brain in 79 per cent of those examined compared to 21 per cent in a matched control group. The authors concluded that the abnormalities were consistent with inflammation or demyelination (loss of the protective sheath that surrounds a nerve cell), and were very similar to findings sometimes observed in patients with multiple sclerosis or HIV infection involving the nervous system.

Interestingly, in nine of these patients, there was a relationship between the site of the MRI brain lesion and clinical symptoms. For example, a 34-year-old woman with severe balance problems had a large cerebellar lesion (the cerebellum is a part of the brain that helps in the control of the brain).

A third American report, from Dr Benjamin Natelson at New Jersey Medical School, found that 52 ME/CFS patients had significantly more abnormal findings on MRI scans than a control group (reference 267).

The first UK study, which compared patients with ME/CFS and a similar number with depression, found no significant differences in the incidence of these abnormalities (reference 259).

A second UK study, from Dr Durval Costa and colleagues at London's Middlesex Hospital, compared MRI findings in 43 ME/CFS patients to a similar number of controls. Abnormalities were found in 32 per cent of the patient group and 28 per cent of the controls. One of the ME/CFS patients had evidence of demyelination (as occurs in multiple sclerosis) on the scan (reference 265).

At present, it is not yet possible to draw any firm conclusions from these findings because similar abnormalities clearly occur in apparently healthy people as well as in a variety of other medical and psychiatric disorders. These UBOs could well represent minute areas of inflammation in brain tissue which have occurred during previous episodes of infection which have entered the central nervous system. However, in view of the occasional presence of larger and deeper lesions within the brain, along with a correlation to clinical symptoms, this is clearly a form of investigation which is worth pursuing.

The routine use of MRI scans in the assessment and diagnosis of ME/CFS is not to be recommended. However, an MRI scan should certainly be carried out if there are prominent or unusual neurological symptoms which suggest the possibility of an alternative diagnosis (e.g. multiple sclerosis).

**SPECT scans** This acronym stands for Single Photon Emission Tomography. SPECT scans make use of the fact that when a small amount of harmless radioactive chemical (isotope) is injected into the body, its uptake by specific body tissues can be measured by monitoring the amount of radiation which is then released. Isotopes can also be attached to other chemicals to allow them to cross the protective blood–brain barrier and so enter various different types of brain tissue. In the case of ME/CFS, SPECT scans are now being used to assess blood flow (perfusion) in a number of different areas within the brain.

Some of the most intriguing SPECT scan results have come from Dr Durval Costa and his team at London's Middlesex Hospital (reference 261). They found a generalised reduction in brain perfusion, which was particularly marked in an area known as the brain stem – a finding which has not been observed in any other medical or psychiatric disorder using this type of investigation. One particular part of the brain stem – known as the reticular formation – may be relevant to ME/CFS because this is an area that is concerned with the control of sleep, movement, behaviour and memory. The reticular formation also contains nerve centres which affect the activity of the heart, lungs and intestines via the autonomic nervous system (see earlier). Similar reports of perfusion abnormalities in the brain stem have now been reported by an Italian research group (reference 272), using a different type of brain scanning technique (PET).

Findings from other research studies using SPECT scans include:

- Perfusion defects in the frontal and temporal lobes, although the parietal and occipital lobes were also affected (reference 266). (These are all well defined areas on the outer part of the brain.)
- Perfusion defects in all regions of the brain with no consistent regional abnormalities (reference 268).
- Perfusion defects which were predominantly in the frontal and temporal lobes. The findings in this American study, which compared ME/CFS patients with those suffering from AIDS, dementia and depression, were said to be *consistent with the hypothesis that chronic fatigue syndrome may be due to a chronic viral encephalitis'* (reference 270).
- In some patients, SPECT abnormalities altered over the course of

time and appeared to correlate with a change in clinical symptoms (reference 269).

- Symmetrical perfusion defects were mainly found in the frontal and parietal regions of the brain (reference 524).

## Neurotransmitter disturbances

The brain and nervous system consist of millions of nerve cells which are separated by minute gaps called synapses. Nervous messages are conducted across these gaps with the aid of chemicals called neurotransmitters. After being released from a nerve ending, the neurotransmitter then locks on to a receptor site on the next nerve, so allowing the message or instruction to be passed to other parts of the nervous system.

Neurotransmitter deficiencies are known to occur in a number of psychiatric and brain disorders, particularly depression (serotonin and noradrenaline) and Parkinson's disease (dopamine), but it has only been recently that researchers have started to look for similar abnormalities in ME/CFS.

The first published report, which came from Professor Mark Demitrack and colleagues at the University of Michigan, USA, found significant reductions in the plasma (part of the blood) level of MHPG (3 methoxy 4-hydroxyphenylglycol) along with an increased level of 5-HIAA (5-hydroxyindolacetic acid). MHPG is a metabolite (by-product) of noradrenaline production, and the finding of decreased levels is compatible with a down-regulation (reduction) in the activity of the sympathetic part of the autonomic nervous system. 5-HIAA is a metabolite of serotonin, and an increased level suggests a possible up-regulation (increase) of serotonin activity in the brain. This latter neurotransmitter helps to control mood, sleep, pain perception and appetite. Both of these results are different from what is normally seen in patients with depression (reference 274).

The most important neurotransmitter abnormality to be reported so far involves acetylcholine, a chemical which helps to regulate a diverse range of brain activities including sleep, memory and concentration. Acetylcholine is also involved in the conduction of messages between nerves and muscles and influences the release of corticotrophic releasing hormone from the hypothalamus (another transmitter which helps to control the release of cortisol).

In an experiment carried out by Professors Peter Behan and Ted Dinan, (reference 273) acetylcholine activity in the brain was assessed by giving patients and controls a drug called pyridostigmine (which acts by increasing the level of acetylcholine in the brain) and then measuring the amount of growth hormone being produced (which acts as a reliable way of checking the resulting increase in acetylcholine activity). There was an exaggerated (increased) response to pyridostigmine in both the ME/CFS patients and a group of patients with an ME/CFS-like illness following exposure to organophosphate pesticides (which are known to act by interfering with acetylcholine activity). These results suggest that people with ME/CFS have an increased sensitivity to acetylcholine, and that this could be affecting various parts of the nervous system where this transmitter plays a role in regulating vital body functions. Specific symptoms which could be related to a disturbance in acetylcholine include abnormal sweating attacks and problems relating to the auto-nomic nerves (see earlier). Treatment with a new drug called galan-thamine hydrobromide, which affects acetylcholine, is currently being assessed in a UK trial (see page 187).

Hormonal studies looking at the release of prolactin in response to agonists such as buspirone and d-fenfluramine (see pages 148–9) suggest that there may be abnormalities relating to both serotonin and dopamine transmission.

Further evidence of a disturbance in serotonin activity comes from work again carried out by Professors Behan and Dinan. They have now found that when 5HT1a (serotonin) receptors in the brain were stimu-lated using an agonist called ipsapirone, there was a significant decrease in blood levels of adrenocorticotrophic stimulating hormone (ACTH) in the ME/CFS patients compared to a control group (reference 275).

If more precise abnormalities can be identified in the activity of neurotransmitters such as acetylcholine, dopamine, noradrenaline and serotonin, these could well have major implications for treatment. However, the use of drugs which increase the level of serotonin in the brain (SSRIs) do not appear to be useful for the majority of people with ME/CFS (see pages 240–1).

# Psychiatry

The role of psychiatric conditions such as depression and anxiety in both the development and perpetuation of ME/CFS is another area where there is a considerable divergence of medical opinion. These differences are discussed in detail in Chapter 12: Mind and Body.

## Psychological testing

Over 20 different research papers have been published on the problems faced by people with ME/CFS in relation to memory, concentration and the ability to maintain attention and process incoming information. Almost all of these research studies have confirmed that such problems genuinely exist, but my own view is that *the results seldom seem to correlate with the severity of symptoms which almost all of my patients report* in relation to their mental functioning (see pages 45–46).

Among the more interesting findings so far reported into what is known as cognitive function are:

- People with multiple sclerosis (MS) and ME/CFS have similar difficulties with mental tasks that require simultaneous processing of complex cognitive information (reference 278).
- The most significant mental impairment involves the speed of processing of incoming information (reference 279).
- Significant differences in cognitive performance occur between those with ME/CFS who have some form of co-existent psychiatric illness (e.g. depression) and those who do not. The cognitive problems in ME/CFS cannot simply be explained by the presence of psychiatric illness (reference 280 and 525).
- There is a decreased ability to process complex information in a simultaneous format, combined with a selective impairment with the processing of auditory (heard) information (reference 283)
- A reduced capacity for maintaining attention which results in an impaired performance to carry out tasks which require planned or self-ordered generation of responses from memory (reference 284).
- Consistent findings involving slower reaction times, poor performance on complex tasks which require memory and attention, and a slowness in the ability to acquire new information (reference 291).
- A significant memory deficit, which is *far worse than implied by CDC diagnostic criteria for CFS*. This pattern of memory deficit is consistent with an abnormality in a part of the brain known as the temperolimbic system and is different from that seen in people suffering from depression (reference 294).
- Problems with mental functioning are more likely to be encountered when performing complex mental tasks which require ME/CFS patients to do two things at once or work at a higher rate of speed than normal (reference 301).

A complete list of research studies which have been carried out into cognitive function in ME/CFS are listed on pages 460–462.

## Sleep

Various types of disturbance, ranging from increased requirements (hypersomnia), especially early on in the illness, through to generalised poor quality sleep patterns are common complaints in ME/CFS.

Several research studies have now examined this aspect in more detail (see references 303–11), but some of the most interesting findings on sleep disturbance in both ME/CFS and fibromyalgia come from Professor Harvey Moldofsky and his colleagues at the University of Toronto in Canada. They have described a particular pattern of sleep rhythm abnormality in which alpha waves, which are typical of an alert, awake state of mind, intrude into the normal delta wave pattern that is characteristically found during periods of deep sleep. A similar type of sleep disturbance is found in some rheumatic disorders and fibromyalgia, but is not seen in depression. Professor Moldofsky has also been examining the possibility that some of these ME/CFS sleep abnormalities could be related to disturbed levels of cytokines (e.g. interleukin 1) and hormones (e.g. corticotrophin releasing factor) in the brain.

Recent research from the UK has found no real evidence to support the hypothesis that people with ME/CFS plus depression or anxiety have any more sleep disturbance than those who do not (reference 309).

It appears that sleep disturbances in ME/CFS form part of the actual disease process rather than being an extension of any underlying psychiatric disorder. A better understanding of this particular aspect would obviously be of considerable benefit when it comes to choosing an appropriate drug therapy aimed at correcting disordered sleep (see pages 77–79).

# Other Types of Research into ME/CFS

## Up-regulation of the 2–5A synthetase RNase L antiviral pathway

This is an antiviral enzyme system which is activated whenever cells in the body are exposed to interferons (immune chemicals). Reports that the system is in a chronic state of overactivity (up-regulation) add support to the hypothesis that persisting viral infection may be involved in ME/CFS. Specific abnormalities in this system appear to be unique to ME/CFS and could form the basis for a diagnostic test. (See references 365 and 366.)

## Serum angiotensin-converting enzyme (ACE)

In a US study, 80 per cent of patients with ME/CFS had raised levels of this enzyme compared to only 9 per cent in a control group (reference 361). Elevations in ACE levels also occur quite frequently in sarcoidosis (see page 102) and may be linked to an overactive immune response.

## Heart problems

In addition to the findings that some people with ME/CFS have neurally mediated hypotension (see earlier), other research studies indicate that a subgroup may have abnormalities involving the heart itself. These include:

- Electrocardiogram (ECG) changes – repetitively negative to flat T waves, alternating with normal T waves in a 24-hour ECG – suggesting that a subtle form of heart disturbance may be contribution to the fatigue in some cases of ME/CFS (reference 360).
- A markedly abbreviated exercise capacity as shown by a slow increase in heart rate and fatigue in the exercising muscles long before a maximum heart rate is achieved (reference 533), a finding which could be compatible with the effects of a latent viral infection affecting the heart and muscles.
- Abnormalities in function of the left ventricle (one of two large chambers of the heart which pump out blood into the circulation) (reference 359).
- Some patients with all the typical features of ME/CFS also have angina-type chest pain which is characteristic of a condition known as syndrome X. Although extensive investigations (including ECGs and coronary artery blood flow studies) are usually normal in syndrome X, these patients have been shown to have abnormalities at a cellular level as demonstrated by the use of radioactive (thallium) scans. This work has been carried out by Professor Behan's group in Glasgow (reference 358).

## Ion channel abnormalities

Research from Australia indicates that people with ME/CFS have lowered levels of potassium (reference 369), an important body salt which helps to regulate all kinds of intracellular activities. Defects in the way that potassium passes in and out of the cells – possibly as the result of a cell membrane defect caused by a viral infection or toxin – could help to explain the presence of syndrome X in some ME/CFS patients as well as the abnormality in resting energy expenditure described below.

It is also interesting to note that ion channel disorders (channelopathies) are now being linked to a number of nerve and muscle diseases, including ciguatera poisoning (see page 106), multiple sclerosis and Guillain-Barré syndrome. The possibility that drugs such as mexilitine and 3,4-diaminopyridine, which help to stabilise the cell membrane defect, could be used as a treatment is also being assessed (reference 526).

## Resting energy expenditure (REE)

This refers to the percentage of available energy which the body uses for maintaining activity inside cells (70 per cent) as opposed to that being used for obvious forms of physical activity. Research by Professor Behan's group has shown that REE in a small group of ME/CFS patients was significantly higher than expected so leaving less energy available for normal forms of physical activity (reference 358).

## Urinary markers

Researchers at the University of Newcastle in New South Wales, Australia, claim to have identified the presence of abnormal levels of certain chemical by-products (metabolites) in the urine of people with ME/CFS. The two compounds so far identified have been named chronic fatigue syndrome urinary marker 1 (CFSUM 1) and 2 (CFSUM 2) Concentrations of CSFUM 2 tend to be lowered. The presence of these urinary markers – whose precise identity has yet to be confirmed – adds weight to the view that some form of biochemical disturbance is occurring at a cellular level. It also raises the possibility of them being used as either a diagnostic test or as a way of assessing illness activity (see references 362 and 363). Details of the Newcastle University research is available on their Internet Home Page:

http://www.newcastle.edu.au/department/bi/birjt/cpruis.

## Homocysteine levels

Increased concentrations of homocysteine (an animo acid) in the cerebrospinal fluid (CFS) have been reported by a group of researchers from Göteborg University in Sweden (reference 364). The researchers have speculated that this finding may be related to lowered levels of vitamin B12 in CFS (concentrations of vitamin B12 in the blood relate inversely to those of homocysteine).

Possible abnormalities in the shape of red blood cells are described on page 23.

Links between ME/CFS and athletic overtraining syndrome, ciguatera poisoning, fibromyalgia, Gulf War Syndrome, organophosphate pesticide exposure and post-polio syndrome are described in Chapter 6: Other Causes of Chronic Fatigue.

# PART 2

# PRACTICAL STEPS TOWARDS COPING WITH ME/CFS

# ME/CFS and your Doctor

My personal experiences over the past 20 years, both as a doctor and as someone who has this illness, have made me appreciate that in many chronic conditions doctors only play a relatively minor role in any recovery process. What is often of far more importance is how patients learn to help themselves.

One of the principal reasons why doctors are frequently so bad at managing patients with chronic illness is that they prefer to concentrate on the purely medical aspects of treatment. Very little attention tends to be paid to other factors – the practical aspects of disability, problems with employment or obtaining benefits, psychological and emotional difficulties – which can be just as important when it comes to trying to cope with something like ME/CFS. Fortunately, a growing number of doctors are now starting to take a much more holistic approach in which the patient, their illness, their family and their environment are all taken into account.

The current trend towards high-tech medical investigations and treatments has also tended to raise expectations of patients when it comes to the diagnosis and management of conditions such as ME/CFS. They often fail to realise that a positive approach to recovery and making appropriate changes in lifestyle, along with practical and sympathetic support from family and friends, may be far more relevant to any recovery process than what a doctor can provide via a prescription pad.

So do bear these difficulties and limitations in mind when it comes to what your doctor may be able to do in terms of providing an accurate diagnosis and helping you to recover from ME/CFS.

## Obtaining a Diagnosis

Why do some doctors find it so difficult to cope with their ME/CFS patients, their diagnosis and management? In order to understand how a doctor sees you – the patient with possible ME/CFS – it's useful to go right back to the onset of your illness.

The first consultation may have been along these lines: 'I had this infection a few weeks ago, but I'm still not feeling any better. I'm tired all the time, I've got painful muscles which quickly tire after exercise and my brain isn't working properly.'

At this point, the doctor's role is essentially one of trying to pin a 'label' on your various symptoms. Only when this has been done can a plan of management be decided. Your doctor would like to successfully treat the newly diagnosed illness, but if that's not possible, at least try to alleviate some of the symptoms. If no firm diagnosis can be made, and there doesn't appear to be anything seriously wrong, a doctor may well end up concluding that you have a 'self-limiting condition' – i.e. it will clear up in its own good time without any specific drug treatment. Hopefully, you and your strange collection of symptoms will disappear – without any further appointments!

Now, if doctors can't actually recognise a particular pattern of symptoms and associate them with a specific illness, they're never going to diagnose that condition. And this why a considerable proportion of people with ME/CFS still have to wait months – sometimes even years – before the correct diagnosis is finally made.

So how should a doctor go about making a diagnosis of ME/CFS? This is largely going to be based on three important components of any good medical consultation: history, examination and investigations.

Taking a good clinical history largely consists of listening to the medical information you provide and asking the right questions. If a possible diagnosis isn't fairly obvious after a patient has given a good description of their main symptoms, then information obtained during the rest of the consultation is unlikely to provide the right answer. With most family doctors only being able to devote about ten minutes to each consultation, it may be a good idea to ask if you can have an extended appointment, possibly outside normal surgery hours. You could also write down some *brief* notes about the sequence of events leading up to the appointment and what your principal symptoms are. If your memory and concentration aren't very good, then ask if you can take a friend or partner along to help answer some of the doctor's questions. This shouldn't cause any problems.

Second is a physical examination, the result of which may reinforce a doctor's believe that there's nothing physically wrong, especially when no obvious abnormalities can be found when the muscles or nerves are examined.

Objective muscle weakness, for example, is usually only found after a period of physical exertion. Actual muscle wasting is fairly unusual in ME/CFS; it seldom occurs unless there has been a period of prolonged immobility.

One nervous-system abnormality that does occur quite frequently involves balance. A doctor will assess balance by what is known as a Romberg test: asking you to stand upright with your eyes closed. My experience is that many people with ME/CFS find this test difficult to carry out, especially when it is made harder by standing on one leg (see pages 55–56).

The only other physical abnormality that may be found is enlargement of lymph glands, particularly those in the neck. Widespread or prominent enlargement of lymph glands will almost certainly require further investigation (e.g. removal of a gland for examination under the microscope) to exclude other medical explanations.

If you feel that you are running a fever – either intermittent or constant – it's helpful to make an accurate diary of any fluctuations (using a reliable thermometer) to show your doctor. Again, this may require further investigation to rule out some form of low-grade chronic infection.

The final part of the consultation will normally involve checking to see if any abnormalities appear on routine blood or urine tests. In the case of ME/CFS, these results are often within normal limits, so their main value is in excluding other possible causes for your symptoms. However, when results from laboratory tests in large numbers of people with ME/CFS have been reviewed, clear abnormalities do occur. The largest study so far reported (reference 367) analysed results from 579 ME/CFS patients and a similar number of healthy controls. The ME/CFS group had raised levels of various immunological markers (e.g. immune complexes, immunoglobulin G and antinuclear antibodies) as well as cholesterol and two enzymes associated with liver upsets (alkaline phosphatase and lactic dehydrogenase, both of which help to convert pyruvic acid to lactic acid).

Unfortunately, when all these blood tests come back as normal, the doctor who doesn't believe in ME/CFS will then be left with a continuing diagnostic problem: a patient with a mysterious collection of symptoms; nothing abnormal on physical examination and a whole range of normal laboratory tests.

## Arranging the correct blood tests

Although I'm not in favour of over-investigating people with ME/CFS, especially when there is a clear history of developing the illness immediately after an infective episode, the following blood tests should *always* be checked before the diagnosis is confirmed:

- ESR or acute phase protein changes (e.g. CRP)
- haemoglobin
- white cell count
- routine biochemistry (urea, electrolytes, calcium, phosphate, etc)
- liver and thyroid function
- oestrogen (women only)

- creatine kinase
- urine test for protein, blood and sugar

The following tests can also reveal useful information in certain circumstances:

- antigliadin antibodies
- autoantibody screen
- cortisol
- folic acid
- rheumatology tests (for SLE, etc)
- tests for specific persistent infections (e.g. HIV, Lyme disease)

Set out below are details of the various different blood tests which may be relevant to either the initial diagnosis or subsequent management of someone with ME/CFS.

*Antigliadin antibodies* These are a useful marker of untreated coeliac disease – a condition which can be mistaken for ME/CFS (see page 84). This diagnosis should always be considered where there is a combination of muscle, nervous system and irritable bowel-type symptoms (reference 81).

*Calcium* Although not strictly relevant to ME/CFS, this is still worth checking if there is any doubt about the diagnosis because a raised level of blood calcium is a rare but recognised cause of chronic fatigue (see page 104). The possibility of sarcoidosis being present may also have to be excluded if the calcium level is raised (see page 102). A lowered level of blood calcium raises the possibility of osteomalacia being present (see page 104).

*Carnitine* Decreased levels of this protein, which plays an essential role in muscle energy production, have been reported in several research studies (see page 140). There is also a report of a correlation between blood levels of carnitine and levels of mental/physical fatigue (reference 235). Measuring the level of carnitine may turn out to be a helpful way of identifying people for whom treatment with a carnitine supplement is worth trying.

At present, there is no indication to recommend that this test is carried out routinely. It should be noted that facilities for measuring levels of carnitine are not readily available.

*Cortisol* A severe deficiency of this stress hormone occurs in a rare condition known as Addison's disease – which has a number of similar symptoms to those found in ME/CFS (see page 86). Researchers in America have found that a *milder* reduction in the level of cortisol also occurs in ME/CFS (see pages 149–50), so it may be worth including a measurement of blood cortisol as part of any routine screening. Raised levels of cortisol occur in depression and Cushing's syndrome (see page 87).

*Enzymes* These are proteins which are released from inside a cell whenever damage or inflammation occurs. Different body tissues all have their own characteristic enzymes which can easily be measured once they spill out into the blood. This means that the actual site(s) of cell damage can sometimes be detected by a simple blood test. For example, viral infections sometimes inflame the liver during the early stages of ME/CFS, so raised levels of specific liver enzymes might be found using such a blood test (see page 166).

Muscle enzymes are released into the blood in various muscle diseases. Creatine kinase is the one most frequently measured and a research study has shown that levels of this enzyme are slightly raised in a minority of ME/CFS patients (reference 319).

*ESR (erythrocyte sedimentation rate)* Healthy people have red blood cells which don't normally stick together. However, in a wide range of illnesses – particularly infections and inflammatory disorders – stickiness can occur so that red cells start to clump together (agglutinate) and hence their ability to sediment increases.

The ESR test measures the distance that red blood cells fall in one hour when placed in a tall glass tube. If abnormal, it indicates that 'something is wrong somewhere'. In ME/CFS, *the ESR is almost always within normal limits* (less than 15mm/hour in men and 20mm/hour in women under the age of 50). Anyone who is found to have a raised ESR (or even one that is on the borderline of normal) almost certainly requires further investigations to look for other possible explanations. An elevated ESR should raise the possibility of Crohn's disease (if gastric symptoms are prominent), Sjögren's syndrome or lupus (if joint pains are present) and polymyalgia rheumatica (widespread pain and stiffness). A similar type of test is known as the plasma viscosity test.

*Folic acid* Decreased levels (less than 3.0 microgm/1) of this important nutrient have been reported in a small research study (see page 278–9). Folate deficiency can also occur in coeliac disease.

*Haemoglobin (Hb)* This is a vital part of the red blood cells which contains iron. If decreased, it indicates that some form of anaemia is present. *People with ME/CFS do not have anaemia as part of this illness*. If you are found to be anaemic, further investigations are required to determine the precise cause. This could be due to dietary deficiency, malabsorption of vitamin B12, blood loss from the bowels or something more unusual such as coeliac disease or Crohn's disease (see also pages 84–5).

## Immunological function tests

- Autoantibodies occur when the body's immune system starts to produce antibodies against its own tissues. Low levels of antinuclear, antithyroid, antismooth muscle and antigastric parietal cell antibodies have all been reported in ME/CFS.
- Immunoglobulins are antibodies in the blood and minor abnormalities are quite often present in ME/CFS. Among the most common ones reported are changes in the level of immunoglobulin G (IgG). A raised level of IgE suggests that some form of allergic condition is present. It can also occur with toxocara infection (see pages 94–5).
- Changes in the levels of cytokines (chemical messengers of the immune system), immune complexes and special white blood cells such as natural killer (NK) cells have all been reported in research studies, but can only be measured at specialist research centres. This type of detailed immunological assessment is seldom relevant to making a diagnosis of ME/CFS.

For more information on all of the above immunological abnormalities see pages 129–136 in Chapter 8: Current Research.

*Liver function tests* These measure the amount of specific liver enzymes and chemicals in the blood such as bilirubin – the pigment that turns the skin yellow during an attack of jaundice.

Raised levels of liver enzymes indicate that some form of inflammation or malfunction is taking place in the liver. Common causes include viral infections, drugs such as antidepressants, some herbal remedies and too much alcohol. In some people with ME/CFS, the changes in liver function are very similar to those seen in a condition known as Gilbert's syndrome – an inherited form of mild liver dysfunction (see pages 96–97). A condition known as primary biliary cirrhosis may also need to be excluded (see page 96).

If your liver function tests remain permanently and significantly abnormal, then it is a good idea to ask to be referred to a specialist who can decide if further investigations are needed. These might include taking a small sample of liver tissue for examination under the microscope or an ultrasound scan to see if there is any form of obstruction taking place.

*Oestradiol* Lowered levels of this female sex hormone have been reported in a small subgroup of people with ME/CFS who were attending a gynaecological clinic. Their symptoms were frequently exacerbated during the premenstrual phase of their cycle or showed improvement during pregnancy. Measuring serum oestradiol levels may be a useful baseline investigation in women who are suspected of having ME/CFS. Hormone replacement therapy (with both oestrogen and progestogen) will have to be considered if the level is low (see page 189).

*Thyroid function tests Anyone suspected of having ME/CFS must have their thyroid function checked.* There are two important reasons for including this in the list of baseline investigations.

First is the fact that in anyone over the age of 45, a partial failure of the thyroid gland may already be starting to occur. This can produce a range of symptoms which have many similarities to ME/CFS, e.g. fatigue, muscle pain, problems with memory/concentration, feeling cold. If there is any co-existent thyroid deficiency, this will inevitably cause an exacerbation of ME/CFS symptoms. Second, although rare, is the fact that viral infections are capable of causing a painful inflammation of the whole thyroid gland (de Quervain's thyroiditis). In the early stages, this results in overactivity of the thyroid (hyperthyroidism), but this can be followed by underactivity (hypothyroidism or myxoedema).

The hypothesis that poor thyroid function occurs in the presence of normal thyroid function tests has been put forward by a group of doctors in the *British Medical Journal* (reference 400) and is discussed in more detail on pages 189–90. I have yet to be convinced that this is the case.

*Urea and electrolytes* The amount of urea in the blood gives a rough and ready guide as to how the kidneys are functioning. Levels of electrolytes (body salts such as sodium and potassium) are measured at the same time. Although all these results should be normal in ME/CFS, one research study from Australia (reference 369) found that the total amount of potassium in the body may be reduced. A raised level of potassium suggests the possibility of Addison's disease being present.

*White blood count (WBC)* measures the number of cells in the blood which are primarily produced to fight off infection. There are several different types including neutrophils, lymphocytes, monocytes and eosinophils. In the early stages of an infection the lymphocytes are often raised in number – a lymphocytosis. As the condition becomes chronic there may be no significant abnormalities, although a few people with ME/CFS go on to have a slight decrease in their white cell count – a leucopenia or lymphopenia. Abnormally shaped lymphocytes (atypical lymphocytes) are sometimes seen under the microscope, particularly in cases of glandular fever. T lymphocyte subsets (see earlier) cannot be found on this type of routine blood test. If there is a rise in the numbers of eosinophils (an eosinophila), then this may indicate some form of allergic response or possible infection with toxocara (see page 94–5).

*Other blood tests* The decision to order further blood tests will largely depend on whether or not there are unusual symptoms present which could be explained by an alternative diagnosis. For example, anyone with a significant degree of joint pain may need tests to exclude the possibility of SLE or specific infections which can produce a mixed syndrome of arthritis plus fatigue (see page 41).

If neurological symptoms point to the possibility of multiple sclerosis, then an MRI scan will probably have to be arranged.

## Testing for the presence of persisting viral infection

In the absence of any conclusive scientific evidence to show the presence of persisting viral infection in ME/CFS, there isn't usually any point in arranging further blood tests which look for antibodies to specific types of infection (e.g. Coxsackie virus).

Antibody tests merely assess whether the body's immune system has reacted (as shown by neutralising antibodies) or is still reacting (as shown by other types of antibody such as IgM) to an infection. These tests are of very limited value and even when positive don't necessarily confirm that someone has developed ME/CFS as a result of a specific infection. At the same time, a negative antibody test will not disprove the diagnosis. Problems associated with the interpretation of antibody tests and the value of new diagnostic procedures (e.g. polymerase chain reaction) are discussed in more detail on pages 127–9.

*The VP1 Test* VP1 stands for viral protein one. It is one of four separate proteins that form the outer capsule of any enterovirus. One specific portion of VP1 is present in all of the 72 different enteroviruses.

Researchers at St Mary's Hospital in London developed a unique antibody which identifies this common portion of VP1 and then used it to develop a blood test. A positive VP1 test may indicate the presence of enterovirus in the blood, but not which one. It is neither a test for ME/CFS nor an indicator of illness activity. A positive test result can also occur in someone who has picked up an enteroviral infection such as a common cold, so the finding must be interpreted with caution.

*Epstein-Barr virus tests* These are much more difficult to interpret because 90 per cent of all adults will have already developed antibodies to this virus by the age of 30 from previous contact with the infection during childhood or adolescence. Any rise in antibody levels may therefore be due to reactivation of a latent viral presence. However, some research studies have shown that a number of people with ME/CFS do have raised levels of certain types of antibody (e.g. anti early antigen/EA), suggesting an increased activity of this latent virus is taking place. The role of Epstein-Barr (glandular fever) virus in ME/CFS is discussed in more detail on page 34 and page 128.

*Other types of chronic infection* In certain cases it may be worth checking for chronic infections such as giardia (requires stool samples), hepatitis B/C, Lyme disease, mycoplasma or HIV. All of these infections can produce a persisting fatigue state which has very similar symptomatology to ME/CFS and may require specific drug treatment (see pages 88–96).

## Other investigations

*X-rays* of the chest and joints are usually perfectly normal.

A trace of the heart rhythm (an *electrocardiogram/ECG*) may reveal abnormalities in those who start off their illness with an infection involving the heart muscle (myocarditis). Research from America indicates that other types of heart rhythm disturbance can occur during continual ECG monitoring (see page 157).

*Tilt-table testing* may be indicated where there are problems with fainting and low blood pressure (see pages 53–54).

The results from a *lumbar puncture* – which drains off a small amount of fluid surrounding the spinal cord – are usually quite normal.

*Electroencephalograms (EEGs)*, which monitor electrical activity in the brain, sometimes reveal minor non-specific abnormalities.

As described in the chapter on Current Research, there is now a wide range of high-technology investigations being used in the assessment of people with ME/CFS. These can identify viral infection in blood or muscle tissue (the polymerase chain reaction), pick up subtle abnormalities in muscle (single fibre EMGs), brain tissue (MRI scans), brain blood flow (SPECT scans), function of the hypothalamus gland (cortisol studies) and the immune system (T lymphocyte analysis). It's important to remember that the results obtained are not always consistent and their significance in ME/CFS has yet to be decided. None can be regarded as being diagnostic and they are seldom available outside specialist teaching hospitals. You are unlikely to be referred for any of these investigations unless you are seeing a specialist who is involved in a particular research project.

At present, *there is no reliable or objective test for confirming that someone has ME/CFS* – this decision is still down to a doctor's basic clinical skills and intuition. The result can sometimes be a very long wait before a diagnosis of ME/CFS is made.

## Other causes of chronic fatigue

ME/CFS is not the only cause of the various symptoms commonly associated with this illness. Other possible explanations must not be overlooked, especially in view of the fact that some of them can be successfully treated. A comprehensive review of the many different causes of chronic fatigue is contained in Chapter 6.

# How to Deal with your Doctor Once ME/CFS has been Diagnosed

People with ME/CFS don't always make easy patients to deal with – you have what is probably going to be a long-term illness that isn't going to be 'cured' by drugs, and you may also have a range of time-consuming social, emotional and benefit problems.

Despite all these difficulties, a growing number of family doctors are now accepting and managing ME/CFS in a perfectly satisfactory manner. This fact is borne out by a survey conducted by Dr Darrel Ho-Yen, a consultant microbiologist in Inverness, who sought the opinions of nearly 200 local general practitioners (reference 17). Overall, 71% accepted that ME/CFS existed, 22% were undecided and 7% did not.

If you are still having difficulty persuading your family doctor or specialist that this is a real illness, then ask the ME Association to send the doctor concerned a copy of my *Guidelines for the Care of Patients* booklet. This contains details of symptoms, research and management. You could also tactfully suggest that the doctor follows up some of the more important research papers mentioned in the booklet.

## *What can your doctor prescribe?*

Although no specific drug treatment yet exists which has been shown to alleviate all the symptoms of ME/CFS, there are a number of prescription drugs which may be worth trying. The next chapter contains a detailed review of all such treatments.

## *Referral to a consultant*

Is there any need for you to be referred to a consultant for further advice? Obviously, yes, if your own doctor has any doubt about the diagnosis, or an unusual new symptom appears, or there are doubts about the most appropriate form of management. Unfortunately, as many people with ME/CFS know from previous experience, this type of referral can end up being counter-productive, and even harmful if you are sent to see a consultant who isn't familiar with this illness.

As ME/CFS symptoms cut across a whole range of medical boundaries (virology, infectious diseases, immunology, neurology, psychiatry, etc), specialists in a wide range of subjects have become involved in seeing hospital patients. It should now be possible, in most parts of the country, to find at least one specialist who is interested in seeing ME/CFS patients. And it doesn't really matter what sort of -ologist you are referred to – the most important thing is that you are sent to see someone who knows what to do.

Your own doctor may know of a suitable local specialist, but this could mean travelling to the nearest teaching hospital. An alternative source of information in these circumstances can be the members of a local ME Association group. They are often well informed about which local specialists are worth going to see – and who is definitely *not* worth going to see!

NHS specialists don't usually like to see private patients unless they're first referred by their NHS family doctor (GP), so it's always best to ask for a proper referral letter. Unfortunately, some GPs become extremely annoyed when patients go off to see private specialists without their knowledge or 'permission' – and they do have a valid point. Even if a specialist is willing to see you without a referral letter, it is still regarded as unethical if they don't then keep your GP fully informed about their diagnostic opinion or treatment.

If you're really not happy about the way your GP is managing your illness, do think very carefully before going off for other medical opinions without discussion, as this will inevitably place a further strain on your doctor–patient relationship.

In Britain, it is also possible for your GP to refer you to an NHS specialist outside your usual health district. However, many health authorities are starting to strongly discourage or even refuse to fund such referrals. The other problem with requesting an outside referral is that those specialists who are interested in ME/CFS, particularly in London, are becoming so overwhelmed by requests that they're no longer able to offer any appointments.

I believe that ME/CFS is a condition which is ideally managed by a good general practitioner and other members of the primary healthcare team – provided you can find a suitable practice!

## Referral to specialist clinics

A growing number of ME/CFS clinics are now operating within the NHS. Most are situated in university teaching hospitals (the ME Association can supply an up-to-date list) where they are staffed by doctors who are carrying out research into various aspects of the illness. The advantage of being seen in one of these clinics is that you'll be given a very thorough assessment – both physical and mental – on your first visit to make sure the diagnosis is correct. One possible disadvantage is that all the doctors involved may follow one particular line of thought about cause and management of ME/CFS.

A smaller number of NHS clinics are starting to be established in district general hospitals, often as a direct result of a local group of the ME Association putting pressure on the health authority to provide such a service. It can be a long slow process, but it's wroth it in the end. The ME Association normally holds information on where such clinics are currently operating as well as giving advice on how to try and set up this type of service.

Waiting lists tend to be extremely long and it may be difficult to obtain funding if you live outside the clinic's normal catchment area. However, if there is no local specialist available to provide advice on diagnosis or management, it's worth contacting your local community health council (or even your local MP and the media) if the health authority refuses to sanction a referral.

The National ME Centre, based at Harold Wood Hospital in Essex, is the only NHS unit to offer a comprehensive service for both in-patient and out-patient care. Assessment and management involve close co-operation between doctors, occupation therapists and various other health professional. For further information see page 402.

## The private medical sector

There are a growing number of private medical practitioners and clinics who claim to specialise in the treatment of ME/CFS. Some are willing to accept referrals without the knowledge of your own GP, but this is neither ethical nor wise. Although their approaches vary considerably, a great deal of emphasis tends to be placed on identifying and treating allergies (using the sort of techniques described in Chapter 13: Alternative and Complementary Approaches), anti-candida regimes and dietary modification. A few are much more orientated towards current psychiatric theories and concentrate on behaviour modification techniques.

Some of the treatments available in the private sector have come in for well deserved criticism and few have been subjected to good clinical trials to assess their value. Remember, there are no tests available in the private sector that can diagnose ME/CFS, and if you decide to be treated outside the NHS, do take advice from your own GP first, and try to find out how much consultations and treatments will cost before making a firm commitment. Unfortunately, there is no doubt that anyone with time and money will eventually find a private doctor who will diagnose and treat their ME/CFS.

## Uninterested doctors

What can you do if your general practitioner isn't sympathetic towards ME/CFS, and can't accept that you feel as ghastly as you claim?

Your doctor may well be one of those who just isn't interested in chronic illnesses, where there's very little that can be done to alleviate symptoms or change the course of the disease by writing out something on the prescription pad. Alternatively, they may not like talking to patients for more than 10 minutes, and may consider that emotional or social problems are not there to be dealt with by the medical profession.

If your doctor fits into this category, with an attitude that doesn't change, then there's probably no other option but to try and find someone else. If you belong to a group practice, it should be quite easy to see another partner, and you may not have to actually change to their individual list. Any good practice should have a flexible policy for patients who find they don't have any rapport with one doctor and want to see another member of the team.

Alternatively, you might try the practice 'trainee' if there is one – a good sign that the practice has come up to standard when it was selected for such a purpose. Trainee general practitioners – sometimes called GP Registrars – have already spent several years in hospital medicine, but are now intending to enter general practice. They work for an introductory year under the supervision of one of the senior partners in the practice. Trainees have more time to devote to individual patients and are encouraged to take on unusual or 'difficult' conditions, even writing them up as part of their examination. Unfortunately, trainees are only usually in post for a period of one year and seldom progress to a job in the same practice, so this isn't a long-term solution.

As a last resort you may have to consider finding another GP altogether. Try and find out from friends and neighbours (or other people with ME/CFS) about local doctors, and ask if the one you choose is prepared to take you on to the list. Your local Community Health Council or FHSA can help you further with the technical details of how to change.

In Britain, it's worth remembering that GPs are paid on a capitation fee system – about £20 every year for each patient on the list, no matter how many consultations you request – so there's no great incentive to encourage people with chronic illnesses to join up! And, as many people with ME/CFS are all too well aware, most doctors tend to be very wary of patients who 'swap' doctors in the same area and may view you as a potential problem. Also, practices have fairly well-defined geographical limits on who they're prepared to take on, so outside large towns such action may be practically very difficult or even impossible.

If you do decide to change doctor, try not to leave it to your Family Health Service Authority (FHSA) to allocate a new practice. This really is the last resort and a very bad start to any new doctor–patient relationship. No doctor likes having patients allocated to them by an anonymous administrator.

The final option is to opt out of the NHS altogether and go privately, but do take advice and think very carefully about who you go and see, or you could end up spending a lot of money on unnecessary drugs and investigations, along with some very poor advice. In many large towns there are a few purely private general practitioners, but you're not supposed to remain on an NHS practitioner's list at the same time. A private GP, although being able to spend more time with you, may not know any more about ME/CFS than your NHS one.

There aren't any easy answers about how to establish a good doctor–patient relationship; a lot depends on pure luck and where you happen to live. At the end of the day it's like any relationship – some doctors just don't hit it off with some of their patients and vice versa. You've really got to treat it like a marriage – if both partners don't contribute, it won't work.

# Some of your 'Rights' from the NHS

Patients don't have many rights when it comes to the NHS – just reasonable requests. Here is a summary of the most important ones:

## General practitioners

Everyone is entitled to join a GP's practice. You can choose from any local NHS general practitioner, provided they are willing to accept you. Some GPs even allow prospective patients to come and have a chat before joining their list to see if both parties are going to be suited! Lists of all local GPs can be found in main post offices, libraries, the local family health service authority (FHSA) or a citizens' advice bureau. All GPs should now be producing a leaflet giving details of their staff, hours of clinics and other services which are provided.

During normal working hours you have a 'right' to be seen by a GP in the practice, but not necessarily your own. If the practice runs an appointment system, you should be given a space as soon as possible, provided the delay isn't harmful.

Patients do not have a 'right' to demand a visit at home from a GP. This depends on the doctor's individual judgement as to whether it is necessary. Doctors are becoming increasingly reluctant to do home visiting for the chronic sick, and prefer patients to visit the surgery whenever possible. However, your GP is obliged, under the NHS contract, to come out and visit in any true emergency.

If you're temporarily away from home, you can visit one of the local GPs and be seen as a temporary resident. This shouldn't cause any problems as it attracts an extra fee!

When you move to another area (or if you become unhappy with your present GP), it should be quite easy to change to another doctor or practice, and you don't have to give any reason for doing so. Ask the new GP if you can be accepted on their list and send your medical card to the FHSA. Equally, it's also possible for GPs to remove patients from their list without giving any reason, although few doctors would do this just because of a chronic illness. The usual reason is a breakdown due to a clash of personalities, or disagreements over treatment. In this case the FHSA must find you another doctor.

## Drugs

As far as drugs are concerned, you can't demand to have a new treatment which you may have heard about, but which your GP isn't yet aware of. Doctors are quite rightly reluctant to start prescribing new drugs until their benefits are proven and any long-term side-effects fully established. If your GP is unfamiliar with the use of a drug such as the gammaglobulin injections or magnesium, they will probably want to discuss this with a specialist before giving it. It seems that expensive legal actions against doctors for side-effects from drugs they've prescribed are going to become increasingly common, so this type of cautious approach is inevitable.

## Hospital treatment

Once again, you don't have any 'right' to a second opinion from a specialist, but it would be unreasonable if a GP were to refuse such a request when there were doubts about either the diagnosis or how the illness should be managed. Under the NHS, you can't choose which specialist you want to be referred to, but there's nothing to stop you suggesting a particular name if you've heard that this consultant is sympathetic to or interested in ME/CFS.

If you are admitted to hospital, you can discharge yourself at any time if you are unhappy with either the treatment or the investigations being carried out. Obviously, this will cause a great deal of upset and won't make you very popular with either the hospital or your GP. The ward staff will almost certainly make you sign a form to say that you left hospital against medical advice. However, this doesn't necessarily relieve them of legal liability if anything goes wrong following such treatment.

You can only be detained in hospital against your will if the doctors decide to use powers granted under the Mental Health Act. This is really only relevant to severe psychiatric illness and does contain an appeal procedure. The best organisation to provide further help in this area is MIND (see Useful Addresses, page 424).

## Consenting to treatment and investigations

All patients should fully understand what their treatment and tests entail before they commence. If you end up being treated or examined without such consent it could, in legal terms, be regarded as assault. This is particularly important where doctors are using treatment regimes which are unproven or as part of clinical trials for new drugs.

In theory, you are free to decide whether or not to accept any particular treatment option, but as we all know different specialists take opposing views as to which is the best way to manage people with ME/CFS. I have no doubt that some people are being pressurised into following advice which they are not happy about and may well be doing them harm.

It's essential that when a specialist wants to involve you in any unusual or risky new treatment/investigation that all possible hazards are fully explained first. Otherwise, doctors could be laying themselves open to legal action if something goes wrong. All large hospitals should now have an ethical committee whose purpose is to examine and approve research projects and clinical trials looking at possible new forms of treatment. For more information contact your local Community Health Council and ask for their leaflet: *Making Choices: Finding Out about your Illness and Consenting to Treatment.*

In large teaching hospitals it's quite likely that you'll be examined by medical students. Most patients are only too happy to co-operate in this learning process, but if you'd rather not, then do tell the consultant.

## Access to medical records

From November 1991 all patients were given the right to inspect their medical records under the 1990 Health Records Act. You also have a previous right under the 1984 Data Protection Act to inspect any health records which are held on computer.

Although far from perfect, this legislation does give patients the opportunity to check what has been written about them by GPs and specialists. In theory, it also provides a means of correcting any inaccuracies. Unfortunately, one of the loopholes in the Act is that the holder of the records does not have to clearly state that part of the information has been withheld, so you may never even know what's been left out!

The Act covers information held by both the NHS and private sectors, except for Northern Ireland, which is covered by a separate law. In theory, you can inspect anything that has been written about you by a doctor, dentist, optician or clinical psychologist. You only have legal access to information recorded after 1 November 1991; before that you will have to rely on the doctor's willingness to comply.

If you wish to make use of the Act, you should apply in writing to your GP, or to the local health authority (health board in Scotland) in the case of NHS hospitals. With 'trust' and private hospitals, you should apply directly.

After this you should be given access to your medical records within 40 days. It is also permissible to ask someone else to look at your notes or for you to take photocopies. If you notice any mistakes, you can ask for them to be corrected. If the holder (doctor or hospital) disagrees with this request, a note of your views should still be recorded.

Access can only be refused on three grounds: where it will cause *serious harm* to your mental or physical health; where it comprises a third party, such as a relative; and where the information was recorded before 1 November 1991.

If you have difficulties in persuading your doctor or hospital to comply, contact your local Community Health Council. There is also a right of appeal to the courts if access is refused; but it may be possible to pursue such a dispute by using established hospital complaints procedures.

If your GP writes a medical report to your employer or an insurance company, you also have a right to see this before it is passed on – unless the doctor decides the information could be harmful. If necessary, you can refuse to let your employer or insurer see this report and may even add your own comments.

## Medical confidentiality

Doctors should never pass on medical information without your permission. The only exceptions are to other health professionals involved in your treatment and in certain circumstances your close relatives. If you don't want a doctor to discuss your condition with a spouse or partner, do make sure that this fact is clearly written down in your medical notes. For more information ask your local Community Health Council for their leaflet *On the Record: Confidentiality and Medical Notes*.

# How to Complain about Services and Treatment Provided by the NHS

First of all you need to decide whether you want (a) an internal investigation aimed at producing an apology or explanation; (b) disciplinary action taken against the doctor concerned; or (c) financial compensation for what has gone wrong. All of these options require a different course of action.

## Local internal investigation

Complaints about GPs or consultants need to be made as soon as possible after the event. Direct contact with the doctor concerned, followed by a discussion about what has happened and what you want done, may well clear the air and lead to a satisfactory resolution of the complaint.

The alternative course, especially if the complaint is of a more serious nature, is to send in a formal written complaint (make sure you keep a copy) to the complaints manager at the relevant hospital trust or health authority (in the case of a GP). Before doing so, ask for a copy of their local complaints procedure leaflet, which should provide clear instructions about procedures and all the information which you need to supply. Your local Community Health Council (see the phone book or Useful Addresses under 'Health Information') can offer detailed advice on dealing with health service complaints, help you draft a letter and send a representative to accompany you to any meetings at which the complaint is then discussed.

A local complaints procedure involves officials examining your medical records and (possibly) arranging a meeting to discuss the complaint in more detail. A lay conciliator might be appointed to discuss the matter with everyone involved. You should receive a written report within 20 working days.

If you're not satisfied, you can then request an independent review panel to look at the complaint, but this must be done within 28 days of you receiving the results of the internal investigation. If the hospital or health authority agrees, a review panel will then examine all the relevant paperwork. Once again, you might be interviewed or asked to meet or all of the parties concerned. An independent review should be completed within three months; you'll then be sent a copy of the draft report to comment on. If you're not satisfied, you still have the option of contacting the General Medical Council, taking legal action or asking the Health Service Commissioner (Ombudsman) to investigate.

Appeals to the Ombudsman (see Useful Addresses, page 399), who is completely independent of the NHS and government, must be made within a fixed time limit. If the Ombudsman agrees to investigate, this will involve an extremely thorough review of all aspects of the case. The Ombudsman currently upholds around 60 per cent of complaints which are investigated, but the process may take around a year to complete.

## Disciplinary action

You can complain to the General Medical Council (see page 418) if you believe that a doctor has behaved unethically or unprofessionally. Doctors found guilty of serious professional misconduct can be removed from the register or suspended from practising. Again, it's worth contacting the General Medical Council for an information booklet before making a formal written complaint.

## Legal action

This is the route to follow if you are seeking some form of financial compensation. However, if the hospital or health authority feels that you have a good case, it's possible that they will try to settle out of court by awarding an 'ex-gratia' compensation payment. Do obtain good advice from a lawyer who's accustomed to dealing with medical negligence cases. Action for Victims of Medical Accidents (see Useful Addresses, page 422) should be able to put you in touch with a suitable expert. Legal aid might be available on the Green Form scheme if you're on a low income.

# Insurance Problems

With an increasing number of claims now being submitted, ME/CFS is starting to cause concern amongst the insurance companies. There are six types of policy in which problems may arise, and where you may need help or advice from your doctor.

## Motor vehicle insurance

Most policies now ask very careful questions about any illness or disability which could impair one's ability to drive. Obviously, the fact that you have ME/CFS cannot be ignored when filling in such a form, and failure to disclose this information could result in problems if an accident occurs – even if it is not your fault. The fact that you have ME/CFS may result in the insurer requesting a medical opinion from your GP on your fitness to drive or asking you to report your circumstances to the medical department at the DVLC in Swansea.

## Life insurance

This is one piece of important financial planning that should not cause any great difficulty. I am not aware that any of the reputable major insurance companies are refusing life cover on the grounds of ME/CFS, although the cost of the policy might be slightly loaded and a medical examination requested if the cover is high. ME/CFS is not a life-threatening condition, although for the small minority who have persisting heart problems following an initial myocarditis, the insurers are likely to be far more cautious (see also pages 121–2).

## Permanent health insurance (PHI)

This type of policy pays out a regular monthly income as long as the policyholder is unfit for work. Because of the high cost of premiums, most PHI policies tend to come into operation after several months of ill health, often when sick pay from an employer has been terminated or reduced.

As long as your GP is willing to issue DSS sick notes confirming that you are 'unfit for work', there shouldn't be any difficulties. However, problems will arise if the DSS stops incapacity benefit or recommends that you are now fit to resume 'suitable alternative work'. In the latter case the policy may be such that it will 'top up' any loss of earnings as a result of switching to lower paid employment or part-time work. When a PHI claim continues for a prolonged period of time the insurer may well ask for an independent medical examination. For details on how to deal with disputes involving PHI policies see pages 234–7.

## Permanent disablement insurance

This type of policy pays out a lump sum or a regular monthly income when the company is fully satisfied that the claimant is *fully and permanently* disabled. In the case of ME/CFS, permanent disablement is not always easy to define, especially in the early stages of the illness when the outcome is very unpredictable. Also, it is not unknown for some degree of recovery to occur even after a prolonged period of ill health. So, in view of the large sums of money often involved, insurers are unlikely to settle unless they are fully satisfied that there is no real chance of recovery taking place. In practice, this almost certainly means that several years of ill health will have to occur before a settlement is reached. It is also quite likely that the insurer will require a specialist medical examination, and this may not always be carried out by a doctor who views the condition favourably. For more information on issues relating to permanency and prognosis see pages 118–121.

## Private medical insurance

Once again, some of the insurers specialising in this type of cover are becoming concerned about the very high cost of investigations and speculative treatments being advocated by private doctors and clinics who claim to treat ME/CFS. I know of one private hospital where bills running into several thousand pounds are not unknown. Some of these insurers are already making it clear that they will no longer reimburse high charges for an ongoing illness like ME/CFS over an indefinite period. So, if you are embarking on expensive private care using insurance cover, it may be wise to check with the company before doing so. It is also possible to purchase private health insurance which covers several types of alternative therapies.

## Travel insurance

Policies which provide medical cover for travel abroad shouldn't cause any problems providing you are *not travelling against medical advice*. However, it's always a good idea to check the small print on any package holiday cover well before departure.

When problems with insurance companies arise with a claim relating to ME/CFS, do make sure that you keep copies of all correspondence with the official involved. If you're not making satisfactory progress, then write to either the Chief General Manager or the Chief Medical Officer and send your letter by recorded delivery. As a last resort you can ask the Insurance Ombudsman (see Useful Addresses, page 421) to intervene.

## Miscellaneous Problems

### *Jury service*

This could involve a very unpredictable amount of time in court and would obviously required periods of sustained concentration, making it a most unsuitable task for anyone with ME/CFS. If you are still unwell and receive such a request to report for jury service, you should write to the court and state that you have ME/CFS. You should also explain that this causes severe problems with any kind of intense or prolonged concentration as well as short-term memory loss. It's highly likely that the court will accept this explanation and not pursue the request. In the unlikely event of the court not accepting your word, it will then be necessary to ask your GP to write out a certificate stating that you are not fit for jury service. This may involve payment of a small fee.

## Further Information on Health and Health Services

A variety of national organisations – the College of Health, community health councils, the NHS Health Information Service, the Patients Association – provide advice and information on all aspects of health care and services which should be available on the NHS. Assistance is also available to anyone involved in disputes with doctors or health authorities. For further details see under 'Health Information' in Useful Addresses.

The 1998 National Task Force report on services for patients with ME/CFS is available from Westcare (see Useful Addresses, page 403).

# Drug Treatments

Although a growing number of drugs are now under investigation, no form of generally effective treatment or cure for ME/CFS has yet been found.

Thirteen drug treatments have now been subjected to properly controlled clinical trials, where volunteers are given either the active treatment under investigation or a placebo (dummy) treatment. Most of these studies have only involved small numbers of patients, and few have been replicated by more than one research group, so the results – positive or negative – *all need to be viewed with a considerable degree of caution.*

Positive results have been reported from trials involving Ampligen, evening primrose oil (Efamol Marine), magnesium sulphate injections, moclobemide (Manerix) and phenelzine (Nardil).

No advantage has been reported from the use of acyclovir, fludrocortisone, fluoxetine (Prozac), hydrocortisone, terfenadine (Triludan), transfer factor and injections of vitamin $B_{12}$.

Conflicting results have been reported from trials involving amantadine and immunoglobulin injections.

At present, there is no orthodox drug treatment which is going to help all the symptoms of ME/CFS. Even so, there are a number of drugs which may be worth trying in certain circumstances as well as others that can be effective in relieving specific symptoms such as pain or sleep disturbances.

Whatever drug is used, it's important to remember that people with ME/CFS seem to be unduly sensitive to a wide range of medications which are either prescribed by a doctor or purchased over the counter. Consequently, it may sometimes be advisable to start with a very low dose (sometimes less than is actually recommended by the manufacturer in their data sheet) and then *gradually increase* this over a period of time.

## Allergy Treatments and Antihistamines

The controversial subject of allergies, their possible role in ME/CFS, the methods of diagnosis and different approaches to management are all covered in more detail on pages 255–60.

## Terfenadine (Triludan)

This antihistamine is the only anti-allergy drug to be properly assessed in ME/CFS. A small American study concluded that this drug was *not* of any benefit (reference 403). Terfenadine also has a number of side-effects (including heart rhythm disturbances), so is probably best avoided by anyone with ME/CFS who requires an antihistamine preparation to relieve allergic symptoms associated with hayfever, etc.

## Histamine (H₂) receptor antagonists

These include drugs such as cimetidine and ranitidine. Although principally used in the management of stomach ulcers, they have also been given as a possible treatment for glandular fever (Epstein-Barr virus) and shingles (herpes zoster).

Experimental studies suggest that a number of important aspects of normal immune function are suppressed by histamine, and this is one explanation why these type of antihistamines could have a role in ME/CFS. Unfortunately, no properly controlled trials have been carried out to prove or disprove this hypothesis.

# Amphetamines

Drugs in this group, which act as powerful stimulants on the central nervous system, are occasionally prescribed for people with ME/CFS. Although they may well produce a temporary increase in energy levels and feelings of well-being, there is a very high risk of addiction occurring. Amphetamines also have a number of potentially serious side-effects. *I believe their use in ME/CFS is most undesirable.*

# Antidepressants

These can undoubtedly be of considerable value when ME/CFS is accompanied by true clinical depression. In addition, a small dose of one of the more sedating tricyclic antidepressants (e.g. amitriptyline 10–25mg or doxepin 10mg at night) can sometimes be helpful in relieving muscle pain and/or insomnia. Otherwise, the use of antidepressants in ME/CFS is highly debatable, as many people are particularly susceptible to their side-effects.

Very few placebo-controlled trials have been carried out to assess the true value of antidepressants in ME/CFS. One such study involving fluoxetine (Prozac) found no benefit whatsoever in patients with or without a depressive component (reference 407).

Three trials have been carried out to assess the value of drugs belonging to a group known as MAOIs. A small open study using moclobemide (Manerix) found a minor reduction in the levels of fatigue and anxiety (reference 410) and limited benefit was reported from a large placebo-controlled study carried out in Australia (reference 388). Some improvement was also noted in a small study involving phenelzine (Nardil), which was carried out in America (reference 394).

It has also been suggested that venlafaxine (Efexor) can produce benefits by reversing immunological disturbances involving natural killer cell activity in ME/CFS (reference 386).

(For a more comprehensive review of antidepressant drugs and their use in ME/CFS see pages 233–241.)

# Antiviral Drugs

In Chapter 8 I reviewed the conflicting scientific evidence surrounding a possible role for *persisting* viral infection in ME/CFS. Despite all these uncertainties, a number of antiviral drugs have been used in American treatment trials.

## Acyclovir

This is an antiviral drug which is extremely active against some forms of herpes virus infections, particularly severe cases of chicken-pox and persistent cold sores. It was assessed in a small study at a time when many American doctors believed that glandular fever (Epstein-Barr) virus could be the cause of some cases of ME/CFS. In a placebo-controlled trial, 46 per cent of those receiving acyclovir reported benefits compared to 41 per cent in the placebo group (reference 404). Despite the fact that reactivation of herpes viruses has been linked to ME/CFS in more recent research, no further studies have been carried out using this drug.

## Amantadine (Symmetrel)

This is a drug which is principally used in the treatment of Parkinson's disease. It also has some antiviral activity, particularly against influenza A virus. Suggestions that it could help to relieve the fatigue associated with multiple sclerosis – which can be similar to that found in ME/CFS – have led to some doctors using it on their ME/CFS patients. Most of the claims for benefit are purely anecdotal, but a small placebo-controlled study from America found substantial improvements in symptoms, particularly fatigue (reference 380). The most frequently reported side-effects included vivid dreams and sleeplessness. However, another American study concluded that amantadine was *'ineffective and poorly tolerated'* (references 396 and 397).

Amantadine has a number of other disturbing side-effects, including depression, tremor and fluid retention. This is a drug which is certainly worthy of further investigation, but its effects may be more to do with the way it enhances dopamine (a chemical transmitter in the brain) activity rather than any antiviral action.

## Ganciclovir

This is a new antiviral drug which is mainly being used to treat cytomegalovirus (CMV) infection in people with AIDS. An American research group used ganciclovir in a small subgroup of ME/CFS patients who all had raised levels of antibodies against CMV infection and abnormalities on their electrocardiograms (heart rhythm tracings). Before being treated with ganciclovir, none of the 18 patients involved could work or carry out household duties. After 24 weeks treatment, 13 returned to their previous level of health. No side-effects were reported (reference 390).

Ganciclovir could turn out to be useful in *carefully selected cases where there is reliable evidence of CMV infection*.

## Kutapressin

This is a substance obtained from pig liver which is claimed to have antiviral effects on herpes viruses. It is mainly used in America and described in more detail on page 286.

At present, there are no antiviral drugs available for human use which have proven effects on enteroviral infections although one product, disoxaril, has been used in animal studies involving persistent enteroviral infection in the nervous system.

# Beta-blockers

These are a group of drugs which are mainly used to treat heart conditions (e.g. high blood pressure, angina, rhythm disturbances), migraine and symptoms of anxiety. Beta-blockers act by reducing the heart rate, so they are quite often used to treat palpitations. It's for this reason that one of the group might be prescribed to someone with ME/CFS.

All beta-blockers need to be used with care in ME/CFS as they have a number of potential side-effects. These include cold hands and feet, sleep disturbances and vivid dreams, fatigue, depression, confusion and dizziness. Some of these side-effects can be minimised by careful choice of which beta-blocker is prescribed. For example, lipid-soluble drugs (which dissolve in body fat and so enter the brain more easily) such as propranolol, metoprolol and oxprenolol are more likely to cause sleep disturbances and fatigue. Water-soluble drugs such as atenolol, nadolol and sotalol (which are less likely to enter the brain) are probably a better choice for someone with ME/CFS.

There are very few indications for using beta-blockers in ME/CFS apart from palpitations and anxiety which fails to respond to other types of medication. If your doctor does decide to prescribe a beta-blocker, make sure this is done with careful consideration of the potential side-effects.

## Calcium Antagonists

Muscle pain (myalgia) occurs in around 75 per cent of people with ME/CFS, sometimes quite severely. Mild to moderate painkillers tend to be ineffective, as do the newer types of non-steroidal anti-inflammatory drugs (NSAIDs). Two reports in the medical literature from the UK suggest that some cases of *muscle pain brought on by exertion* may be helped by the use of drugs which affect the way that calcium ions move across the muscle cell membrane and influence mitochondrial activity (see pages 138–140). The calcium antagonist used in both these studies was verapamil, another drug which may be worth trying when muscle pain fails to respond to any other form of treatment (references 389 and 409).

In America, the use of calcium antagonists has become quite popular, especially for the management of problems with mental functioning. Some American physicians prescribe nimodipine (reference 372), but this drug is normally only used in the UK for the treatment of neurological problems following a brain haemorrhage.

No properly controlled clinical trials have been carried out to validate the alleged benefits of calcium antagonists in ME/CFS, and until they have *these drugs should be used with caution*, as one of their principal actions is to cause a fall in blood pressure.

## Essential Fatty Acids (EFAs)

The two main EFAs in our diet are linoleic acid and alpha-linolenic acid. In order to become active inside the body they have to be converted into other acids, including gamma-linolenic acid (GLA) and eicosapentaenoic acid (EPA), along with various prostaglandins (chemicals responsible for inflammation) and cytokines (immune system chemicals). Viral infections have been shown to cause EFA deficiencies, possibly by blocking this conversion process. Any consequent deficiency of EFAs could well lead to problems at a cellular level in a variety of chronic illness.

To date, the only published study on the use of EFA supplementation in ME/CFS involved 63 patients who received either a placebo or capsules of Efamol Marine – a combination of 80 per cent evening primrose oil (as a source of GLA) and 20 per cent fish oil (as a source of EPA). The patients took eight capsules per day of either the active treatment or the dummy capsules. After three months assessment, 85 per cent taking Efamol Marine rated themselves better compared to only 17 per cent taking the placebo. Levels of fatty acids in the blood, which had been significantly reduced at the beginning, returned towards normal in those receiving Efamol Marine (reference 376).

This is clearly one form of treatment which is both safe and worth trying for a couple of months.

## Galanthamine Hydrobromide

One of the most significant research findings in the area of brain chemical transmitter disturbances in ME/CFS involves acetylcholine, a chemical which helps to regulate a wide range of body functions, including sleep patterns, mental activity, heart rate, blood pressure, and muscle movement (see also page 153–4).

Clinical trials are now underway in several UK hospitals to assess the possible value of a drug called galanthamine hydrobromide, which is obtained from a species of snowdrop (*Galanthus nivalis*). Galanthamine acts by inhibiting an enzyme called acetylcholinesterase (which normally helps to remove acetylcholine from the nervous system), and so helps to increase the level of acetylcholine.

A small trial into the use of galanthamine (reference 402) found that 33 out of 43 patients taking this drug reported a significant decrease in fatigue and muscle pain. Improvement in sleep patterns was one of the most striking observations and in some cases the overall benefits were described as being 'dramatic'. Only one patient in the placebo treated group showed any real improvement. The main side-effects associated with galanthamine were nausea, headaches, dizziness and a mild skin rash.

There are several possible explanations as to why galanthamine might be effective in ME/CFS. First is the way in which it has pain-relieving properties, possibly by increasing the release of brain chemicals called endorphins (the body's own naturally produced painkillers). Secondly, by increasing the release of cortisol releasing hormone by the hypothalamus it stimulates the adrenal glands to produce more cortisol (see pages 149–50). Thirdly, it reverses some of the abnormal sleep patterns that are commonly found in ME/CFS.

# Hormones

In Chapter 8 I discussed how a number of studies have shown lowered levels of key body hormones including cortisol, growth hormone and oestradiol. These findings have led some doctors to speculate that treatment with various types of hormone replacement could be beneficial.

## Cortisol

The most significant deficiency so far described involves cortisol – a stress hormone produced by the adrenal glands. Very low levels of cortisol are found in a condition known as Addison's disease, which has a number of similar symptoms to that found in ME/CFS. Addison's disease requires life-long treatment with hydrocortisone, and a number of research groups in both the UK and USA are now assessing the possible benefits of using low doses of hydrocortisone in people with ME/CFS who are known to have a mild form of cortisol deficiency (see also pages 149–50). Early results suggest minor benefits along with potentially dangerous suppression of the body's natural cortisol output (reference 544).

Liquorice has been reported as being another way of increasing levels of cortisol. Dr Richard Baschetti, writing about his own personal experiences, claimed that a significant degree of improvement occurred after taking liquorice dissolved in milk (reference 374). As with other plant-based medicines, excessive doses can produce side-effects. More serious ones include worsening of depression, increasing blood pressure and lowered levels of potassium.

It is generally agreed that *high* doses of steroids should *not* be used as a treatment for ME/CFS. These drugs can cause a marked depression of the body's immune system responses and serious long-term side-effects.

## DHEA (dehydroepiandrosterone)

This is another adrenal gland hormone which is widely available in the UK and USA without the need for a doctor's prescription. Claims have been made that it can build up muscle mass, strengthen the immune system and even prevent the natural process of growing old!

The only research looking at levels of DHEA in people with chronic fatigue found this hormone to be raised (reference 384), so increasing the level still further seems unwise and unnecessary. Interestingly, treatment with steroids (either prenisolone or dexamethasone) resulted in reduced levels of fatigue in the small group of patients.

As far as side-effects of DHEA are concerned, there are disturbing reports of liver inflammation occurring, but what is far more worrying is the way in which large doses of DHEA are converted into masculinising hormones such as testosterone. This raises the possibility that chronic inappropriate use of DHEA could lead to an increased risk of ovarian or prostatic cancer. An editorial in the *American Journal of Medicine* (reference 401) pointed out that *'It would be unwise for people younger than 30 years to take DHEA because the supplement might suppress the body's natural production of the hormone'*, and then went on to warn about the lack of satisfactory regulation over potency and purity of commercial supplements containing DHEA.

My view is that *DHEA should not be used as a treatment for ME/CFS* until properly controlled trials have been carried out to assess any possible benefits, and until concerns over long-term safety have been resolved.

## Fludrocortisone

This another important adrenal hormone concerned with maintaining normal levels of body salts. Fludrocortisone is also used in the treatment of Addison's disease to help raise lowered blood pressure. Studies in ME/CFS indicate that there may be a subgroup of patients with low blood pressure and symptoms such as fainting episodes and feeling dizzy when standing up (see pages 144–45), reference 379. The only placebo-controlled trial involving fludrocortisone found no significant benefits (reference 534).

## Sex hormones

A small research study reported in *The Lancet* (reference 406) found that a group of women with ME/CFS, especially those who noticed a pre-menstrual exacerbation of symptoms or improvement during pregnancy (when oestrogen levels start to increase), had lowered levels of the sex hormone oestrogen. This finding suggests that chronic oestrogen deficiency may be a factor in some cases of women who develop ME/CFS (see also pages 29–30).

Significant improvement was reported in 80 per cent of this group when they were treated with oestrogen skin patches (200 microgram dose) and cyclical progesterone. Unfortunately, no other research studies have looked at levels of oestrogen and progesterone in women with ME/CFS.

(For information on the use of the contraceptive pill and menopausal hormone replacement therapy in ME/CFS see pages 68–69.)

## Thyroxine

Conventional medical opinion has always believed that anyone with normal thyroid function tests (see page 167) shouldn't have any symptoms of thyroid gland disease. This position has recently been challenged by a group of doctors who feel that some people (not necessarily those with a diagnosis of ME/CFS) have a problem with their thyroid gland, yet still have perfectly normal laboratory results when the function is assessed using standard blood tests (reference 400).

No proper research has yet been carried out into this particular aspect of hormonal control in ME/CFS, so it is difficult to say whether thyroid dysfunction is more common than in the normal population. My feeling is that there is no real difference, and that in the absence of such evidence it is *unwise and potentially quite dangerous* for doctors to pre-scribe thyroxine supplements as a possible treatment. Too much thy-roxine in the blood can lead to serious side-effects, including fatal heart rhythm disturbances in anyone who has a pre-existing heart complaint. Long-term inappropriate use of thyroxine will cause a further increase in the risk of developing osteoporosis (brittle bone disease). It could also lead to a permanent disruption to the complex hormonal feedback mech-anisms acting on the hypothalamus (the gland in the brain which con-trols the output of all body hormones).

Thyroid supplementation must always be administered with great care to anyone with evidence of cortisol deficiency (as can occur in ME/CFS) as the adrenal gland may not be able to cope with the result-ing increase in the body's metabolic activities.

## Immunotherapy

A wide variety of speculative treatments aimed at correcting distur-bances in the body's immune system response in ME/CFS have been assessed in clinical trials carried out in America, Australia and the UK. Most of these drugs are costly, of limited availability outside research centres and may involve unpleasant side-effects. The results from a small number of treatment trials so far carried out are not very impressive. At the moment I would not recommend this particular approach to treat-ment unless it is being supervised by a reputable specialist (preferably in immunology or infectious diseases) who has a good working knowl-edge of the immune system abnormalities so far reported in ME/CFS (see pages 129–136).

There appears to be no advantage in using plasma exchange (a method for removing immune complexes from the blood), thymic hor-mone (as a way of stimulating T lymphocyte production) or inosine pra-nobex/Imunovir (a drug with antiviral actions as well). High doses of oral steroids (e.g. prednisolone), plus or minus other powerful drugs which depress the immune system (e.g. azathioprine), have not been found to be helpful in a small uncontrolled trial (reference 377).

## Ampligen (mismatched doubled-stranded RNA)

This is an experimental drug, developed in America from a compound which was originally used in the treatment of cancer. It is claimed to have antiviral activity as well as being capable of altering the body's immune response by stimulating cellular defence mechanisms and inducing the production of interferon. If the immune system is already down-regulated (under performing), then Ampligen is claimed to be able to up-regulate the response (hence its possible value in the treatment of conditions like AIDS). If the immune system is already in a state of up-regulation (being overactive), as may be the case in ME/CFS, then Ampligen is claimed to down-regulate the response.

The possibility that Ampligen could be useful in ME/CFS is currently being assessed in America, Belgium and Canada. Issues relating to cost (over £10,000 for one year's supply), effectiveness and safety profile mean that Ampligen is unlikely to become available in the UK till properly controlled clinical trials have firmly established that this is a safe and effective form of treatment.

Results from a double-blind, placebo-controlled trial involving 92 American patients with ME/CFS were published in 1994 (reference 405). After 24 weeks' treatment, those receiving Ampligen had a significant increase in their Karnofsky performance scores (a disability rating scale similar to the one on page 117) along with improved exercise tolerance and a decrease in problems with memory and concentration. Treatment with Ampligen was also reported to have reversed abnormalities in the 2–5A synthase/RNase L antiviral pathway (see page 156). What remains uncertain is the percentage of patients who then maintained their positive progress without any further treatment with Ampligen.

As with any new experimental drug (especially one as unique as this), concerns have rightly been expressed about both short-term and long-term adverse effects. The experience so far suggests that Ampligen is reasonably well tolerated, and that the main short-term side-effects are limited to dizziness, skin rashes, fever and mild disturbances in liver function. No serious long-term adverse effects have been reported from patients involved in the clinical trials of Ampligen. However, the theoretical risk that this drug could interfere with cellular genetic material (DNA) means that extremely careful follow-up studies need to be carried out over a prolonged period of time to ensure that Ampligen is perfectly safe.

Ampligen is produced in America by:

Hemispherx Biopharma Inc.

1 Penn Centre 660

1617 JFK Boulevard

Philadelphia, PA 19103
USA
Tel: (USA) 215 988 0080
Fax: (USA) 215 988 1739
Internet information on Ampligen is available from:
HEMISPHERx BIOPHARMA INC
*Homepage*: http://www.hemispherx.com/
*Ampligen and CFS*: http://www.cais.net/cfs-news/ampligen.htm

## Immunoglobulin

Immunoglobulin (IgG) is a form of immunotherapy which has been used in several different disorders where there are clear disturbances in the body's immune system response. In the case of ME/CFS it is possible that immunoglobulin acts by helping to neutralise a persisting viral presence or by correcting a subtle defect in the immune system.

A number of doctors in the UK and Australia give injections containing small amounts (dose = 750mg) of human gammaglobulin (the same as used for protection against hepatitis A infection) into the muscle. Doctors who recommend this form of treatment claim that patients who respond often show an exacerbation of symptoms after about five days, followed by an improvement lasting for three to six weeks. Further injections are then spaced close enough together to prevent a further relapse by the time of reinjection. Unfortunately, no properly controlled trials have ever been published on the use of intramuscular immunoglobulin.

My own feedback is that a minority of users do gain benefit and sometimes this is quite significant. However, others feel worse after these injections. A double-blind placebo-controlled trial would clearly help to resolve the uncertainty over this controversial form of treatment.

In 1990, the *American Journal of Medicine* published the results of two separate trials which both used high doses of immunoglobulin G given directly into a vein. The results were conflicting. Dr Andrew Lloyd's Australian trial (reference 391) involved 49 patients who were given three monthly injections (dose = 2g/kg) or a placebo. Improvement in physical, psychological and immune status occurred in 10 out of 23 being actively treated compared to only three out of 26 in the placebo group. Dr Dan Peterson's American trial (reference 395) involved 30 adults who were given six injections monthly (dose = 1g/kg) of either immunoglobulin or placebo. About 25 per cent in each group reported some improvement.

A further study from Dr Andrew Lloyd's group was reported in 1997 (reference 408). This study involved 99 patients in a randomised placebo-controlled trial. They received either intravenous immunoglobulin (at doses of either 0.5, 1 or 2g/kg) or placebo (1% albumin) at monthly intervals for three months. None of the above doses were found to be of any more benefit than the placebo and adverse reactions were reported by over 70 per cent of those receiving immunoglobulin. These included headaches, worsening fatigue, malaise, problems with concentration and disturbances in liver function. The research group concluded that *this form of treatment cannot, at present, be recommended to people with ME/CFS.*

The only double-blind trial involving the use of immunoglobulin in children has also been carried out in Australia. This involved 71 adolescents aged 11–18 years, who were given either 1g/kg of immunoglobulin or a placebo solution. There was a significant degree of improvement in both groups at the six-month follow up. Adverse effects were also quite common in both groups (reference 398).

One of the major problems of using high doses of intravenous immunoglobulin is that it is extremely costly and not without side-effects, although the risk of transmitting viruses such as hepatitis C is unlikely. Before administration, checks should be made for IgA antibody deficiency because this could result in the subsequent development of harmful anti-IgA antibodies. Anyone in this situation will require immunoglobulin with minimal amounts of IgA. Adrenaline and hydrocortisone should also be readily available in case of an allergic reaction.

Despite the conflicting results from properly controlled trials, I still feel that this form of treatment should not be dismissed. It may turn out that a subgroup of people with specific immune system abnormalities are the ones who benefit.

## *Interferon*

This is another costly form of immunotherapy which is currently being assessed in both America and the UK. Results from clinical trials so far reported are once again conflicting. One group of patients given subcutaneous (under the skin) injections of alpha interferon reported exacerbations in myalgia (muscle pain), arthralgia (joint pain) and palpitations, with no long-term benefits (reference 393).

In a second report, interferon alpha was tested on 19 ME/CFS patients at the Royal Free Hospital in London (reference 381). Three megaunits of interferon alpha-2b were again given subcutaneously thrice weekly for three months. Side-effects were reported as minimal, and although the numbers reporting improvement were too small to draw any firm conclusions, the results indicated that further studies on this approach to treatment need to be carried out. The Royal Free researchers felt that the benefits could be due to either the suppression of viral replication or an immunostimulatory effect of interferon.

An American trial, reported in 1996 (reference 399) looked at four separate subgroups of ME/CFS patients and their response to 12 weeks' treatment with interferon alpha-2a (dose = 3 million units three times per week). The only subgroup to show any significant benefit were those with an isolated decrease in their natural killer (NK) cell function.

### Lantinan

This is an immunomodulatory drug which is thought to be able to increase the activity of natural killer (NK) cells (see page 132). One report found it to be an effective form of treatment for a small group of patients (reference 373).

### Transfer factor

This is a type of immune chemical present in white blood cells which can be extracted from a close relative and then transferred to a patient with ME/CFS. In theory, this should then transfer some degree of natural immunity from one person to another, hence the name transfer factor.

The first properly controlled clinical trial of transfer factor was carried out by Dr Andrew Lloyd's team in Australia (reference 392). Ninety patients received either the active treatment or a placebo. After a follow-up period of three months there was no difference between the two groups.

Four further reports from researchers in America, Czechoslovakia and Italy (reference: Biotherapy, 1996, 9, 77–95) have now examined the way in which transfer factor with specific activity against herpes viruses might be of use in ME/CFS.

## Magnesium

Injections of magnesium sulphate remain a highly controversial form of treatment. Although a properly controlled trial, the results of which were published in The Lancet (reference 383), reported both magnesium deficiency and positive responses to treatment with magnesium via injection, most doctors remain unconvinced by these claims. And with several other research groups being unable to demonstrate magnesium deficiency I, too, feel that this is an extremely speculative form of treatment. (For more information on magnesium supplementation see pages 271–3)

## Pain Relief

Muscle pain (myalgia) affects up to 75 per cent of people with ME/CFS. It can become one of the most prominent and distressing symptoms in the whole illness. At first, the pain may just be confined to the shoulders, neck or chest muscles, but later on it can become much more gener-alised. Pain can also involve the tendons (which connect muscles to bones) and the joints themselves (arthralgia). Some people only experience muscle pain and cramp after physical activity, but in a small minority the pain takes on a more severe and intractable quality, result-ing in loss of sleep and reactive depression.

Until we understand more about the mechanisms involved in pain production within both the brain and muscle (where it may be connected to a build up of lactic acid), it seems unlikely that any form of really effec-tive drug treatment will be found. At present, the options to help with pain relief are quite limited. Those which are worth considering include:

## Mild analgesics

The response to mild over-the-counter painkillers tends to be disap-pointing.

*Aspirin* remains an excellent anti-inflammatory drug, provided you don't have any problems with side-effects, so do use it if it helps. Taking aspirin tablets after food will help to minimise stomach irritation, as do enteric-coated tablets. Do remember, though, that prolonged use of aspirin can lead to bleeding from the stomach lining, and that this drug should *never be given to children under the age of 12*. Some preparations of aspirin have a slow onset of action; these can be useful in providing pain relief during the night.

*Paracetamol* This is the main alternative to aspirin, but has little in the way of anti-inflammatory action, making it less effective in the control of this type of muscle or joint pain. The maximum safe dose of paracetamol for an adult is 8 x 500mg tablets over 24 hours – never exceed this or take such quantities for prolonged periods of time, because it is now known that some individuals are extremely sensitive to even quite low doses. Fatal overdoses are quite regularly reported in association with parac-etamol.

*Codeine* This is another analgesic, sometimes combined with aspirin or paracetamol, which may be useful for mild to moderate pain relief. However, it is too constipating for long-term use and may cause dizzi-ness, sedation or nausea.

Commonly used combination products include Co-Codamol (paraceta-mol and codeine) and Co-Codaprin (aspirin and codeine). These can both be purchased without a prescription. The cheapest way of buying simple analgesics like aspirin or paracetamol is to ask your pharmacist for one of their own-brand products.

*Caffeine* is a weak stimulant that is still occasionally added to analgesic tablets; it doesn't have any pain-killing action and may aggravate gastric problems. It is best avoided.

## Stronger analgesics

Although these type of painkillers – which are only available with a doctor's prescription – may be more effective, I believe that their use in ME/CFS should generally be discouraged.

Drugs such as dextropropoxyphene (e.g. Distalgesic), dihydro-codeine (e.g. DF 118) and meptazinol (Meptid) are usually only given to people with chronic pain associated with illnesses such as cancer. This is because they can cause a variety of disturbing side-effects as well as creating problems with tolerance and addiction.

Tramadol (Zamadol or Zydol) is a new type of strong analgesic with a potency which lies midway between codeine and morphine. It probably acts through its effects on brain chemical transmitters such as nora-drenaline and serotonin. Several studies have shown that this drug can be helpful in the relief of muscular pain, and it seems to cause less in the way of sedation and constipation than others in this group. It would be a reasonable choice for anyone with ME/CFS who requires a short course of a more effective pain reliever.

## Anti-inflammatory drugs

Non-steroidal anti-inflammatory drugs (NSAIDs) are another type of mild analgesic which can help with muscle and join pain, as well as headaches. Ibuprofen is sold over the counter as Brufen, or obtainable on prescription. As with any analgesic, the risk of side-effects needs to be taken into consideration, and these include stomach irritation and bleeding, rashes and blood problems. Some people are unduly sensitive to these gastric side-effects, so *NSAIDs must be used with care if you have any history of a possible stomach ulcer*. More worrying is research that suggests that long-term use can result in thinning of the bones (osteo-porosis).

NSAIDs are also available as ointments (worth trying for localised pain relief) or suppositories (for use at night to relieve morning stiff-ness).

When pain becomes more severe and continuous, analgesics may have to be taken more frequently in order to build up and maintain an ade-quate level in the body, but you still need to take care because one side-effect of all the analgesics – especially mixed ones containing aspirin or paracetamol in combination with another drug – is that larger daily doses can aggravate headaches (see pages 49–50).

## Other drugs

Some other drugs which are sometimes used to relieve muscle and joint pain include low doses of sedating tricyclic antidepressants, calcium antagonists and evening primrose oil (as described earlier in this chapter).

The new experimental drug galanthamine has also been reported as producing a significant degree of relief from muscle pain.

Drugs used in the treatment of muscle cramp are described on page 74.

Headaches and their management are described on pages 49–50.

## Self-help measures

These include:

- The use of locally applied heat in the form of a hot water bottle or a warm bath.
- Massage to the affected area using an embrocation such as Deep Heat (popular with runners for muscle pains); some even find horse linament to be effective!
- Spray-on pain-relief aerosols – these tend to provide only temporary relief.
- Good footwear with shock-absorbing insoles and a good arch support for the relief of activity-induced pain.

## Alternative approaches

Approaches such as acupuncture, aromatherapy, massage by an osteopath or chiropractor, or even hypnosis may be worth considering. These are all covered in Chapter 13: Alternative and Complementary Approaches.

## Pain clinics

When pain becomes a continuous and disabling part of your illness, unrelieved by any of the above forms of treatment, it may be worth asking your GP to refer you to an NHS pain clinic. Most large district general hospitals now have such clinics, often run by anaesthetists, but with help from neurologists, psychologists and physiotherapists. Sometimes they offer alternative approaches such as acupuncture as part of the treatment package.

One of the most effective non-drug forms of pain relief which is widely used at such clinics is a TENS (transcutaneous electrical nerve stimulation) machine. Treatment with this device involves applying small padded electrodes on to the skin directly over the site of chronic pain. A small current is then passed, which is thought to stimulate the production of endorphins – the body's own natural painkillers. TENS machines can be hired out from pain clinics and if you find this approach helpful then it may be worth purchasing one from a reputable manufacturer. A growing number of GPs are starting to make use of TENS machines – there may even be one at your local practice.

*The Pain Clinic Directory*, produced by the College of Health, (see Useful Addresses, page 418) lists the various forms of treatment on offer at over 200 centres in the UK. You could also contact The Pain Society (see Useful Addresses, page 428) for more information.

### Psychological treatments

These may form part of a treatment package at a pain clinic and involve the use of what is known as cognitive behaviour therapy (see pages 242–45). The advice may be rather controversial and involve you 'pushing on' despite increasing pain. This is based on the assumption that decreasing activity which normally produces pain is counter-productive and only results in a further deterioration in pain tolerance. Even so, I have no doubt that input from a psychologist who fully understands ME/CFS can be helpful in certain circumstances.

## Sleeping Tablets

Sleep disturbance is an extremely common feature of ME/CFS. Initially, this may involve excessive sleep requirements (hypersomnia), but as the illness becomes more chronic, a variety of other sleep disturbances occur. Sedating-type sleeping tablets have to be used with great care and should only be prescribed for very short periods (days rather than weeks). A more preferable form of treatment involves the use of one of the sedating type tricyclic antidepressant drugs (see earlier in this chapter). Sleep disturbances and their management are covered in more detail on pages 72–80.

## Supplements

Even though health magazines and newspaper articles frequently claim that health supplements can boost energy production or increase mental functioning, I know of no such products which have ever turned out to be beneficial in the case of ME/CFS. Most of these costly supplements are far more effective at relieving savings rather than suffering!

There are, however, three commercially available supplements – carnitine, co-enzyme Q10 and creatine – whose possible value in ME/CFS deserves further assessment.

## Carnitine

Researchers in both Japan and the UK have found lowered blood levels of carnitine in people with ME/CFS (see page 140). As carnitine is a substance which plays a key role in muscle (mitochondrial) energy production, there is considerable interest as to whether commercially available supplements could help to reduce the muscle fatigue and pain associated with ME/CFS.

As yet, no properly controlled trials have been carried out to assess its value in ME/CFS. However, an American research group has reported that 1 gram of carnitine given three times a day improved mental and physical performance in a small group of ME/CFS patients. No significant adverse effects were noted during the eight-week trial period. The only contra-indication to using carnitine appears to be kidney dialysis (reference 397).

Carnitine can be obtained from several health supplement manufacturers. Some combine carnitine with coenzyme Q10 because although these two substances act in different ways, their role in energy production is complementary. You may also find that your local pharmacy is able to obtain a suitable product. Carnitine supplements are not yet available on an NHS prescription.

## Coenzyme Q10

This is one of the body's essential enzymes which is present in all human cells, particularly the muscle mitochondria, where it acts as an igniting force in energy production. Coenzyme Q10 may also have a role in neutralising harmful oxidants which lead to cell damage and degeneration. Natural sources include foods such as meat, fish and vegetable oils. Inside the body coenzyme Q10 is manufactured in the liver.

There is no doubt about the theoretical value of coenzyme Q10, and there is some published evidence to show that supplementation can influence mitochondrial function in some muscle disorders (reference 378). However, there is no such evidence to show that it is effective in relieving any of the muscle fatigue symptoms associated with ME/CFS. Quite a few people claim that taking two or three 30mg tablets/capsules per day helps, and a properly controlled clinical trial using one of the commercial supplements would certainly be worthwhile.

Coenzyme Q10 should *not* be taken by pregnant or lactating women.

## Creatine

This is a substance which is naturally obtained from both fresh fish and meat in the diet. Inside the body it is also made in the liver.

Commercially available supplements contain about the same amount of creatine as could be obtained from eating eight pounds of steak – far in excess of what is normally consumed in a day. These supplements are now being used by athletes to increase their performance. Whether or not they work remains unproven, but the athletic governing bodies are far from happy about the increasing use of creatine in sport.

Physiologists who have studied creatine believe that it could genuinely aid muscle performance in several different ways. First, by providing a reserve source of energy on which the whole muscle can draw when its supplies of ATP – the energy producing molecule – become exhausted. Second, by rapidly replacing phosphates which are consumed when ATP is broken down. Third, by neutralising harmful acids that accumulate in muscle during exercise. Fourth, by aiding the transfer of energy into proteins which make muscles contract.

Although research has suggested that ME/CFS may involve a defect in the way that muscle cells produce energy (see pages 141–143), nobody has yet assessed the use of creatine as a possible treatment. One study found that it could help to improve the performance of failing heart muscle, so there are theoretical reasons why creatine might be of benefit.

Serious concerns about the safety of creatine supplements wre reported in *The Lancet* (1998: 351, 1252–3) following the deaths of three American sportsmen who had regularly been taking 2 gms per day.

## Symptomatic Relief

Drugs used in the treatment of other symptoms which may be associated with ME/CFS are covered elsewhere:

- anxiety on pages 245–9
- bladder problems on pages 56–7
- dizziness on pages 55–6
- headaches on pages 49–50
- joint pain on pages 70–71
- menopause and osteoporosis on pages 68–8
- irritable bowel symptomatology on pages 62–4
- sore throats on page 72.

## Vitamins and Minerals

Apart from the possible use of folic acid supplementation (see page 278) there is no published evidence to indicate that large doses of vitamins or minerals are of any value in ME/CFS. Remember, too, that megadosing vitamins can produce side-effects (see pages 275–80). It should also be noted that the NHS regards most of the commercially available vitamin and mineral supplements as being 'borderline substances', meaning that they cannot be dispensed on a doctor's prescription.

## New and Experimental Drugs

As we start to learn more about the causes of ME/CFS and the resulting disturbances involving hormones, brain chemical transmitters, immune system function, etc, it seems that new forms of drug treatment are highly likely to emerge over the next few years.

The converse is also quite possible, in that the results from carefully supervised clinical trials involving novel or experimental forms of treatment that act on muscle (e.g. carnitine), the immune system (e.g. interferon) or brain chemicals (e.g. galanthamine) may well provide useful information on the underlying disease process in ME/CFS.

It's equally feasible that research into effective treatments for symptoms such as sleep disturbance in depression or fatigue in multiple sclerosis could produce drugs which will help to alleviate the same symptoms when they occur in ME/CFS.

Finally, it may be worth reassessing the possible role of some of the drugs which have previously been dismissed as being of no value in ME/CFS on the basis of small or unsatisfactory clinical trials. The only way forward in the assessment of any drug in ME/CFS is for large-scale trials to take place, preferably involving more than one research centre, in order to try and reduce the bias that sometimes occurs when different specialists tend to see patients who may or may not have co-existent psychiatric problems.

I very much doubt that one drug will appear that is effective in alleviating the majority of ME/CFS symptoms. I do, however, believe that drugs which relieve individual symptoms will be found.

As you can see, it's not easy for doctors when someone with ME/CFS demands that 'something must be done' in the form of drug treatment. There are a limited number of drugs currently available which do seem to help with some specific symptoms in some people with ME/CFS. Unfortunately, for others, all they experience are the side-effects and no form of drug therapy seems to help.

## Sources of Information on Drugs

The best source for reliable information on common drugs is your local community pharmacist. Most large hospitals now have a drug information pharmacist in their pharmacy. These pharmacists are usually extremely helpful, even when it comes to unusual queries, but they are not always willing to respond to queries from members of the general public.

The most useful books providing information on drugs are:

- *Martindale: The Extra Pharmacopoeia* (The Pharmaceutical Society Press) This is *the* reference book for anyone seeking up-to-date information on drugs. It is particularly useful for details of side-effects, precautions, interactions and how drugs work. There are numerous references to medical papers and summaries of original articles describing how a specific drug has been used to treat various conditions. *Martindale* is very expensive to buy, but it may be available in large libraries. All large hospitals should have the most recent edition. Your local pharmacist may have an older copy if you ask nicely!
- *The British National Formulary* (British Medical Association and the Royal Pharmaceutical Society) This is concise and fully revised every six months. The *BNF* provides a good guide to costs, side-effects, drug interactions and comparisons of drugs used for treating specific conditions (but not ME/CFS!).
- *Which Medicine?* (The Consumers' Association and Hodder & Stoughton) Contains details of over 1,500 prescription medicines as well as ones available over the counter.

A full list of medical references describing all the various treatment trials described in this chapter can be found on pages 467–9.

# Self-Help

So long as conventional medicine remains relatively ineffective at altering the natural course of recovery in ME/CFS, the onus lies on patients themselves to try and create the optimum conditions for progress to take place.

Coming to terms with the many restrictions imposed by this illness, remaining positive about the chances of recovery, and adopting sensible changes in lifestyle are the three most important aspects of self-help which require careful consideration. Inevitably, this will mean 'redefining your boundaries' in all areas of everyday life, and not pushing yourself to the point of physical or mental exhaustion. For many previously fit young adults, these are changes in lifestyle which aren't easy to accept or put into practice – as I know all too well from personal experience.

## Rest and Activity

Striking the correct balance between rest and activity – both physical and mental – is one of the most difficult aspects of coming to terms with ME/CFS. On one hand is the need to take an appropriate amount of rest and relaxation, especially during the early stages. A period of slow steady convalescence is in fact essential during the very early stages – something which has largely gone out of fashion in modern medical practice. But this has to then be balanced by the need to try and *gradually* increase activity within individual limitations. It's not easy achieving the correct mix, particularly when you realise that although inactivity brings considerable relief from symptoms, it can also lead to frustration and anger at not being able to carry on with a normal way of life. Equally, just taking relatively small amounts of exercise can cause an exacerbation of symptoms, and this is very obvious when too much activity on a 'good day' leads to post-exertional malaise (to use medical jargon) the following morning. Finding the correct balance – which is not unlike learning how to make mayonnaise – really comes down to using up your variable daily energy quotient in a planned and sensible manner. However, the two most important variables to take into consideration when planning an individual rest/activity programme are (a) what stage you've reached in the illness and (b) how severely affected you are.

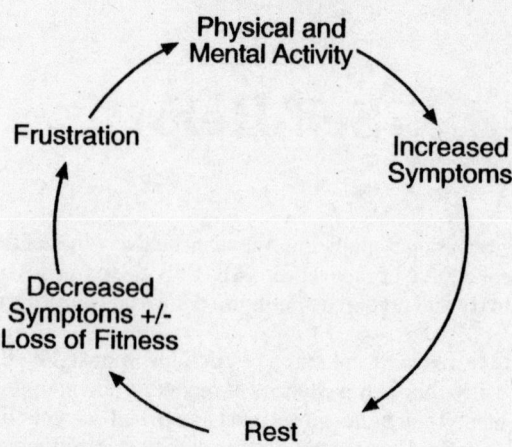

## *The pros and cons of rest*

Rest is definitely the most important factor in promoting recovery during the *very early stages*, especially when there has been an acute onset to your ME/CFS following an infection or vaccination. Without an adequate period of rest, recovery will not start to occur, and those who struggle on, either at home or work, to the point of regularly reaching mental or physical exhaustion stand very little chance of ever making any progress.

Rest means not only relaxing physically, but mentally as well. Every single day needs to be planned ahead to make sure that activities are spaced out to allow a period of rest in between. Ideally, rest periods should be taken in quiet surroundings where there is freedom from interruption. Take the phone off the hook for a while; let friends and neighbours know that you don't want to be disturbed, and probably won't answer the door.

Nobody should feel guilty about taking a short period of morning and afternoon rest at this stage in the illness. For many it will be the only way they can manage to complete the day. You don't have to go to bed, just have a quiet lie down for an hour or so and maybe listen to a radio or tape. You could also make this the time for carrying out relaxation techniques described on pages 247–8.

In the immediate aftermath of a triggering infective illness I have no hesitation in recommending a short period of bed rest before gradually returning to more normal activities. This may mean a week or so in bed, followed by a much longer period of carefully planned convalescence. By doing this you may be able to avoid the progression of ME/CFS into a long-term disabling illness.

However, prolonged bed rest can also damage your health. Besides the obvious problem of constipation, prolonged inactivity in bed can produce far more serious consequences. Doctors now refer to an 'immobility syndrome' which occurs after extended periods of lying in bed, with decreased oxygen intake to the lungs, the risk of venous thrombosis in the legs (another good reason for taking some passive exercises in bed) and loss of calcium (which in turn increases the risk of osteoporosis). If a perfectly healthy person is placed on strict bed rest for a few weeks, they will feel extremely weak, so it's hardly surprising that people with ME/CFS experience similar difficulties when trying to return to normal. This progressive loss of physical fitness associated with prolonged bed rest is what doctors refer to as 'deconditioning'.

The only times when I would recommend a period of complete bed rest is at the very start of ME/CFS or during a significant period of relapse (e.g. following a further infection). At the time of such a relapse I myself generally go to bed and try to rest as much as possible for around 48 hours. I then start to plan a gradual recovery process even if this only means getting out of bed to sit in a chair for short periods. I appreciate that it's not always possible to follow this advice, but the longer you stay in bed during a relapse, the harder it's going to be to return to relative normality.

Some people may find themselves confined to bed for quite long periods. If this is so, try to make sure that either you or a family member carries out some passive arm and leg movements. It can also be quite comforting to carry out this type of exercise whilst in the bath. If you're not sure about what to do, a physiotherapist might be able to come in and advise.

If you are having to spend long periods in the bedroom, then consider making some alterations to the layout to change it into an all-purpose room in which you can eat, work and see visitors, as well as have time to relax and sleep. Have a cupboard or table close by to keep books, telephone and other essential items on. Transfer a few kitchen essentials upstairs, so you don't have to continually go up and down stairs for drinks or food. This may all seem rather strange to friends, relatives and visitors, but it is a practical solution for difficult circumstances.

If you can afford it, invest in a comfortable firm mattress and good quality pillows for the bed – after all, you're probably spending more of your life here than anywhere else. It's also helpful to have a comfortable armchair in the room, so you can still sit out of bed for a while, even if you don't wish to go downstairs.

Try not to feel bothered about seeing visitors in the bedroom. If the room is large enough, have a couple of spare chairs for them to use. Socialising with friends and relatives can be a tiring experience when you're not feeling well; this could be a compromise to not seeing them at all.

During more stable periods you may still need to take some rest during the day. If you wake up in the morning and feel awful, knowing that body and mind aren't going to function properly that day, try resting for a while or even going back to bed for an hour or a morning, then starting all over again after lunch. Don't try to struggle on with what you were intending to do if you feel dreadful – you'll only end up making mistakes and feel worse as a result. On the other hand, if you start the day feeling reasonably well and then accomplish all you intended to do, follow this by carefully considering how much extra you can cope with. It's far better trying to build up your level of activity on a step-by-step basis during a good spell, than to overdo things on the first few days and then end up feeling awful because you tried to do too much.

No two days are likely to be the same with ME/CFS. Predicting how you're going to feel tomorrow or the following week is almost impossible. This is why forward planning of any kind of activity becomes so difficult and arrangements have to be cancelled at the last moment.

Finally, try making a written list of all your planned activities for the coming week – nothing too ambitious to start with – and tick them off as you go along. It can be a tremendous boost to your self-confidence if you plan to do something and then carry it out. Keep a diary of what you've been achieving, even though it may only be a shadow of your previous performance.

## Activity and exercise

Exactly the same principle of achieving the right balance between taking too much and too little rest applies to physical activity and exercise. All too often, one hears about people with ME/CFS – and here I include myself – who, in the earliest stages, before a diagnosis has been made, have tried to get better by overdoing exercise and not taking sufficient rest.

| REST | | ACTIVITY |
|---|---|---|
| Essential for initial recovery but can be counter-productive if prolonged |  | Beneficial, provided you keep within individual limitations – excess can produce a relapse |

So how much exercise should you be taking and what sort of activity is advisable? Like everything else, exercise tolerance will vary considerably from person to person, but each individual soon learns to recognise their own personal limitations. The cardinal rule when taking part in any kind of physical activity is to avoid pushing yourself to the point of fatigue, and *never to the stage of exhaustion.*

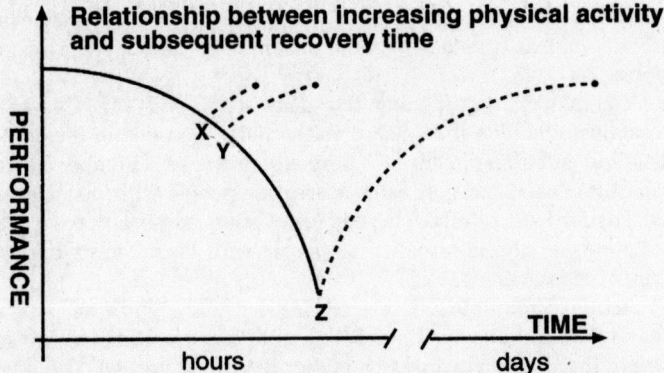

**Relationship between increasing physical activity and subsequent recovery time**

You will already know from experience that after starting to go for a walk you can carry on at a fairly steady pace till you reach point X (see graph above) – when muscles start to tire and obvious fatigue sets in. For some people with ME/CFS, this may only be about 100 yards, but for others it could be half a mile or so. If you then decide to push on beyond point X the fatigue becomes steadily worse, till you reach point Y, where it's becoming extremely difficult to go much further (by this point your brain may also be starting to feel rather confused as well). If you carry on beyond point Y there is further quite rapid deterioration and you're soon feeling exhausted, which forces a complete cessation of physical (and sometimes mental) activity – point Z.

The aim of all physical activity must, therefore, be to learn just how much you can usefully achieve on a day-to-day basis before reaching the points of fatigue and exhaustion, and to *keep to your limits* at all times. If you stop activity at or before the point of fatigue, your recovery period back to normal should be fairly short. Proceeding to the point of exhaustion will probably mean that it will take several days before you feel ready to undertake any more physical activity.

## What sort of activity is helpful?

Very few people with ME/CFS find that they can participate in any form of active sport, and certainly nothing that involves a combination of mental and physical activity. But the real danger is that when you're going through a good patch, you decide to go for a run around the park. Within a very short period of time you're forced to stop and may even be heading for another relapse. There are, however, some physical activities which can still be carried out so long as you're feeling reasonably well, provided you stick to your limitations.

If you like walking, try going on 'circular tours' so that you always end up back home again. Don't set off and reach your point of fatigue halfway round – unless someone is going to come and collect you by car at this point!

You may enjoy gardening, but many people with ME/CFS have had to almost abandon this pleasurable activity, because of the amount of bending and lifting involved. There are, however, a number of practical aids that can make gardening easier for people with disabilities. The Society for Horticultural Therapy (see Useful Addresses, page 422) provides advice and information to people with disabilities who find this type of activity enjoyable.

Another enjoyable form of exercise is swimming in a warm pool. You may find that your local swimming pool has a special weekly session where the water is heated to a higher level than normal. The buoyancy of water in a swimming pool makes it an ideal medium in which to exercise weakened muscles in a gentle fashion and mobilise any painful joints. Local hospitals often have a hydrotherapy pool – a physiotherapist or occupational therapist may be able to arrange regular sessions on the NHS. The Association of Swimming Therapy (see Useful Addresses, page 421) promotes and teaches the art of swimming to people with disabilities.

Some people find that yoga is a beneficial form of gentle exercise, but do take guidance from an experienced teacher and stick to positions which are comfortable.

In the end, it all comes down to listening to what your body is telling you to do. If you're going through a good patch, don't overdo things, but gradually try to increase all forms of activity on a day-by-day basis. Don't push yourself forward at a faster pace than you can cope with, or you'll just end up back in relapse.

## Hitting the glass ceiling

Most people with ME/CFS have no difficulty in accepting that once their condition becomes fairly stable, it's a sensible idea to try to gradually increase their amount of physical and mental activity. You may well find that during a really good patch it's quite easy to improve your level of functioning by 10 or even 20 per cent on a disability rating scale.

However, it then becomes impossible to make any further progress, no matter how hard you try. This impasse has been very aptly described as 'hitting the glass ceiling' and I know from personal experience that if I try to go beyond my own upper limit, such efforts generally tend to be a waste of time and may even be counter-productive.

The presence of this 'glass ceiling' – above which lies a further but unobtainable degree of recovery – is one of the reasons why I remain extremely sceptical about claims for 10 or 20 per cent improvements in functioning following treatment with graded exercise programmes or cognitive behaviour therapy. All that may be happening during a course of such therapy is that people who are functioning on a day-to-day basis at a level where they feel comfortable are then pushing themselves up to the maximum level of ability, i.e. hitting their own glass ceiling.

I have no easy solutions as to how you can make any further progress once you've reached what seems to be your maximum level of ability. There is certainly no point in pushing on beyond your limitations. Nor does the answer seem to lie in drugs, over-enthusiastic exercise regimes or psychotherapy.

The presence of this glass ceiling on recovery adds further weight to the view that whatever psychological or social factors may be having an adverse effect, there is an underlying *biological defect* in this illness.

## Research into the role of rest and exercise

Although some doctors, particularly psychiatrists, believe that people with ME/CFS take far too much rest and not enough exercise, very few scientific studies have been carried out to assess this controversial aspect of lifestyle management.

In 1997, the *British Medical Journal* reported on the results of a properly controlled study involving 66 ME/CFS patients with no evidence of significant sleep disturbance or psychiatric component to their illness (reference 413). The group enrolled on to an exercise programme and were given 12 weekly sessions of supervised aerobic activities (i.e. exercises such as walking, swimming and even cycling, which increased oxygen uptake by the lungs) along with home exercises for at least five days each week between the hospital appointments. Their activity was gradually increased, from 10- to 30-minute sessions, in accordance with each individual's response. The control group were given a treatment programme consisting of simple stretching and relaxation exercises.

Out of 29 patients in the exercise group, 16 rated themselves to be 'much' or 'very much' better after 12 weeks' treatment. This compared to only eight out of 30 in the relaxation group who reported any benefit. Various other assessments were taken (e.g oxygen consumption, heart rate, muscle strength) to assess the response to treatment.

The results of this small study need to be viewed with caution as it excluded severely affected patients and those in the very early stages of being ill. A number of doctors later wrote in to the *Journal* to criticise the way in which patients were both selected and followed up.

And even though the authors pointed out that each exercise programme was individually tailored, and increases in activity were gradual, some doctors went on to interpret graded exercise as meaning a progressive increase in physical activity on a day-to-day basis, which takes no account of how the patient is feeling.

It is worth noting that doctors have now been warned by their medical defence insurers that they have to take just as much care when recommending exercise programmes as they do when prescribing powerful drugs. Patients who subsequently relapse or experience a significant increase in symptoms as a result of inappropriate exercise programmes may well have a case for taking legal action.

The *American Journal of Medicine* also carried an extremely informative report on the effects of excessive exercise on people with ME/CFS shortly after the *BMJ* paper appeared (reference 414). The author, Dr Charles Lapp from the Duke University Medical Centre in North Carolina, carried out exercise testing using a braked bicycle and reported that '*74 per cent [of patients in the study] experienced worsening fatigue and 26 per cent stayed about the same after maximal exercise. None improved. The average relapse rate lasted 8.82 days, although 22 per cent were still in relapse when the study ended at 12 days. Interestingly, we found similar changes with exercise in lymph [glandular] pain, depression, abdominal pain, sleep quality, joint and muscle pain, headache and sore throat . . . The data would suggest that when PWCs [people with Chronic Fatigue Syndrome] are pushed to maximal exertion, they frequently relapse for long periods of time.*'

*Dr Lapp concluded with the comment that 'PWCs can perform mild to moderate exercise (or work) without relapse, providing they have frequent rest periods. This concept forms the basis of our current activity recommendations to limit exercise to less than 5 minutes followed by rest. This work–rest cycle may be repeated several times daily in order to maintain strength, flexibility and conditioning.*'

These are views which I would thoroughly endorse, especially the advice that it is far better to split activity into regular small sessions throughout the day rather than carrying on with one or two prolonged periods of activity.

For details of other research studies into rest and exercise see page 241 and references 415–6 and 538.

# Nutrition

It goes without saying that all aspects of healthy eating should always be encouraged, taking into account any personal allergies or sensitivities to foods.

A wide variety of digestive problems can become a part of ME/CFS, but the cause remains uncertain. Possible explanations include the presence of a persisting infection in the bowel which, in turn, interferes with enzymes that aid the digestion of food. One well-recognised after-effect of a gastrointestinal infection is the development of milk intolerance. This is because the infection reduces the lining mucosa's ability to produce an enzyme called lactase, which helps to break down milk and aid its absorption. Common symptoms include pain, wind and diarrhoea. The diagnosis of lactase deficiency can be confirmed by finding what are known as reducing sugars in the motions. There should then be a dramatic improvement in symptoms so long as milk and all milk products are removed from the diet.

Disturbances involving the chemical transmitter serotonin, which is involved in digestive function, could provide a further explanation (reference 63).

It has also been suggested that bowel problems such as bloating, pain and diarrhoea may be connected with a chronic candida infection, but the evidence here is not at all convincing (see pages 262–266). Another explanation, put forward in *The Lancet* (1991, 338, 495–6) by Dr John Hunter from Addenbrooke's Hospital in Cambridge, is that food residues are broken down by organisms in the gut to produce chemicals which, in susceptible people, are not properly dealt with by liver enzymes and so pass into the general circulation to produce symptoms – a so-called 'enterometabolic disorder'.

Problems with the absorption of vitamins, amino acids and trace elements, such as magnesium and zinc, are often quoted, but there is no reliable published evidence to back up such claims. Vitamin and mineral supplements won't do any harm provided they are from a reputable manufacturer and not taken in excess (see pages 270–280).

A well-balance diet should be low in sugar and fat as well as containing plenty of fish, fruit and vegetables. Try to eat regular meals of energy-rich foods which contain good quality protein, fibre, vitamins and minerals. Good examples include wholemeal bread, pasta, brown rice, peas, beans, lentils, nuts and dried fruit. Foods which contain complex carbohydrates are digested slowly and so release a constant supply of energy into the blood which minimises the risk of hypoglycaemia. Again, hypoglycaemia is frequently quoted as an important feature of ME/CFS, but the evidence to support this is very flimsy (see page 66).

Green vegetables, citrus fruits, tomatoes, potatoes and dried apricots all provide essential vitamins, minerals and fibre. Much of the goodness lies in the skin, but I'd recommend that fresh fruits are always peeled. Citrus fruits and fruit juices are excellent sources of vitamin C. Bananas are very useful as a between-meal snack and are often used by cyclists because they allow a slow release of fructose into the body. They're also a good source of fibre and contain an essential amino acid called tryptophan, which has a calming effect on the brain.

Some alternative therapists now advocate a much more radical change in diet, but this is not without its dangers and should only be carried out under strict supervision. I have now seen several patients who have made themselves very ill on such a regime. My own feeling is that people with ME/CFS have quite enough restrictions placed on their lives without adding a vast range of foods to that list. Equally, I would never recommend fasting as a treatment for ME/CFS.

The relationship between food allergy and ME/CFS remains a very controversial topic and most doctors feel that it is all too often being diagnosed by tests which are not reliable (see pages 255–260). Even so, many people with ME/CFS believe that they have multiple food allergies and cut out dairy produce and wheat in particular. As far as wheat is concerned, I know a few patients who seem to have benefited quite considerably, and it may be that this subgroup are really suffering from unrecognised adult-onset coeliac disease (see page 84).

If you go on to remove all dairy produce from the diet, there is inevitably going to be a severe lack of calcium. This, along with physical inactivity, is an important risk factor in the development of osteoporosis (thinning of the bones) in later life. So, it is essential for anyone under the age of 40, especially if you are female, to make sure that there is an adequate intake of calcium in the diet. Calcium supplementation may well be advisable here, usually with tablets, although milk, sardines and shellfish are excellent sources of natural calcium. If you do take calcium tablets, *never* exceed the recommended dose as too much can be just as dangerous as too little (see pages 68–9).

Lastly, as I've already pointed out in Chapter 6, anyone with a large number of gastric symptoms may need investigations to rule out the possibility of coeliac disease or giardia infection. The specific management of irritable bowel symptomatology is dealt with on pages 63–4.

## How to gain weight

Some people with ME/CFS find that they start to put on extra pounds as the illness progresses. Others lose significant amounts of weight during the very early stages following an infection and then find it extremely difficult to return to their normal body weight.

For anyone who's already genetically programmed to be thin, adding a few extra pounds in weight can be a very frustrating task, especially if you're mainly trying to increase muscle bulk. Here are a few dos and don'ts which might just help:

- Do check with your doctor that there are no other medical reasons which could explain your weight loss (e.g. thyroid disease, gut disorders such as coeliac or Crohn's disease).
- Do try to have at least three proper meals a day.
- Do eat plenty of starchy foods such as bread, pasta and potatoes, as well as several portions of fruit and vegetables each day.
- Do feel free to have plenty of between-meal snacks with unsalted nuts, dried fruits or milkshakes.
- Don't try to put on weight or increase muscle bulk by eating excessive amounts of high-protein foods. This is not an effective way of increasing weight and can place extra strain on the kidneys.
- Don't worry about temporarily increasing the amount of vegetable oils, fried foods, pies, chocolate and dairy produce, because fat is the most concentrated form of calorie intake. Do, however, try to return to a rather more healthy balanced diet once you've managed to put some weight on.
- Don't bother with expensive supplements and nutritional drinks which are claimed to help athletes put on weight. They're no more effective than eating the right sort of food, and much more expensive.

# Hobbies

Family and friends may wonder how some with ME/CFS manages to keep themselves occupied throughout their long days stuck at home. A non-energetic hobby can be both entertaining and rewarding.

Before I became ill, many of my interests had started to gather dust, but the stamp collection has been sorted out, and I've become interested in photography again. Creative writing isn't the sort of thing that everyone can do easily, but I know quite a few people who have taken this up – it's the sort of activity you can do without much physical effort. Some people have invested in a word processor or computer, which can be great fun as well as being extremely useful at correcting one's mistakes!

Starting a new academic course from home might be something to think about. Open University courses can be taken over a period of several years, and the organisers are keen to help people with disabilities wherever possible (see page 422).

Pets are a very good source of companionship. They don't chatter away all day, but can be there as a friend. Remember, a dog will need exercising. A cat (Siamese are great companions), budgie or even a small furry animal would do just as well.

# Avoiding a Relapse

Whatever the current state of your illness, be it static, recovering, or in remission, there's always the possibility that a relapse may occur. Most people with ME/CFS quickly learn to recognise those things which are almost guaranteed to worsen their condition, but avoiding them isn't always easy. Undue physical and mental stress are probably the commonest causes of relapse, and these factors, along with the adverse effects of temperature extremes have already been covered. However, there are several other important causes of relapse which you need to be aware of.

## Alcohol

Alcohol intolerance is extremely common in ME/CFS. I rarely see a patient who doesn't volunteer this fact, and if you're not affected by large amounts of alcohol, then ME/CFS seems an unlikely diagnosis.

Some people who previously enjoyed and tolerated regular consumption of alcohol without any adverse effects, now find that even small amounts make them extremely unwell. This isn't an allergy but a hypersensitivity to the effects of alcohol, possibly related to several different actions.

First, the soporific effects of alcohol are partly explained by the fact that it increases the effects of one of the brain's chemicals (neurotransmitters) – gamma amino butyric acid (GABA). This, in turn, reduces the availability of calcium, which is responsible for triggering nerve cell activity, and so brain function is depressed.

New research from America suggests that a compound produced by alcohol-soaked brain cells – a fatty acid ethyl ester – is capable of inhibiting the release of other types of neurotransmitters. The way in which this mysterious compound acts at a cellular level – particularly in a part of the brain known as the hippocampus – is to speed up the release of potassium ions from the brain cells. This, in turn, inhibits the release of the vital neurotransmitters. Any slowing down of neurotransmitter release will inevitably result in an exacerbation of brain symptoms – including clumsiness and problems with memory or concentration – associated with ME/CFS.

Alcohol can also dilate small blood vessels in the skin, so it helps to divert blood flow away from the brain. Anyone who is particularly susceptible to the autonomic symptoms of ME/CFS (feeling faint or dizzy on standing up) will probably find these are made worse after alcohol.

It's difficult to say whether alcohol consumption, even in moderation, causes any real harm in ME/CFS. If there's any evidence of inflammation in the liver, then alcohol should be avoided altogether. However, most people find that they no longer want to drink any alcohol at all, so the problem doesn't arise. As recovery starts to occur, it's quite often reported that tolerance to alcohol starts to increase and you may well find yourself being able to enjoy an occasional glass of wine or beer.

I have also come across the occasional person who misuses alcohol to try and 'blot out' their symptoms, but this is alcohol abuse. It's a very dangerous path to start on – you only end up feeling ten times worse the next morning and run a serious risk of becoming an alcoholic.

One final reason for avoiding alcohol is the fact that it can damage muscle, but this is usually only associated with heavy drinking.

## Cigarettes and environmental pollution

Any form of environmental pollution, and that means both active smoking and inhaling other people's smoke (passive smoking) is best avoided if at all possible. Do explain to friends and relatives that *their* smoking might be damaging *your* health, and try to make your house or office a no-smoking zone.

Smoking cigarettes decreases the capability of red blood cells to carry vital oxygen around the body in an efficient manner. Research into ME/CFS indicates that there may be problems with the red cells themselves, as well as lack of oxygen to vital muscle and nerve cells. It doesn't seem sensible to exacerbate this problem further.

Most people with ME/CFS feel a lot better in a non-polluted atmosphere – so why not clean up the environment at home by banning the use of aerosols and spray-on chemicals?

## Drugs

All medication, both prescribed by your doctor, or purchased over the counter (and this includes vitamins, minerals and herbal preparations) should be taken with caution, and only with good reason. This is because an increased sensitivity to a wide range of drugs seems to occur quite commonly in ME/CFS. As with alcohol intolerance, this doesn't appear to be due to an allergic reaction. It may, in fact, have more to do with the way drugs are broken down in the body and the way they can affect chemical transmitters in the brain.

Antibiotic sensitivity can occasionally be a problem, but if you have a serious infection which requires treatment with a specific type of antibiotic, then do take the course – unless, of course, you have a genuine allergy to something such as penicillin.

## Table 7: Drugs and ME/CFS

1.  *Drugs which may exacerbate pre-existing symptoms:*

| Antidepressants | worsen autonomic/vasomotor symptoms can cause further sedation |
| Tranquillisers | increased sedation |
| Beta-blockers | fatigue in higher doses may worsen cold hands and feet |
| Some asthma drugs | worsen autonomic symptoms |

2.  *Drugs to which people with ME/CFS may be more sensitive:*
    Antibiotics
    Some analgesics and NSAIDs

3.  *Drugs which are best avoided unless really necessary for other reasons:*

| Steroids | depress the immune system |

## Infections

Picking up any new infection will almost certainly cause some form of temporary setback or relapse, and for anyone in regular contact with small children, this can become a frequent problem. It's obviously sensible to try and avoid close contact with relatives, friends, colleagues at work, etc, who already have an infection, but this is something that's easier said than done!

Good dental care with regular check-ups is also important, as a grumbling gum or tooth infection is likely to make anyone feel ill and debilitated.

If you pick up any sort of infection and start to feel unwell, rest and perhaps go back to bed for a short while till you're starting to feel less 'flu-like.

If you develop an infection and temperature and are not sure why, it's advisable to check with your GP after about 48 hours. There may be a chest or urinary infection present which is producing little in the way of obvious symptoms, but still requires treatment with an antibiotic. Before starting a course of antibiotics, it's always a good idea to ask if a sample of sputum or urine can be sent off to the hospital laboratory so that the exact infection can be identified and the most appropriate type of antibiotic prescribed.

A severe infection is likely to leave anyone with ME/CFS feeling extra-debilitated for several weeks, even months, so do try to be patient while a gradual return to your normal state of health occurs.

## Stress

Just as excessive or chronic stress – both physical and mental – may be a factor in predisposing or precipitating a case of ME/CFS, so it can also play an important role in maintaining or exacerbating this illness.

Earlier in this chapter I described how excessive amounts of physical activity can produce an exacerbation in both fatigue and a number of other common symptoms associated with ME/CFS. Excessive amounts of mental stress can also produce a very similar adverse effect on symptoms – a fact which is particularly relevant when someone tries to return to work and the employer fails to take any account of their new circumstances. Fortunately, the Disability Discrimination Act (see pages 344–6) makes it quite clear that employers can no longer ignore the needs of employees with chronic health problems, and may well be contravening the Act if they continue to expect an employee with ME/CFS to simply carry on with their normal workload.

A further situation in which stress can exacerbate ME/CFS involves what is termed 'traumatic stress' following some form of major accident or incident. This aspect has been highlighted by a number of cases involving people whose condition has markedly deteriorated following the physical and mental stress associated with a road traffic accident. In one famous case, which eventually came before both the Court of Appeal and the House of Lords, a man with ME/CFS was awarded £162,000 in damages for an exacerbation of his pre-existing condition following the 'nervous shock' he experienced in a road accident (reference: *The Lancet*, 1996, 347, 824).

There are a number of possible explanations as to why undue stress may cause a relapse or exacerbation of ME/CFS. My own view is that the most likely one involves the fact that this illness probably involves a defect in normal stress responses which is a result of disturbances in hypothalamic function and lowered levels of cortisol described in Chapter 8: Current Research. Whatever the true cause, it is important to make sure that your stress levels don't become excessive.

## Surgical operations and general anaesthetics

For anyone with ME/CFS, having to go into hospital for an operation will be a major event, so do try to do everything possible to minimise the upheaval. To start with, make sure that you're in the best physical state possible and rest as much as you can in the days preceding admission.

It's important to let your consultant and anaesthetist know in advance about the effects that ME/CFS has on your physical and mental functioning. Almost everyone feels weak and tired after an operation, but people with ME/CFS will probably experience increased fatigue and problems with memory/concentration for a much longer period of time.

The explanation could involve two separate factors. First is the way in which blood flow to the brain can be significantly reduced during both surgery and the immediate post-operative recovery period. Second is the use of various drugs during surgery, particularly those to correct a low heart rate or reverse muscle paralysis. Some of these drugs act on a brain chemical transmitter known as acetylcholine, levels of which appear to be affected in ME/CFS (reference 273).

If the surgeon or anaesthetist seems rather sceptical about ME/CFS being exacerbated by surgery, you could tactfully refer them to the above research which has been carried out into disturbed cholinergic transmission. It's possible that more careful use of anaesthetic drugs during and after an operation could reduce the severity of these side-effects. You could also ask if oxygen levels are going to be monitored during the operation using what's known as pulse oximetry.

The actual surgery is probably inevitable, but there is a trend now towards using less drastic procedures wherever possible. Kidney stones, for example, can now be removed by lithotripter – a machine which breaks them up using shock waves and doesn't involve open surgery – while some types of gallstone can be dissolved using drugs. Such alternatives aren't available for every surgical problem, but do ask your consultant if the operation is really necessary, and whether there are any alternative approaches – such as 'keyhole surgery' – suitable for your particular complaint.

Local anaesthesia is being increasingly used for a whole range of operations (some of them quite major); this is another option you may wish to discuss with the anaesthetist.

Explain to the nursing sister on the surgical ward that you have ME/CFS, so that all the staff are aware of the problems which might occur during your stay. It's quite possible that the nurses haven't looked after anyone with ME/CFS before and consequently know very little about the illness. It might even be worth taking in some medical information for them to read – but I can't guarantee the response will be positive!

Your post-operative recovery may well be much slower than for a normal healthy person. Hopefully, the ward will be sympathetic and not attempt to push you forward at a pace you can't cope with. If you're not happy about the way things are going, do speak to the sister or one of the doctors.

Back home, you're likely to need a great deal of practical help from other members of the family and/or the community nursing services. Try and make sure that this is properly organised *well before* you go into hospital. Everything should then run smoothly when you finally arrive back home.

## *Vaccinations*

Besides triggering a small minority of cases of ME/CFS, vaccination may also cause a further exacerbation of symptoms in some people, who are already affected by the illness. This seems to be particularly so for those whose illness was precipitated by a clear cut infection (or vaccination) and still have a number of continuing 'flu-like symptoms (e.g. sore throats, enlarged glands, temperature-control problems). So, it's always a good idea to arrange with your doctor for any necessary vaccination to be given at a time when you're feeling in a reasonably good state of health and can take things easy over the following few days. In the case of children, this may mean postponing a non-essential booster till they've improved or the school holidays have arrived.

Obviously, any such risk from a vaccination will always have to be carefully balanced against the chances of contracting whatever infection the vaccine is designed to protect you from. For example, maintaining up-to-date protection against tetanus would be *vital* for anyone who is working on a farm or regularly messing about in the garden. For those whose job places them at extra risk from catching hepatitis B infection (e.g. theatre nurses), vaccination against this potentially fatal liver disease must be seriously considered, even though the vaccine does appear to act as a trigger in the development of a number of cases of ME/CFS (see pages 35–7). I know of several instances where 'flu vaccine has triggered a significant relapse, frequently in people who experience ongoing 'flu-like symptoms. A nasty dose of 'flu is also quite likely to cause a relapse, so this vaccine may be worth considering, especially if you've already received a dose whilst being ill and suffered no ill effects. Anyone with pre-existing heart, kidney or chest disease should certainly consider having this protection.

Foreign travel occasionally involves a number of compulsory vaccinations as well as those which are just recommended. Don't rely on travel agents or travel brochures for advice or information as to which vaccinations may be necessary. The best source of information is either your GP (who should have an up-to-date chart from *Pulse* or *GP* magazine listing all the common holiday destinations along with relevant health risks) or MASTA (tel: 0891 224100), an organisation which can also provide individual advice. The need for a specific vaccination might be affected by whether you intend to stay in a reputable resort hotel or travel into remoter parts of the country in question. It's also important to try and plan your course of holiday vaccinations well in advance, so do make sure you're not having any final boosters the day before you actually set off!

Here are some basic guidelines:

- **Polio** is still a common disease in underdeveloped countries and it would be *extremely unwise* to visit a high-risk area without adequate protection. There is no evidence that polio vaccine can cause a relapse of ME/CFS (reference 338).
- **Diphtheria** is now being reported in some parts of Eastern Europe. A further booster may be necessary if you're going to a high-risk area.
- **Hepatitis A** protection, using immunoglobulin, doesn't usually cause any problems for people with ME/CFS. It provides a high degree of short-term protection for those travelling to anywhere with unsatisfactory levels of sanitation. Up to ten years' protection against hepatitis A can be obtained from a new vaccine against this liver disease.
- **Cholera** vaccine offers very little protection and is seldom recommended or made a compulsory requirement for entry.
- **Typhoid** vaccine isn't 100% effective, but it would be foolish to avoid having this protection if you are travelling to an area where cases have recently been reported. Typhoid vaccination certainly causes adverse reactions in perfectly healthy people, so it's worth asking your doctor about an oral form of protection against typhoid (Vivotif capsules), as this may reduce the incidence of side-effects. Please note that Vivotif is contra-indicated in people who are immunosuppressed and is inactivated by some antibiotics. It should not be given at exactly the same time as an oral polio vaccine or within twelve hours of giving or receiving mefloquine (an antimalarial). Taking sensible precautions with food, drinking water and where you bathe is just as important in preventing illnesses like hepatitis, cholera and typhoid as the relevant vaccines.
- Antimalarial tablets *must* be taken if advised.

For travel to more exotic locations, you may need (or even be required) to be vaccinated against encephalitis, meningitis, rabies and yellow fever.

## Summary of how to cope with a relapse

- Try to avoid any of the factors which are known to worsen ME/CFS.
- At the first sign of a relapse, start to increase your ratio of rest to activity. If you've developed an infection and temperature, go to bed. Aspirin is still a very good drug to use, provided you can tolerate it (not for under-12s though).
- If you have a serious infection, let your general practitioner know. Do take any antibiotics which are prescribed.
- Organise your bedroom into a living area, so you're not struggling up and down the stairs all day.
- Try not to prolong bed rest for more than a few days and don't be

afraid to commence a gradual rehabilitation programme, keeping within your limitations.

- Try to do some muscle exercises during bed rest, either by yourself or with help from a member of the family. Don't repeat any exercise to the point of fatigue. Don't exercise painful muscles and joints – let them settle down first.
- Don't neglect your diet – if you can't face solid food try to take some liquid nourishment (e.g. Complan) and don't let your fluid intake fall.
- Organise the family, friends, neighbours into helping out as much as possible.

Your body can recover from a relapse, but you must give it the best possible circumstances in which to do so. Remember, it's far better to regard relapses as setbacks on your road to recovery, rather than 'another step down the ladder'.

# Further Reading

## Nutrition

*Foods that Harm, Foods that Heal* (Reader's Digest) Describes the nutritional benefits and drawbacks of all widely available foods and drinks. Specific topics include additives, allergies, minerals and vitamins.

## Travel

*Traveller's Health* by Dr Richard Dawood (Oxford University Press) Covers all aspects of healthcare abroad.

# Mind and Body

'If you don't think that you're ever going to get better, then you probably never will.'

Taken literally, such a dramatic statement is not entirely applicable to something like ME/CFS, but there's more than a grain of truth in it. Attitude of mind – both positive and negative – is going to have a very significant effect on many aspects of living with this illness.

The primary effect may simply be on your 'coping mechanisms' – i.e. how you're able to deal with all the frustrations, anxieties and problems associated with ME/CFS. It's also quite likely that some of the physical symptoms associated with ME/CFS will be affected by your mental attitude towards them, and there's accumulating evidence that the body's immune system can be either strengthened or weakened by the effects of 'the psyche'. This is not to say that ME/CFS is a psychosomatic condition, where physical symptoms are *largely* under the control of the mind. But there is, for *some* people, a psychosomatic component, just as in other physical illnesses like asthma, where both physical factors (infections and allergies) can combine with emotional ones to exacerbate or cause relapse.

## Mind–Body Interactions

The relationship between mood, brain function and immune system responses is highly complex, and only just beginning to be understood by scientists interested in the subject – which has become known as psychoneuroimmunology. Several studies have now shown that T lymphocytes are often reduced in number in patients with severe depression and that natural killer cell activity is altered by stressful life events. Equally, the amount of the stress hormone cortisol, regulated by the hypothalamus (see pages 149–50), plays a role in immune system regulation. The reverse process can also occur – what's known as somatopsychic illness, where physical symptoms start to affect the emotional state, causing anxiety and depression as additional problems. These interrelationships between mind and body are highly complicated, but in illnesses such as ME/CFS they both probably occur in varying degrees of severity.

# A Positive Approach to Recovery

But how can this knowledge be applied to helping someone who already has ME/CFS? The obvious first step must be to try and take a 'positive approach'. I know it's not easy being optimistic when everything seems to be going wrong, but it's essential not to let your mind slip into the 'I'm never going to get better' approach, even when things are at their lowest ebb. Patients with HIV infection (AIDS) are now being taught to 'think positive' ('body positive'), even to the extent of imagining that cells from their immune system are being released 'into battle' against the persisting HIV infection and killing off the virus (a technique called 'imaging'). There's no scientific proof that this approach actually reverses any of the immunodeficiency changes seen in AIDS, but it does stimulate a very positive approach of mind. I'm not suggesting that people with ME/CFS should start taking the same approach but what I do advocate is that everyone tries to adopt a positive attitude towards recovery. You *can* and *will* get better, even if it takes a very long time to do so.

ME/CFS is a very individual illness in its presentation, symptoms, the secondary problems it causes and the way it progresses. If you talk to a group of people with ME/CFS, each one will probably have a symptom or problem that no one else has. This is why an individual approach to all aspects of management – physical, psychological and social – is essential.

In the early stages (and this means anything up to the first two years or so after the illness started) it's much easier to remain optimistic, hoping that the mysterious symptoms will go away by themselves, given time. However, as time goes by and symptoms don't improve, anxieties naturally increase, especially if there has been a long delay in obtaining a diagnosis.

Once a diagnosis is made there is inevitably a tremendous sense of relief. At long last there's an explanation for all your bizarre symptoms and you have a 'genuine illness', something to be believed by your general practitioner (hopefully), your family and your friends. You now have some idea of what's going wrong with your body, why you feel so ill all the time and the sort of actions you should be taking to try to recover. Most importantly, you're no longer quite so alone. There are an awful lot of other people suffering in a similar manner, who also find a trip to the supermarket a major effort, and have equal difficulties with friends and family when they're 'non-visibly' disabled.

This feeling of relief may only be temporary. Once the diagnosis has been made and the resulting consequences have started to sink in, a further change in attitude may then start to occur. At this point, it's quite easy to feel depressed and pessimistic about what may lie ahead. You start to realise that you're going to have to come to terms with the possibility of living with a long-term illness with a very unpredictable outcome. You and your family may have to consider making some very major changes in the way you live.

All kinds of questions now arise: what to do about work, whether to put off starting or adding to the family, whether or not to move home. Making the correct decisions isn't going to be easy. At this point it's often quite helpful to talk to someone else with ME/CFS who can provide the sort of sensible practical advice which your doctor may be unable to give. Afterwards, you can keep in touch – even if this is only by phone or letter – with someone who really understands how you feel, and can offer sound advice when nobody else seems to know what to do.

If you're in an occupation such as teaching or nursing, talking to someone in the same job about how to cope with difficulties at work or with sick leave, can also be helpful, just as mothers with young children can pick up useful advice from others in the same position. If you're having difficulty finding someone in the same occupation, the ME Association may be able to help.

If you're having trouble with social security benefits, then talking to someone who's experienced the same difficulties and won in the end can be very supporting. Try not to feel fed up and just give in to the system. It doesn't help you and it won't help other people who find themselves facing similar hassles in future.

You may also be wondering about whether to start or extend a family. ME/CFS often comes along at an age when this sort of decision is often about to be made. For a woman this can be a very difficult decision to make – just how long should one keep on avoiding pregnancy in the hope that a significant degree of recovery will occur? Once again, talking things through with someone who's become pregnant is the most useful advice that can be offered (see also pages 310–315).

At times when things aren't going too well, or you're experiencing a relapse or exacerbation of symptoms, try to think of this as being a setback on the road to recovery – something that's only going to be temporary, which you *will* get over, not an irreversible change for the worse.

# Psychiatric and Emotional Problems in ME/CFS: Depression, Anxiety and Emotional Lability

There's no doubt that ME/CFS is capable of producing a wide range of psychiatric and emotional problems. For a few people these become an increasingly distressing part of their illness, and when doctors or specialists have missed the diagnosis of ME/CFS, these aspects may even start to dominate their lives.

Understandably, true clinical depression certainly occurs in ME/CFS, and probably affects between a quarter and a third of people at some stage. Anyone who suffers from depression is likely to feel 'tired' as well, but this isn't the type of overwhelming exercise-induced muscle fatigue and weakness experienced in ME/CFS. Problems with memory and concentration can also form part of any depressive illness, but mixing up words, carrying out inappropriate actions, lack of co-ordination and clumsiness, all of which tend to be brought on by physical or mental exertion, are *not* characteristic of a depressive illness.

Another key group of ME/CFS symptoms – those associated with autonomic nervous system dysfunction – are, as described earlier (see pages 50–4), thought to be due to overactivity of the sympathetic nerves. Unfortunately, these are also a part of the nervous system that can be affected in anxiety, so some symptoms are similar to both conditions. Not surprisingly, if symptoms such as palpitations, sweating and feeling faint are prominent in a case of ME/CFS, the result can be a misdiagnosis of anxiety. Once again, there shouldn't be any confusion between the two when other classic features of ME/CFS are included. The unusual problems with temperature control and ongoing 'flu-like symptoms in ME/CFS are not seen in anxiety states.

One particular feature, which does seem to be an integral part of ME/CFS in some cases, is what doctors refer to as 'emotional lability'. Here, the emotional state and mood may start to fluctuate widely, often for no apparent reason, but sometimes related to frustrations imposed by the illness. Those who experience emotional lability may find themselves bursting into tears, feeling extremely low or depressed or becoming uncharacteristically irritable with friends or family members. Not everyone with ME/CFS experiences this type of emotional lability, but it can occur in people who would have regarded themselves as being stable individuals, not usually subject to showing their emotions so publicly, before the onset of their ME/CFS.

Do remember that it's a perfectly normal human reaction to periodically feel fed up with ME/CFS, especially when you're going through a difficult patch. Who wouldn't, with such a frustrating illness that imposes so many restrictions on your lifestyle? The important thing is to differentiate being fed up from being truly depressed, and not allowing your feelings of inner anger to radiate out and make everyone else feel miserable as well.

## Explaining Psychiatric Symptoms

So why do some people with ME/CFS develop significant emotional and psychiatric problems, whereas others don't? The most important underlying reason is probably connected with your underlying personality before the illness occurred. By this I mean to what extent you used to be a 'coper' – how you used to react to life's major upsets and crises. Those who were used to 'sailing through' before, not letting things get them down too much, and having a generally optimistic view of life and the future are probably going to fare much better from the emotional point of view than the opposite type of personality. For people who don't cope as well, the problems associated with having ME/CFS may well tip the balance and trigger any underlying susceptibility to developing anxiety or depressive illness – especially if this has already occurred in the past.

There is some evidence that women are more likely to succumb to these aspects of ME/CFS, especially when they're part of a conventional family grouping. Women with ME/CFS often find it impossible to properly rest when they are still trying to cope with bringing up children, doing housework and providing meals at the end of the day. In this situation, they are not being given a chance to even start their recovery process.

In contrast, the conventional husband who develops ME/CFS is still likely to be at work. If he then goes on sick leave, problems with the children and the home can be delegated while he initiates the major changes in lifestyle so necessary for recovery.

Although your underlying personality may well be the central factor in deciding how you manage to cope, a number of other factors may then start to interact and form a vicious circle which exacerbates the basic emotional problems.

Initiating this circle of events is the fact that parts of the underlying disease process – particularly any triggering infection – could be having a direct effect on parts of the brain which control mood and emotions. It's a well-recognised fact that one important cause of a true depressive illness is the aftermath of a viral infection. One possible explanation for this involves the way in which levels of brain chemical transmitters (neurotransmitters) in key areas of the nervous system have become severely depleted. Secondly, a viral infection may upset the production of various immune chemicals and brain hormones – substances which are capable of having direct effects on various aspects of mood, emotions and normal mental functioning.

Proceeding round this circle, the frustrating and disabling physical symptoms, and the constant feeling of being unwell are depressing in themselves. This can only be increased in those who are still trying to obtain a diagnosis. The circle is completed, as time goes on, by the social, family and financial problems which so commonly become part of ME/CFS. And these in turn aren't helped by battles with the authorities to obtain various sickness and disability benefits. All these factors

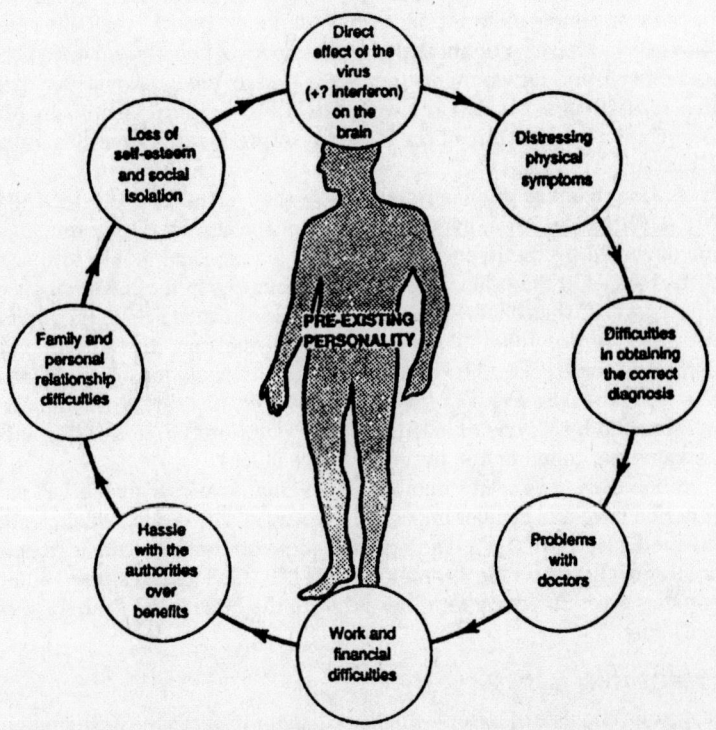

interact and place a great strain, not only on the person with ME/CFS, but also on their family. A resultant loss of self-esteem, even feelings of worthlessness, when all aspects of one's life seem to be falling apart, can place tremendous pressure on the most stoic of individuals, who may eventually find they just can't cope any longer.

So, it's not surprising that some people with ME/CFS pass from a state of just being 'fed up' from time to time, into true clinical depression. They may even develop suicidal feelings, which should never be ignored.

## How Psychiatrists View ME/CFS

Following publication of several research papers during the mid-1980s, the media once again became interested in this controversial illness. When I discussed ME/CFS on Radio 4's *Medicine Now* programme, the BBC received well over 1,000 letters requesting further information; and an article by Sue Finlay in the *Observer* brought in over 6,000 letters – all from people who believed that they might have ME/CFS. What had become an almost unknown illness was suddenly back in the public eye. As a result, I have no doubt that large numbers of people who were tired and unwell, and for whom doctors could find no obvious cause for their ill health, became labelled as having ME/CFS. Not surprisingly, the ME Association became one of the fastest growing medical charities in the UK.

Although most psychiatrists had by then dismissed the idea that ME/CFS was hysteria, hypochondriasis or malingering, they remained unconvinced by the hypothesis that it was a physical illness involving disturbances in the brain, muscle and immune system. In March 1988, three psychiatrists challenged this hypothesis in an article in the *British Medical Journal* titled 'Postviral fatigue syndrome: time for a new approach' (reference 133). The psychiatrists' explanation, to quote from a letter to the *New England Journal of Medicine*, was that 'symptoms are perpetuated by a cycle of inactivity and a deterioration in the tolerance for exercise, compounded by a depressive illness'.

Since then, a growing number of psychiatrists in both the UK and America have had a major impact on the way in which other doctors and the media view ME/CFS. Their current ideas on cause and management are largely based on the assumption that ME/CFS involves three different stages which are rather different from the hypothesis I put forward in Chapter 3.

## Predisposing factors

Stage one consists of factors which predispose towards the development of ME/CFS in susceptible individuals. The belief here is that an individual is far more likely to succumb to ME/CFS in later life if they have a previous history of emotional distress or psychiatric illness, particularly depression or a tendency to somatise, i.e. develop physical symptoms which are psychological in origin.

My own view is that much of the research data used to support this theory is nowhere near as reliable as claimed. Equally, studies which have found that people with ME/CFS are no more likely to have had a psychiatric diagnosis before the onset of their illness than the general population (references 53 and 440) are largely ignored.

## Precipitating factors

Stage two involves events which then trigger the onset of ME/CFS. Although many psychiatrists do now accept that infections can act as triggers, they are far more sceptical about a possible role for vaccinations, pesticides, toxins or any other immune system stressors. Psychiatrists also maintain that the presence of a viral infection at the very start of ME/CFS is analogous to a broken leg following a road traffic accident. The reasoning is that although the car/virus may have caused someone to break their leg/develop ME/CFS, the course of the fracture/subsequent ME/CFS from then on is dictated by events which have nothing to do with what precipitated it (i.e. the car/virus). In other words, they see no possibility of persisting infection playing a role in maintaining the symptoms of ME/CFS.

## Perpetuating factors

The third stage involves those factors which maintain ill health and disability. As well as questioning the role of persisting infection, psychiatrists have been extremely critical of much of the published research involving abnormalities in muscle and the immune system. They argue that these changes are more likely to be due to inactivity (muscle) or the way in which emotional and psychiatric illness can affect the immune system's response. When it comes to research into various aspects of brain function (e.g. SPECT scans, hypothalamic function studies), they agree that these findings are interesting, but point out that disturbances in blood flow to the brain and changes in the levels of various hormones can also be found in various psychiatric disorders affecting mood.

The main factors which influence outcome in ME/CFS – according to many psychiatrists – are (a) lack of physical fitness (deconditioning), (b) the development of co-existent psychiatric conditions such as depression, anxiety or somatisation and (c) what is termed 'abnormal illness behaviour', meaning unhelpful beliefs or attitudes about the cause of ME/CFS and inappropriate ways of managing the illness.

Some degree of physical unfitness is, I agree, an inevitable consequence whenever a previously fit young adult dramatically reduces their level of physical activity. However, most people with ME/CFS do not (as many psychiatrists believe) spend their days resting in bed. The vast majority remain up and about, trying to do all they can to progressively increase levels of physical and mental activity.

Again, depression certainly occurs in a significant number of people with ME/CFS, but I believe it is nowhere near the figure of over 50 per cent, which is frequently quoted. The disagreement with psychiatrists over the role of depression in ME/CFS has, unfortunately, led to accusations that this is an attempt to stigmatise psychiatric illness. Nothing could be further from the truth -- psychiatric illnesses such as depression are just as real and horrible as ME/CFS, but there is no point in labelling ME/CFS as some form of 'atypical depression' when it is clear that the symptoms, hormonal changes (particularly low cortisol) and response to antidepressant therapy are very different from those seen in depression.

Negative and unhelpful beliefs (or 'attributions' in medical jargon) about both cause and management of ME/CFS are now thought by many psychiatrists to be the major stumbling block on the road to recovery. In particular, they maintain that patients who hold a strong belief in a viral or 'physical' cause for their illness are far less likely to make any improvement. But could it not be that people whose illness follows a clear-cut infection have a very different condition from those whose fatigue is largely psychological or social in origin? There is also a strong acceptance among psychiatrists that a significant number (perhaps 10 per cent or more) of people with ME/CFS, particularly those who have a large number of physical symptoms, are actually suffering from somatisation rather than any form of organic illness. Whilst agreeing that there are people labelled as having ME/CFS whose real cause of ill health is somatisation, I cannot accept the view that anyone who has more than a handful of different symptoms is probably suffering from this condition.

Equally, the idea that you can become well again by reprogramming your psyche and removing 'negative thoughts' about distressing symptoms shows no understanding of ME/CFS whatsoever.

Not surprisingly, psychiatrists tend to recommend management programmes which emphasise psychological rather than physical explanations for the various symptoms. Approaches to treatment may well involve a course of graded aerobic exercises (see pages 209–210) to counteract the effects of physical inactivity/deconditioning. Cognitive behaviour therapy (CBT) is frequently included to challenge 'unhelpful beliefs' about either what caused the illness or how it should be managed (see later). Antidepressant medication may also be prescribed, even though you are not showing any signs of obvious depression.

I wouldn't dispute that these approaches to management can be helpful for *some* people with ME/CFS, especially those who have emotional and/or psychiatric problems and are not approaching lifestyle management in an appropriate manner. I don't, however, believe that they offer a solution for well-motivated people whose ongoing ill health is not being caused by a psychiatric problem – even the psychiatrists acknowledge that *between one-quarter and one-third of those who fulfil [diagnostic] criteria for CFS do not fulfil any criteria for psychiatric disorder'* (reference: Royal Colleges' report into CFS, para 7.6).

Going to see a psychiatrist who understands and takes an open-minded view about ME/CFS can be extremely helpful in some instances. But if you're well motivated, not depressed and taking sensible attitude to changes in lifestyle, then such a referral is unlikely to be of any real value.

The case put forward by psychiatrists can be followed up in further detail by referring to the research papers on pages 470–3 and reading the Royal Colleges' report into CFS (see pages 438–9).

# Recognising Depression in ME/CFS

The big danger for anyone suffering from a depressive illness is not being able to recognise that it is occurring. It may be all too obvious to family and friends, but not to the person whose mental health is steadily deteriorating. So, how can true clinical depression be separated from just feeling 'fed up' as a result of having ME/CFS?

There are a number of distinct features which are characteristic to all depressive illnesses. Three of them – namely fatigue, memory and/or concentration problems and sleep disturbances – are all recognised features of ME/CFS. However, the exercise-induced fatigue and post-exertional malaise experienced by people with ME/CFS aren't usually the sort of symptoms mentioned by people with mild to moderate depression. By comparison, their fatigue tends to be constant in nature and primarily stems from a lack of motivation or interest in doing any sort of physical activity. As far as problems with memory and concentration are concerned (cognitive function), I've already described the results of various complicated types of psychological testing (see pages 155) which indicate that there are some important differences between ME/CFS and depression. Equally, the type of sleep disturbances commonly found in ME/CFS (particularly the alpha wave intrusion) differ from those seen in depression (see page 156).

Other important clinical features which help to differentiate ME/CFS from depression include:

- A very sudden onset to ME/CFS, whereas depression tends to appear in a more gradual fashion.
- The presence of symptoms such as sore throats, enlarged glands, muscle twitchings, joint pain, night sweats and disturbances in temperature control, which are common in ME/CFS but are not at all characteristic of depression.
- The absence of any of the core symptoms of depression (e.g. anhedonia (a total and complete loss of interest in all forms of activity), guilt, worthlessness, hopelessness and lack of motivation) in ME/CFS – unless, of course, the person concerned has also become clinically depressed.
- People with ME/CFS are frustrated by their inability to participate in work, hobbies or family pursuits which involve physical activity, but are still able to enjoy more passive pursuits. By contrast, those with depression usually experience anhedonia.
- Symptoms in ME/CFS are always exacerbated when people push

themselves beyond their limits of physical or mental capability. Depressed people don't usually experience any ill-effects from exercise; on the contrary, they often feel better as a result.

- The highly characteristic phenomenon whereby physical or mental activity produces both physical and mental fatigue in ME/CFS is not a finding that is remarked upon by depressed patients.
- A neurological component to ME/CFS consisting of clumsiness and unsteadiness is not characteristic of straightforward depression.

In addition, there are also a number of important research findings which indicate that the biological abnormalities in ME/CFS are quite different from those found in depression. These include:

- Lowered levels of cortisol in ME/CFS but raised levels in depression (see pages 149–50).
- Enhanced prolactin production following the administration of buspirone is found in ME/CFS but not in depression (see pages 148–9).
- Different types of neurotransmitter abnormalities in ME/CFS compared to depression (see pages 153–4).
- Significant hypoperfusion to the brain stem (as demonstrated by SPECT scans) in ME/CFS but not in depression (see pages 152–3).
- Different types of immunological abnormalities in ME/CFS compared to depression (see pages 132–6).
- The failure of ME/CFS patients – with or without depression – to respond to an SSRI antidepressant (see pages 240–1).

Even so, there are some important mood changes which would strongly suggest that someone with ME/CFS was becoming depressed. A combination of *three or more* of the following, occurring as 'new' symptoms, for more than two weeks, would indicate the need for urgent professional help:

- Recent loss of appetite and/or weight.
- Change in sleep pattern to early morning wakening.
- Sudden loss of interest in sex.
- Apathy and complete withdrawal from social contacts and friends.
- Pessimism, hopelessness and a complete loss of self-confidence.
- Feelings of guilt.
- Inability to enjoy or sustain interest in passive activities.
- Suicidal ideas or plans – which *must* be taken seriously even as an isolated symptom.

# Management of Depression

One of the major problems with any type of depressive illness is the fact that it can create its own vicious circle. It's all too easy to spend vast amounts of time dwelling on your difficulties and negative thoughts – which will only make you feel even more depressed. Although the vast majority of people with true clinical depression gain considerable benefit from the type of drugs I describe later in this chapter, there are also some important self-help measures that can go a long way towards breaking the hold that depression so often creates. These include:

- Not dwelling on what's going on 'in your mind'. Try taking up some new interests which could temporarily remove your thoughts away from being depressed.
- Taking some actions which will make you feel better about yourself. Don't neglect your appearance and leave the house untidy.
- A break from your usual daily routine. Consider taking a short break away from home or a holiday – we all need something to look forward to.
- Not bottling up feelings: if you need to cry or get angry then do so, but preferably in the company of someone who understands your situation.
- Not being afraid to ask for help from friends, family and health professionals – the longer a depressive state goes untreated the worse it becomes.

## *Drug treatment for depression*

Doctors can now choose from a wide variety of effective antidepressant drugs. They all act by increasing levels of various chemicals in the brain (neurotransmitters) which are thought to be depleted in depression. The two most important neurotransmitters are called noradrenaline and serotonin.

Interestingly, there is also some research which suggests that these drugs may act on the body's immune response by affecting natural killer cell function or histamine receptor activity. A further intriguing possibility is that part of their action could be to lower levels of cortisol (a hormone which is frequently raised in depression but reduced in ME/CFS) (see also reference 169).

Benefits from antidepressants don't usually start to occur till several weeks after commencing treatment. The first features to respond are lowered mood, lack of interest, hopelessness and suicidal intentions, followed by low self-esteem, sleep disturbances, and anhedonia; guilt feelings, anger, hostility, lowered sexual drive and anxiety tend to respond more slowly.

Deciding on how long to continue treatment with any antidepressant isn't always easy. People who have responded adequately to a drug should probably be maintained on a full dose for at least six months. Stopping treatment earlier than this results in relapse rates of more than 50 per cent, as compared to around 20 per cent in those who continue with medication. Another six months' treatment is then advisable, especially in anyone who has had more than one previous episode of depression, and the dose should not be significantly reduced unless side-effects are troublesome. If symptoms are still present at the end of a drug treatment phase, then relapse is always likely if the drug is reduced or discontinued.

Withdrawal symptoms, consisting of nausea, headache, sleep disturbances and anxiety, may occur after stopping any antidepressant. Although there is no certain way of preventing this happening, it's always a good idea to *gradually decrease* the dose over a period of about four weeks, particularly if the dosage is high or if the antidepressant has been given for more than two or three months. If withdrawal symptoms do occur, they should be managed by restarting the drug in question and then withdrawing it over a much longer period of time.

All antidepressants are best avoided during pregnancy, if at all possible. The safest drugs to use appear to be the tricyclics, but if another type of antidepressant is already in use, it may be better to carry on with that particular one.

*Tricyclic antidepressants* These are still the most widely used drugs in the management of depression. Some of them are sedating (useful for anyone who has associated anxiety or difficulty with sleep), whereas others have a mild stimulating effect (more appropriate where someone has become withdrawn and lethargic). A few are combined with tranquillisers, but most psychiatrists feel that this is not a good idea, as it makes adjustments in dosage more difficult.

Tricyclic antidepressants can interact with a variety of other drugs, sometimes causing quite serious adverse reactions. The main drugs involved are other types of antidepressant medication (especially MAOIs), epilepsy treatments, adrenaline and some anaesthetics (treatment with a tricyclic drug may need to be stopped before you have a general anaesthetic). Always check with your doctor or pharmacist if in doubt about the advisability of combining other drugs (even some over-the-counter ones) with a tricyclic antidepressant.

## Table 8: Side-effects of tricyclic antidepressants

| | |
|---|---|
| Gastrointestinal | nausea + |
| | dry mouth + |
| | weight gain + |
| | constipation + |
| | stomach upsets |
| | liver function disturbances |
| Heart | fall in blood pressure or fainting |
| | palpitations and irregular heartbeats |
| Nervous system | dizziness + |
| | nervousness |
| | tremor + |
| | exacerbation of epilepsy |
| Miscellaneous | increased sweating |
| | allergic skin reactions |
| | poor diabetes control |
| | blurred vision |
| | difficulty passing urine |
| | impotence or premature ejaculation |

+ = common ones

A common problem with all tricyclic antidepressants is that they have unpleasant side-effects to which people with ME/CFS seem particularly susceptible. These tend to occur almost as soon as treatment is commenced, so it's not unknown for people to stop taking their antidepressant before any benefits start to accrue. Side-effects can often be reduced by commencing treatment with a low dose, which is then *gradually increased* over a few weeks to build up a tolerance. Taking the entire daily dose at night may be helpful, but do check with your doctor first.

Side-effects mean that tricyclic antidepressants must be used cautiously by anyone who has pre-existing heart disease, liver or thyroid problems, as well as conditions such as glaucoma, diabetes and prostate gland enlargement.

At the start of treatment they can produce raised levels of liver enzymes, but these usually return to normal. Even so, they should be used with extreme care in anyone who started their illness with an infection in the liver (hepatitis); regular checks on liver function should be made.

*New tricyclic antidepressants* In the past few years a 'new wave' of tricyclic drugs has been developed (e.g. lofepramine/Gamanil) which appear to have a faster onset of action and fewer side-effects (particularly on the heart) than the 'older' tricyclics. Although these drugs are considerably more expensive than original tricyclics such as amitriptyline, their relative lack of side-effects may make them a more appropriate choice for people with ME/CFS.

## Table 9: Classification of tricyclic antidepressants

| Type of drug | Generic name | Trade name | Comments |
| --- | --- | --- | --- |
| original tricyclics | amitriptyline | Lentizol | sedating + |
| | | Tryptizol | sedating + |
| | clomipramine | Anafranil | non sedating and useful if phobias or obsessional features are present. Must *not* be combined with an SSRI. |
| | dothiepin | Prothiaden | sedating + |
| | doxepin | Sinequan | sedating + |
| | imipramine | Tofranil | non sedating |
| | nortriptyline | Allegron | non sedating |
| | protriptyline | Concordin | non sedating |
| | trimipramine | Surmontil | sedating |
| new tricyclics | lofepramine | Gamanil | non sedating |
| combinations | nortriptyline + phenothiazine | Motipress | |
| | nortriptyline + fluphenazine | Motival | |
| | amitriptyline + phenothiazine | Triptafen | |

*Monoamine oxidase inhibitors (MAOIs)* MAOIs act by inhibiting the action of an enzyme called monoamine oxidase (MAO). This, in turn, raises the levels of three important brain chemical transmitters: noradrenaline, dopamine and serotonin. MAOIs have rarely been given in the past as first-choice antidepressants because their use involves major dietary restrictions which many people find difficulty in complying with. These drugs are, however, useful in cases of depression where fatigue, increased sleep or increased appetite are prominent features.

Common side-effects include dizziness, headache, fluid retention, postural hypotension (fall in blood pressure on standing), sexual problems and sleep disturbances. Parnate is chemically related to amphetamine, so it has a potential for abuse.

The original types of MAOIs – phenelzine (Nardil), isocarboxazid (Marplan) and tranylcypromine (Parnate) – are gradually being phased out by most psychiatrists. Instead, they are increasingly making use of a new type of MAOI called moclobemide (Manerix). This is because moclobemide is much safer to use in cases where an MAOI is thought to be worth trying.

The main problem with older MAOIs is that foods rich in tyramine (e.g. cheese, yeast extracts (Bovril, Oxo, Marmite), alcohol (red wine, beer, sherry), along with cough mixtures, cold cures and some prescription drugs can produce a potentially fatal reaction (involving raised blood pressure, headache, vomiting, palpitations) when taken together with a MAOI.

MAOIs should *never* be combined with selective serotonin reuptake inhibitor (SSRI) antidepressants, and only *very cautiously* with a tricyclic antidepressant (and *never* with clomipramine/Anafranil). After stopping an MAOI, there should always be a two-week gap before starting any other type of antidepressant. In some cases this may need to be even longer (five weeks in the case of fluoxetine/Prozac).

The big advantage with moclobemide (Manerix) is that dietary restrictions involving tyramine-rich foods are far less severe. It's also much easier to change to another antidepressant if necessary. Manerix is a drug which is certainly worth trying in cases of depression which have failed to respond to other drugs, particularly where panic attacks or phobias are present as well. The commonest problems with Manerix include insomnia, headache, dizziness and nausea. Care needs to be taken when it is used together with cimetidine (for stomach complaints) or opiod painkillers (whose effects are increased).

*Selective serotonin reuptake inhibitors (SSRIs)* These are a relatively new group of antidepressant drugs which act by increasing the level of a brain chemical transmitter called serotonin. SSRIs appear to be as effective as the older tricyclics and may cause fewer side-effects. They can be particularly helpful when depression is associated with anxiety or obsessional thoughts.

The most commonly prescribed SSRIs are:

- citalopram (Cipramil)
- fluoxetine (Prozac)
- fluvoxamine (Faverin)
- nefazodone (Dutonin)
- paroxetine (Seroxat)
- sertraline (Lustral)

Commonly reported side-effects include nausea, weight loss (which can be a benefit in some cases), diarrhoea, headaches, sweating, dizziness and visual disturbances. Problems with male sexual function sometimes occur and then persist until treatment is discontinued. A number of other more unusual side-effects have now been noted. These include disorders of body movement and tremor, lowered levels of body sodium (causing drowsiness and confusion), and a dangerous reaction involving tremor, confusion and high fever.

Other problems with individual SSRIs include:

- Minor birth defects associated with fluoxetine (*New England Journal of Medicine*, 1996, 335, 1010–15).
- Liver inflammation with paroxetine (*British Medical Journal*, 1997, 314, 1387).
- Behavioural symptoms, aggression and suicidal intentions following withdrawal of paroxetine (*The Lancet*, 1995, 346, 57).
- Episodes of fainting exacerbated by fluoxetine and sertraline (*The Lancet*, 1997, 349, 1145).
- Blood disorders including bleeding problems, low levels of neutrophils (neutropenia) and aplastic anaemia with fluoxetine (*The Lancet*, 1998, 351, 1031).

SSRIs should *not* be combined with MAOI antidepressants and a gap of at least two weeks (five for Prozac) should be left if a MAOI is being changed to an SSRI.

My personal experience is that *a number of people with ME/CFS are extremely sensitive to SSRI antidepressants*, something which may be related to the fact that research studies have found evidence of abnormalities involving serotonin transmission in ME/CFS (see page 154). Even at half the normal recommended daily starting dose, I know of people who have quickly experienced a range of disturbing side-effects (in particular sweating, diarrhoea and depersonalisation) and have been unable to continue the course. However, I still believe that it can be worth trying an SSRI because some people do seem to gain genuine benefits.

## Other types of antidepressants

- **Amoxapine (Asendis)** has a similar degree of effectiveness and range of side-effects to the tricyclics. It can, occasionally, cause *disturbing neurological side-effects* and what is known as 'the neuroleptic malignant syndrome' (a life-threatening condition with fever, confusion and muscle rigidity).
- **Fluanxol (flupenthixol)** is a drug which has antidepressant properties when used in low doses (1–3mg daily) but is mainly used in the treatment of psychotic illnesses such as schizophrenia. *This is not a drug that I would usually recommend in the case of ME/CFS* although I know that some doctors use it as part of a pain management plan. Side-effects include restlessness, insomnia, dizziness, tremor, visual disturbances, headache and Parkinson's disease-like symptoms.
- **Mianserin (Bolvidon)** affects the level of serotonin in the brain. It is as effective as other types of antidepressants and *can be useful in*

*treating resistant cases of depression* when combined with a tricyclic drug. Drowsiness is the most common side-effect, but its general use tends to be limited because it can cause bone marrow depression. Consequently, regular blood tests should be carried out every four weeks for the first three months and *immediately* if symptoms such as a sore throat occur.

- **Mirtazapine (Zispin)** is the first of a new class of antidepressant drugs. In clinical trials it has been shown to be just as effective as tricyclic antidepressants and faster in onset than drugs such as Prozac. Mirtazapine is *claimed to have a good safety profile* and doesn't appear to produce troublesome interactions when used in combination with other drugs. It works by increasing the level of two important brain chemicals: serotonin and noradrenaline. Side-effects found with SSRI drugs (e.g. nausea, sexual dysfunction, insomnia) generally seem to be avoided, and the only problems so far reported include weight gain and sedation. It remains to be seen whether this is a useful drug for people with ME/CFS who require an antidepressant.

- **Nefazodone (Dutonin)** affects levels of serotonin, and is said to be particularly effective in the *treatment of major depression associated with sleep disturbance*. It is generally quite well tolerated, with dry mouth, nausea and dizziness being the most frequent side-effects. Postural hypotension (lowered blood pressure when standing up) is unusual.

- **Reboxetine (Edronax)** is the first of another new class of antidepressant drugs (noradrenaline reuptake inhibitors/NARIs) which selectively increase the level of noradrenaline in the brain.

  Early results from clinical trials suggest that some *severely depressed patients respond better* to this type of drug than with an SSRI. Side-effects so far reported include insomnia, sweating, dizziness, low blood pressure, paraesthesiae, dry mouth, constipation and urinary problems.

- **Trazodone (Molipaxin)** affects the level of serotonin and is used in cases of *severe depression where anxiety is a prominent feature*. Common side-effects include drowsiness and postural hypotension.

- **Tryptophan (Optimax)** is an essential amino acid, but it also has antidepressant properties. The drug has now been *withdrawn from general use* following the discovery that it can cause a potentially fatal condition known as eosinophilia-myalgia syndrome. It is, however, available for use by hospital specialists for occasional use in severe and intractable cases of depression.

- **Venlafaxine (Efexor)** affects levels of both serotonin and noradrenaline. It may be more effective than other drugs in some cases of severe depression. Side-effects include nausea, sleep disturbances, sexual problems and postural hypotension. One report has suggested that venlafaxine may produce benefits in ME/CFS by reversing immunological disturbances involving natural killer cell activity (reference 386).

- **Viloxazine (Vivalan)** is an antidepressant which is chemically related to the beta-blocker group of drugs (see pages 185–6). It is generally well tolerated, although nausea and vomiting can sometimes be troublesome.

## Clinical trials involving antidepressants in ME/CFS

A small number of placebo-controlled trials have been carried out to assess the possible value of antidepressant drugs in ME/CFS. Relevant findings are summarised below:

*Tricyclics* Although there is general agreement that a low dose of a sedating tricyclic antidepressant can be of value in relieving muscle pain and insomnia, no clinical trials have been carried out.

*MAOIs* A placebo-controlled trial using a low dose (= 15mg per day) of *phenelzine (Nardil)* was carried out in America (reference 394). Nine patients in each group were assessed after six weeks' treatment. Some of those receiving phenelzine reported a 'significant pattern of improvement', but a number had to drop out because of unpleasant side-effects.

An open study (i.e. no control group present) using up to 600mg of moclobemide (Manerix) per day for up to six weeks has been carried out in the UK (reference 410). Three patients dropped out because of adverse side-effects but otherwise these were minimal. Overall, there was a small reduction in levels of fatigue and anxiety. The greatest improvement occurred in patients with a co-existent depression, 50 per cent of whom rated themselves to be 'much better' after six weeks.

Limited evidence of benefit was observed in a large double-blind placebo-controlled trial in Australia using moclobemide (reference 388). An improvement in the subjective sense of energy was not associated with any alteration in mood.

*SSRIs* A placebo-controlled trial of fluoxetine (Prozac) has been carried out in the Netherlands (reference 407). This involved 44 ME/CFS patients with depression and 52 patients with no evidence of depression. After eight weeks' treatment (dose = 20mg/day) it was found that fluoxetine had 'no beneficial effect on any symptom associated with CFS' (including depression). Fifteen per cent of those being treated with fluoxetine had to withdraw from the trial because of side-effects (common ones being tremor and increased sweating). The failure of fluoxetine to even improve depressive symptoms suggests that this ME/CFS subgroup may have chemical changes in the brain which are not quite the same as those found in other types of depression.

A further trial involved the use of Prozac and graded exercise (reference 542). Those taking Prozac reported a modest reduction in their depressive symptoms, but this was not sustained. Graded exercise produced only limited improvements with a very high dropout rate (14 out of 33 patients).

An uncontrolled trial of sertraline (Lustral) has been carried out by Professor Behan's group in Glasgow (reference 375). This involved 79 patients with ME/CFS, none of whom had any symptoms of major depression. Sixty-five per cent of those who completed the trial reported benefits (particularly regarding levels of fatigue, muscle pain and sleep disturbance). Fifteen per cent complained of side-effects, mainly nausea, diarrhoea and impaired sexual function. The average time for a positive response to occur was 53 days.

## Alternative and complementary approaches

Many people with mild forms of depression or anxiety obtain a degree of relief from alternative therapies such as aromatherapy, massage, meditation or relaxation. The use of alternative therapies in more severe forms of mental illness is much more controversial, and hypnosis can certainly exacerbate depression, so such measures need to be used carefully. The mental health charity MIND publishes a useful booklet on alternative therapies (see end of this chapter).

One alternative therapy which is currently receiving a great deal of attention amongst psychiatrists is the use of a herbal medicine known as *Hypericum perforatum* (St John's Wort). Extracts from the herb have been frequently used in Germany for the treatment of depression, and a *British Medical Journal* review (reference 483) of all the current evidence concluded that it was more effective than a placebo in the treatment of mild to moderate depression.

At present, there is no satisfactory explanation as to why hypericum works in depression. One possibility is that it contains an ingredient called hypericin, which inhibits an enzyme called monamine oxidase. This, in turn, increases the levels of chemical transmitters in the brain which are depleted in depression. However, hypericum probably contains a number of other active ingredients which have yet to be identified.

No serious drug interactions have been reported with hypericum and the incidence of side-effects (around 20 per cent) is much lower than seen with conventional antidepressant drugs (around 60 per cent). The most commonly reported ones are stomach upsets, allergic reactions and fatigue (obviously relevant to ME/CFS).

In the UK, hypericum is available in a low-dose tablet form called Kira (manufactured by Lichtwer Pharmaceuticals). The recommended daily dose in Germany is up to 900mg of hypericum extract per day. As with ordinary antidepressants, it appears that the herb needs to be taken for several weeks before any possible benefits occur. This herbal remedy is certainly worthy of further scientific assessment. It is worth a try if you need to take an antidepressant and cannot cope with the side-effects from orthodox drugs.

## Psychologically based treatments

Antidepressants are undoubtedly a quick, easy and effective way of treating many types of depressive illness. However, they cannot be used in isolation, especially in the case of ME/CFS, where several different factors may be contributing to the development of depression, and they won't have any effect on problems with the DSS, doctors or employers – all of which can become very depressing! Neither can they help to resolve a family or financial crisis. If practical difficulties exist and remain unresolved, there is no way that antidepressant drugs are going to be effective on their own.

In addition to drugs, some doctors make use of various kinds of 'talking treatments' or psychotherapy. With a GP, this is unlikely to be anything deeper than problem-solving counselling, which gives the depressed patient an opportunity to talk through their difficulties, fears or frustrations. Other forms of counselling can be much more intense and prolonged, especially when they involve coming to terms with distressing events in the past which are still having a negative impact on your life. Building up a good relationship with a professional counsellor is essential if such an approach is going to be successful.

Psychiatrists are more likely to employ a technique known as cognitive behaviour therapy (CBT).

### Cognitive behaviour therapy (CBT)

CBT is a relatively new and fashionable form of short-term psychotherapy. It is claimed to be effective across a wide range of common psychiatric disorders, along with medical conditions where there may be significant psychological problems. Examples of both include depression, phobias, panic attacks, insomnia, compulsive forms of behaviour and irritable bowel syndrome. CBT can be used alone or in combination with drugs such as antidepressants – the decision is based on the severity and nature of the symptoms being treated.

The underlying theory behind CBT is that it deals with 'here and now' problems rather than delving into underlying conflicts, which may even date right back to childhood. Cognitions describe the way in which we interpret events, thoughts and attitudes to everyday life. By changing (and even challenging) the way in which someone thinks about their circumstances, the aim of CBT is to alter what is known in psychiatric jargon as 'self-defeating beliefs' about illness/disability and the various restrictions – both physical and mental – which they may impose on someone's normal way of life.

CBT also aims to encourage various practical coping strategies to help alleviate fears or anxieties about performing physical or mental tasks. Consequently, a gradual re-exposure to physical activity, without the premature cessation due to fatigue or pain, may well form a key part to the exercise component of a CBT rehabilitation programme. A course of CBT is likely to include therapist and patient agreeing on a list of specific daily or weekly targets covering a wide range of mental and physical activities (e.g. walking, reading, visiting the shops, swimming, returning to some form of part-time work). Particular attention will be paid to sleep routines, and this may involve rising at a specific time each morning, reducing the amount of time spent in bed or resting during the day and retiring to bed later in the evening.

A course of CBT is likely to consist of up to 15 regular hourly sessions at weekly or fortnightly intervals with a hospital-based cognitive behaviour therapist. You'll be asked to monitor your week-by-week progress by keeping a diary with details of progress and how you feel. This will be reviewed at each clinic attendance.

The CBT approach is clearly based on the assumption that symptoms and disability in ME/CFS are far more likely to be due to the psychosocial model of this illness (as already described on pages 227–31) than any underlying organic cause. It may, therefore, be of benefit to people with chronic fatigue who clearly have these type of problems.

Results from a number of clinical trials using CBT in ME/CFS have now been published in the medical journals. Relevant findings include:

- The first UK trial (reference 450) produced some positive results, but was criticised for its high dropout rate, the lack of any control group and no independent assessment of outcome. The design failed to permit the effects of concurrent antidepressant therapy to be satisfactorily distinguished from purely psychological treatments.
- A large Australian trial (reference 454) concluded that a CBT 'rehabilitation programme' conducted in an out-patient setting provided no more benefit in global well-being, physical capacity or functional status than attendance at an ordinary medical clinic.
- An American study (reference 453) concluded that a small subgroup of ME/CFS patients, with a clear depressive component to their illness, might benefit from a course of CBT.

- A second UK trial carried out in Oxford (reference 455) divided a group of 60 ME/CFS patients into 30 receiving CBT and 30 who were given 'no further explanation or advice' about their illness – apart from being advised to increase their level of activity (described as 'medical care alone'). Twenty-two out of the 30 receiving CBT achieved what was described as a 'satisfactory outcome' – a change in their Karnofsky score (a similar type of disability assessment to the one described on page 117) of more than 10 points, 12 months later. Only eight of the 30 receiving 'medical care alone' achieved a similar degree of improvement. Deterioration was reported in four of the CBT group and three of the control group. Of particular interest was the fact that *a significant number of patients in both groups were suffering from a depressive, anxiety or somatisation disorder.* The authors failed to provide any information on which factors might have helped to predict a favourable outcome.

- The most recent UK trial of CBT, carried out at King's College Hospital in London (reference 451), involved 60 ME/CFS patients who were given either 13 sessions of CBT (graded exercise and what was termed 'cognitive restructuring') or muscle relaxation therapy. The researchers claimed that 70 per cent of those who completed the CBT programme achieved 'good outcomes' compared to only 19 per cent in the relaxation group.

- The only study so far carried out in primary care involved general practitioners who treated a group of patients with either a specific behaviour management programme or normal management guidelines for a period of one year. At the end of the study there was little difference in outcome (as measured by levels of fatigue, functioning or mental health) between the two groups (reference: *GP* magazine, 10 April 1998, page 39).

My conclusions about the value of CBT is that it may be a useful form of therapy for a subgroup of people with ME/CFS who are not managing their lifestyle readjustment in an appropriate manner (and this may mean doing too much or doing too little) or who have unhelpful rigid beliefs about the cause(s) of their illness and how this affects their management. It may also be of help to those with co-existent depression or those who are experiencing considerable difficulties in coping socially or psychologically.

If you feel that CBT could be of benefit to you, then this is a matter which needs to be discussed with your GP. Referral can then be made to a specialist unit which has therapists with the necessary expertise. For people with ME/CFS who are coping perfectly well with their lifestyle management and have no psychiatric or emotional problems, I don't believe that CBT has any benefits to offer. I am also aware of disturbing instances where inappropriate (and sometimes quite harmful advice) from a therapist has had adverse effects, so do make sure that you are referred to someone (preferably within the NHS) who fully understands this illness.

# Other Psychiatric and Emotional Problems

Relationship difficulties, which may be directly or indirectly attributed to ME/CFS, can often be helped by talking them through with an experienced counsellor at Relate (see Useful Addresses, page 430). Equally, the ME Association's Listening Ear Service has volunteers available each evening who are willing to talk in confidence and give whatever support they can.

Unfortunately, for a small group of people with ME/CFS, their depression and despair at ever making any improvement becomes severe, a feeling of total worthlessness develops, even to the point of considering suicide. At this point, professional help is essential, possibly involving a short spell in hospital during such a 'crisis period'.

If you ever start feeling this low, and there doesn't seem to be anyone you can turn to, then do phone the Samaritans (in the phone book or see Useful Addresses, page 425). Trained volunteers are available 24 hours a day to provide confidential help and advice (see also pages 121–22).

## *Anxiety*

Anxiety is a common and quite normal response to any stressful situation. Many public performers have palpitations as they go on stage and anyone's pulse rate will rapidly rise if, for example, they have a near miss in traffic. It's only when these symptoms become commonplace and out of all proportion to whatever an individual feels worried about, that a state of anxiety exists.

As already mentioned, differentiating some of the symptoms of anxiety from those of ME/CFS may not be easy, even for an experienced doctor, and in those who are naturally prone to anxiety there may be a combination of both.

### Common symptoms of anxiety
*Psychological:*
    Irritability and restlessness; difficulty getting to sleep
    Poor concentration
    Increased sensitivity to noise
*Physical:*
    Overactive autonomic nerves:

palpitations, sweating, diarrhoea, frequently passing urine,
impotence
From overbreathing (hyperventilation):
dizziness, paraesthesiae ('pins and needles'), fainting
From muscle spasm:
headaches, aches/tension in the neck or back

Some doctors are still far too keen on immediately treating anyone who
has anxiety with a benzodiazepine tranquilliser such as diazepam
(Valium). These drugs act by dampening down nervous activity in the
brain and in my experience at least one-third of all long-term ME/CFS
patients have been given a tranquilliser to try at some stage in their illness.

On the whole, these drugs should be avoided in ME/CFS as they
have *no effect whatsoever* on the underlying disease process, and as they
'numb the mind' still further and exacerbate fatigue, they may well make
things worse. The only time to consider using them is for a very short
period (i.e. days, not weeks or months) to deal with an acutely stressful
event. Using them to blot out stress or anxiety is *not* a solution in
ME/CFS and can lead to the problem of long-term dependence.

There are still far too many people with ME/CFS taking tranquillisers on a long-term basis, and in most cases this isn't helping them to
recover. Once you've taken a tranquilliser for more than a few weeks, it's
hard to stop, as many people then experience a withdrawal syndrome,
very similar to the problems seen with other drugs such as alcohol.
Many of the original symptoms of anxiety return as soon as there's no
trace of the tranquilliser left in the body, and some of the withdrawal feelings can be very disturbing and frightening, such as increased sensitivity to noise, feelings of depersonalisation or being 'unreal', and
occasionally hallucinations or delusions. These feelings can persist for
weeks or months, becoming quite unbearable, so it's tempting for both
doctor and patient to just restart the drug again.

Anyone with ME/CFS who is taking long-term tranquillisers should
seriously consider taking steps to 'come off', but as a withdrawal process
isn't easy, it must be done under medical supervision. If your general
practitioner isn't keen to help, it may be necessary to ask for advice from
a psychiatrist. Self-help groups such as Panic/No Panic (see Useful
Addresses, page 425) provide useful counselling, and can put you in
touch with someone locally who has been through the withdrawal
process. The dose must be reduced *very slowly* – over a period of four to
12 weeks, sometimes longer – to lessen any rebound anxiety taking
place. Using one of the beta-blocking drugs during this withdrawal
period can help to reduce some of these unpleasant rebound anxiety
symptoms.

If drug treatment is really thought to be necessary with anxiety – especially if there are a lot of symptoms connected with autonomic over-activity – one of the beta-blocking drugs may be helpful, but the exact one should be chosen with care (see pages 185–6).

Buspar (buspirone) is a new type of drug which is claimed to be just as effective as benzodiazepines in relieving anxiety, but without impairing mental functioning or causing dependence. Exactly how it acts on the brain remains uncertain, but there don't appear to be any muscle relaxant or sleep-inducing effects. Although side-effects are claimed to be fewer than seen with conventional tranquillisers, Buspar can produce headaches, dizziness, nausea, light-headedness, fatigue and nervousness. As with many of the antidepressant drugs, it usually takes several weeks before any benefit accrues.

At present, the role of Buspar in the management of anxiety associated with ME/CFS seems very limited. In view of the experiments conducted with this drug on hormonal control (see pages 148–9), it would appear that people with ME/CFS may be more susceptible, so I would suggest that its use is still viewed with caution.

A much better approach to managing stress and anxiety is by self-help relaxation techniques, by which you learn how to relax both body and mind – what some people refer to as their 'instant dose of Valium'. You can discover how to do this from reading, learning from a cassette tape or going to a relaxation class, but it does have to be carried out on a regular basis to be effective. Relaxation techniques can also be of help when you have difficulty in going off to sleep.

## A General Relaxation Technique

- Set aside a quiet period each day, preferably for about 20 minutes or so, when you know you're not going to be disturbed.
- Sit comfortably in your favourite chair, or lie down quietly on the bed. Take the phone off the hook to prevent any interruptions.
- Close your eyes, relax and take in slow deep breaths at a regular pace. Don't overbreathe though!
- Allow your mind to wander on to some pleasant thought, sound or experience – whatever you feel appropriate. Listening to some tranquil music at the same time can be very soothing.
- **For muscular tension** This can be particularly useful for dealing with areas of muscular tension in the neck, shoulders, etc, when associated with stress. However, it's *not advisable* to follow this part of the method for muscles which are painful and weak.
- Learning to tense an area of muscle to the point of maximum tension

and then having to relax it can be very beneficial. First, make a firm clenched fist and notice the feeling of tension in the area. Then, let the fist suddenly relax and see how a warm feeling follows – indicating that it's now become fully relaxed. This process can be repeated in other 'trouble spots' around the body where muscle spasm/ tension seems to be a problem, using the same principle of artificially producing tension followed by sudden relaxation.

By the end of the session you should be feeling totally relaxed, and your breathing should be slow and regular. Have a few minutes doing nothing and then get up again.

If you're using these techniques to help you get off to sleep at night, they can be carried out shortly before retiring.

Relaxation tape cassettes can be obtained from either the British Holistic Medical Association, Relaxation for Living or Lifeskills (see Useful Addresses). The latter organisation produce:

- *Relax – And Enjoy It!* – a comprehensive course in deep, quick relaxation techniques.
- *Control Your Tension* – teaches the skills of anxiety management and is particularly useful where anxiety is associated with phobias.

Anyone with anxiety problems may also find other alternative approaches such as yoga or meditation helpful (see Alternative and Complementary Approaches, pages 287 and 293).

## Panic attacks

For anyone who is already experiencing anxiety, panic attacks can be a further incapacitating problem. These attacks are brought on by fear, which is out of all proportion to the stressful situation.

Fears of going into public places or crowds of people in the course of using public transport or shopping in a busy supermarket are common causes. In some severe cases an attack can be caused simply by the fear of going out of the house.

To appreciate what such an attack is like, imagine how it feels when you've just stepped off the kerb and nearly been knocked down by a bus – a panic attack produces exactly the same sort of symptoms, but not for just a few seconds. The incapacity can last for up to half an hour. During such an attack a victim will feel unreal and start to tremble or shake. This is invariably accompanied by palpitations, chest pains and shortness of breath – even a feeling of choking. Rapid overbreathing (hyperventilation) washes out carbon dioxide from the blood and causes a sensation of pins and needles (paraesthesiae) in the skin. Other common symptoms include dizziness, sweating or flushing. Once an attack is over the victim feels thoroughly exhausted and apprehensive.

Successful treatment of panic attacks often requires expert profes-sional help. Benzodiazepine-type tranquillisers are generally best avoided, but a fast-acting tranquilliser, such as alprazolam/Xanax, can be useful if symptoms are severe. Tricyclic antidepressants and SSRIs (both of which can exacerbate symptoms of anxiety to begin with), at lower doses than are used to treat depression, have also been shown to be helpful in treating panic attacks.

Drug treatment, however, won't succeed by itself, and sufferers have to learn to control their bodies, especially the overbreathing during an attack. The relaxation techniques already described to help anxiety may be useful here, and a further approach known as behaviour therapy can also be tried.

Behaviour therapy involves people being gradually exposed to the sort of situations they fear. In the case of crowds and open spaces, this may first involve just looking at pictures and thinking about the situa-tions for short periods. This is then followed by short trips outside the house in the company of a friend or counsellor, until eventually the per-son feels confident enough to confront what they fear most. This is a slow, time-consuming approach, which requires practical assistance from an experienced therapist, but can be very effective in reducing phobic anxiety. Further self-help advice can be obtained from Panic/No Panic (see Useful Addresses, page 425).

## Hyperventilation

Hyperventilation, or chronic overbreathing, is frequently associated with anxiety and panic attacks.

One group of specialists has consistently maintained that the major-ity of people with ME/CFS also hyperventilate (references 458, 460 and 461). These claims were widely reported in the media and resulted in further adverse publicity for ME/CFS, one particularly bad example being 'Yuppie flu is all in the mind' (*Sunday Times*, 17 July 1988).

The theory is that following an initial stressful event, such as a viral infection, the body reacts by chronically overbreathing (hyperventilat-ing), even though both patient and doctor may be completely unaware that this is happening. The result is that too much carbon dioxide is washed out from the lungs alongside a rise in the level of stress hormone adrenaline. A vicious circle quickly develops with changes in blood chemistry causing symptoms due to overexcitability of the nerves (pal-pitations, dizziness, pins and needles) and constriction of the blood ves-sels (cold extremities). Other common symptoms include shortness of breath, tremors, chest pains, muscle weakness and feelings of unreality.

Chronic borderline hyperventilation is not easy to diagnosis, even using some of the most sophisticated lung function tests which are now available. One very simple test for hyperventilation is to lie down, place one hand on your stomach and the other on your chest. If you are hyperventilating, the upper hand on the chest should be moving far quicker than the lower one.

As far as ME/CFS is concerned, an association with hyperventilation has not been confirmed by any other research group. Dr David McCluskey from Belfast, in a *British Medical Journal* paper (reference 248) concluded that 'Patients with chronic fatigue syndrome do not hyperventilate' and researchers from King's College Hospital in London found that 'there is only a weak association between hyperventilation and CFS.' When present, hyperventilation is usually related to known causes of respiratory stimulation such as asthma or panic (reference 462). Researchers from the Netherlands have also concluded that 'hyperventilation in CFS should probably be regarded as an epiphenomenon'* (reference 457).

The case for hyperventilation being the main cause of ME/CFS was further discredited when one of its advocates attempted to sue a Channel 4 television programme which had used undercover filming to examine the way in which the doctor in question was diagnosing hyperventilation. Having admitted in the High Court that his research papers contained serious defects, the doctor concerned withdrew his action and agreed to pay over £750,000 in costs to Channel 4 (reference: *British Medical Journal*, 1997, 314, 1501).

Where hyperventilation is confirmed, the principal treatment involves breathing exercises which are taught by a physiotherapist. Drugs have very little role in the management of this disorder, although some doctors use a controversial regime which involves initial sedation with large doses of tranquillisers such as Valium. This approach has come in for much criticism because of the serious risk of dependency.

My view is that hyperventilation syndrome certainly exists and is probably under-diagnosed by doctors. I suspect that it is the true cause of ill health for a *small number* of people who have been wrongly labelled as having ME/CFS. However, *hyperventilation is not the cause of ME/CFS, and inappropriate treatment with drugs such as Valium could end up doing far more harm than good.*

If you require further advice or information on any aspect of mental health, I would suggest contacting either MIND or the education depart-

---

* A secondary symptom, which is neither the cause nor the result of the main condition.

ment at the Royal College of Psychiatrists (see Useful Addresses, page 425). They both provide useful leaflets; MIND acts as a pressure group on behalf of all people with mental health problems.

## Further Reading

The mental health charity MIND (see Useful Addresses, page 424) produces a large number of publications on all aspects of mental health. Among the most useful are:

Booklets in the *Understanding* . . . series, including anxiety, depression, phobias and obsessions, seasonal affective disorder, and talking treatments.
Their *How to* . . . series contains advice on coping with loneliness, panic attacks, relationship breakdown and suicidal thoughts.
Their *Making Sense of Treatments and Drugs* series, which includes booklets on antidepressants and tranquillisers.
*The A–Z of Complementary and Alternative Therapies* – a useful guide to those which may or may not be helpful in mental illness.
*MIND Guide to Managing Stress* – how to cope with the symptoms of stress.
*Tranquillisers: The MIND Guide to Where to Get Help* – a national directory of services for people who want to come off tranquillisers.

Other useful publications on mental health problems include:

*Anxiety, Phobias and Panic Attacks* by Elaine Sheehan (Element Books) – provides practical advice on ways to keep anxiety under control and the various sources of help available.
*Depression: The Way Out of your Prison* by Dorothy Rowe (Routledge) – a radical approach to overcoming depression.
*Stress and Relaxation* by Jane Madders (Macdonald Optima) – a self-help guide to coping with stress and nervous tension.

The Royal College of Psychiatrists (see Useful Addresses, page 425) also has publications on all aspects of mental health.

# Alternative and Complementary Approaches to the Management of ME/CFS

In view of conventional medicine's current inability to provide any really effective treatment for ME/CFS, it is hardly surprising that many people decide to opt for alternative approaches. Whilst remaining open-minded about alternative medicine, I feel that I can only recommend those therapies which seem to offer genuine benefit and advise extreme caution about many of the others.

You may also find that your GP has strong opinions about alternative therapies. Some are well informed and supportive, whereas others are hostile and negative. Whatever view your own doctor takes, it is always a good idea to discuss any specific treatment before going ahead, especially if this involves taking drugs, unusual supplements or having injections.

Many alternative practitioners now like to use the term 'complementary medicine' because they would prefer working with your own doctor rather than in isolation. Unfortunately, this type of co-operation is not always made easy when exaggerated and unsubstantiated claims are made by some alternative practitioners and 'pill pushing' manufacturers about 'breakthrough' treatments. There are no miracle cures for this illness.

Furthermore, do remember that so-called 'natural medicines' are not always harmless, as the scandal with germanium illustrated. This expensive mineral supplement was successfully targetted at people with ME/CFS and AIDS during 1989 with claims that it could 'boost the immune system'. Germanium turned out to be harmful to the kidneys and muscle (reference: *Clinical Nephrology*, 1988, 30, 341–5), and the Department of Health had to withdraw it from sale.

Many people with ME/CFS undoubtedly find alternative approaches to be helpful, but exactly why remains open to debate. It may, of course, be due to the fact that the therapy is beneficial. However, what could be just as important is the fact that, at last, you are doing something positive to improve your health. Alternative treatments aren't generally subjected to the same type of rigorously controlled trials as conventional drugs, so it is difficult to rule out a placebo effect as well. The fact that you are taking, and paying for, something which you've been told will help, can have a very positive effect. It is also quite likely that the sympathetic and optimistic approach of most alternative practitioners may be having an equal or even more powerful effect than their therapy!

So, if you're going to experiment with alternative medicine, what sort of questions should you be asking before going ahead?

- Is the therapist recommended and do they have any worthwhile qualifications? This sort of information is not always easy for a lay person to evaluate so long as dubious diplomas are issued from unrecognised Colleges and Institutes.
- How much is a course of treatment going to cost? Some forms of therapy, especially from private medical clinics, can be very expensive. Bills of hundreds, even thousands, of pounds are not unknown.
- Does the treatment have any possible adverse effects? (Particularly important in allergy treatments.)
- How is the treatment supposed to work? Has it been subjected to any form of objective and impartial trial? Very few have. Remember that there are many different views as to 'what is going wrong' in ME/CFS amongst alternative therapists.
- Will the therapist be informing your own GP about their findings and treatment?
- Does the therapist have any professional indemnity insurance?

It is obviously not possible to describe all the different types of alternative therapies currently available. However, the following is an A–Z guide through some of the most popular amongst people with ME/CFS.

## Acupuncture

Acupuncture is a traditional Chinese technique which involves the insertion of very fine needles into specific points of the body – the acupuncture points.

The Chinese view of health and disease differs markedly from that of conventional Western medicine. They feel that our bodies are in a state of flux between what they refer to as yin (passivity) and yang (activity). The healthy body is 'in balance', but the unhealthy body is 'out of balance' between these two vital forces. The aim of acupuncture is to restore balance, and so return the body to normal.

An essential part of Chinese philosophy is that energy (*qi*) flows through the body in channels, each channel corresponding to one of the vital organs such as the heart, brain, etc. If there is disease present in that part of the body, then energy flow in that specific channel is disrupted. By selecting sites where these channels of energy pass, and applying an acupuncture needle, the aim is to correct any dysfunction in energy flow. These channels don't exist in terms of conventional anatomy. They can't be found at dissection, like nerves or blood vessels, and this is why conventional medicine finds this theory hard to understand.

The acupuncturist decides which parts of the body are unhealthy by first carrying out a clinical examination, not dissimilar to a normal doctor. Particular attention is paid to the pulse and the state of the tongue – considered to be key indicators of health by the Chinese.

## Can acupuncture help ME/CFS?

Conventional medicine accepts that part of the therapeutic effect of acupuncture involves the release of morphine-like substances (endorphins) in the body, which is why it can be effective in pain relief and even anaesthesia. There is also the suggestion that acupuncture needles are capable of stimulating tiny nerve fibres which send messages back to the brain to control activity in other pain relief centres. Perhaps acupuncture might be a good alternative for someone with ME/CFS who requires an anaesthetic during pregnancy.

Anyone who has particular problems with localised bone or muscle pain which is unrelieved by ordinary painkillers might well consider making use of this approach. Some people find that electroacupuncture is particularly effective in relieving pain and one properly controlled trial of its use in fibromyalgia (reference 463) supports this view.

Another effect of acupuncture is on the autonomic nervous system. Anyone experiencing symptoms of autonomic overactivity (see pages 50–4) such as palpitations might find acupuncture worth trying. Acupressure at the wrist may also help in the control of sickness.

Acupuncture can't 'cure' something like ME/CFS, but it can help with some symptoms. In China, acupuncture is a true form of complementary medicine, with acupuncturists working alongside colleagues in hospitals and clinics who practise traditional forms of medicine. Acupuncture usually needs to be given in a course of treatments if it's going to have any effect; you won't gain benefit from a one-off treatment. Benefits may not start to occur for several weeks or months, and further treatment may be necessary at a later date.

This therapy can now be obtained on the NHS, but with difficulty. A few general practitioners have become interested and use it on their patients, but they are still few in number, and there's not much financial incentive for them to do it. Some NHS pain clinics now use acupuncture as part of a multidisciplinary approach.

For patients, though, it means going privately. For those who do, make sure that you find a reputable practitioner because side-effects have been reported. Fortunately, they appear to be quite rare and the more serious ones are entirely preventable. Relatively minor ones include fainting during treatment, vomiting and increased pain. Serious side-effects include the transmission of infections such as hepatitis B and HIV (through the use of unsterilised equipment) and a punctured lung (reference 464).

For details of how to find a reputable acupuncturist see Useful Addresses, pages 407–8.

## Alexander Technique

This aims to improve all aspects of general health by paying particular attention to posture and good breathing. The technique has to be learned by practical instruction from a teacher who has undertaken a three-year training course. An introductory session allows you to experience the process at first hand and then to ask any questions. For further details on how to find a therapist see Useful Addresses, page 408.

## Algae

Blue-green algae supplements are made from a layer of algae which grows on the surface of Lake Klamath in the American state of Oregon. This new fashionable 'superfood' is claimed to be full of nutrients which increase vitality and memory, as well as being useful in the treatment of a wide range of medical disorders.

There is very little scientific evidence to support any of these claims and none at all to show that algae supplements are helpful for people with ME/CFS. Of far greater concern is the fact that some of these algae supplements contain small amounts of harmful toxins which can damage both the liver and nervous system (reference: *Health Which*, October 1997, 166–7).

Orthodox medicines have to pass extremely strict assessments of safety, efficacy and quality control, but food supplements are largely exempt from such procedures. *The presence of these toxins means that this is one of a large number of alternative supplements that I would not recommend using.*

## Allergies

These are included in this chapter on alternative approaches because there is no real evidence to support the view that ME/CFS is an 'allergic disease' like asthma or hayfever. Although some people do go on to develop secondary allergies as part of their illness (and I've developed mild hayfever since becoming ill), around 15 per cent of the population suffer from allergies, so any association with ME/CFS could just be pure coincidence. However, research into this possible association indicates that there does seem to be an increased incidence of skin sensitivity to a variety of common allergens (reference 467) and some people with ME/CFS have raised levels of IgE, an antibody found in the blood that can be associated with allergic responses (reference 465). This latter study also found that lymphocytes (white blood cells) from people with ME/CFS reacted more strongly than normal when exposed to allergens.

A number of interesting suggestions have been put forward as to why allergies might be more common in ME/CFS. One possibility is that people with this illness have an immune system which reacts excessively to all kinds of challenges, not just allergic ones. One part of this abnormal response might be the actual development of ME/CFS following exposure to an infection, vaccination or toxin. The second part of the immune system response might then be the development of new allergies or the exacerbation of pre-existing ones. Another intriguing idea is that lowered levels of the stress hormone cortisol (see pages 149–50) could help to trigger allergic reactions (cortisol is used as a treatment for allergic disorders because it dampens down the body's normal immune responses).

Whatever the true cause and actual incidence of allergies in ME/CFS, it is worrying to find that people who have no evidence of true allergic reactions are spending vast amounts of money at private allergy clinics trying to find out what they are allergic to.

Of all the alternative approaches to the management of ME/CFS, allergies are probably the most confusing. Allergy, in medical terms, is simply a way of describing an over-enthusiastic response by the immune system to factors which most people would regard as harmless. The allergic symptoms then occur whenever a sensitive (allergic) patient comes in contact with that substance – the allergen. A comprehensive list of all known allergens would be endless, but many of them are normal everyday constituents of our environment: pollens, furs, foods and drugs. Some truly allergic patients have allergies which change in the course of time. So, identifying which particular allergen(s) are involved in any one individual isn't always easy.

Symptoms result from inflammatory responses taking place in different parts of the body. Inhaled allergens can cause asthma, chemicals on the skin can cause eczema and foods can produce varied symptoms: abdominal pain, changes in bowel habit, etc. When an allergic patient comes into contact with an allergen, the immune system responds by releasing chemicals such as histamine which cause an immediate inflammatory response in the particular target tissue.

Both doctors and patients experience a considerable degree of confusion and misunderstanding over the distinction between allergy and sensitivity, and this might be particularly relevant in the case of ME/CFS to foods. Certainly, some people have a true allergic response to certain foods – especially milk and dairy products, wheat and nuts – but just because a certain food makes you feel unwell doesn't mean that you're allergic to it. Caffeine, for example, in coffee will quickly upset some people due to its direct effect on the nervous system, causing palpitations, tremor and a headache. But this is a direct effect of the caffeine – there is no allergic response taking place.

Many people seem to suffer from digestive problems once they've developed ME/CFS, but if an infection has disturbed the lining mucosa of the bowel wall, this could be causing a type of food sensitivity right there in the gut, as opposed to a more generalised type of allergic reaction.

Whatever mechanisms are involved – allergic or increased sensitivity – the most reliable way of detecting a 'culprit' food is by an exclusion diet, followed by challenge with the suspected food, but this must be done with the help of a doctor or dietician. This type of diet involves a strict regime of what are known as 'non-allergic foods' for a week or so. These could consist of spring water, a source of protein such as lamb and a source of carbohydrate such as rice. Foods can then be slowly introduced in groups (e.g. wheat products) to see which one(s) produce a recurrence of symptoms. If no significant improvement has occurred at the end of the strict exclusion, it would seem that food sensitivity or allergy is *not* the cause of the problem.

## Allergy testing

Many alternative therapists believe that a whole range of allergies can be quickly and simply diagnosed by 'allergy tests', but this isn't so. Conventional medicine tends to rely on the result of skin (provocation) tests and blood tests. These can be obtained on the NHS by referral to an allergy clinic at one of the larger district general hospitals.

**Skin tests** A small amount of very dilute allergen is pricked into the skin, and the inflammatory response – due to histamine release – measured. This type of testing is particularly useful for inhaled allergens causing asthma and for skin eczema, but only for a few food allergies (e.g. egg). For the majority of foods it's probably of little value as they don't tend to produce this type of response in such a short time.

**Blood tests** These measure the levels of specific antibodies which allergic patients make in response to specific allergens. (This is known as the RAST test – standing for Radio Allego Sorbant Test.) These results again have to be carefully interpreted, as not all foods produce this type of response.

A wide variety of other allergy tests are now available, but conventional allergists regard the majority of them as being of dubious value; consequently, they are seldom available on the NHS. Even so, I know of desperate people who have spent hundreds, even thousands of pounds searching for 'hidden allergies', using techniques which are reducing savings rather than suffering.

At one end of the spectrum are perfectly respectable private doctors and clinics. At the other are naïve amateurs and charlatans with no recognised qualifications operating via adverts in various health magazines. Their advice ranges from the bizarre to the positively harmful.

Unfortunately, many people still believe, with some justification, that orthodox medicine regards allergy as a 'no go area'. Hence the current boom in private and alternative services of which your own GP probably has very little working knowledge. Here is a brief guide to the most popular forms of allergy tests used by alternative practitioners:

**Cytotoxic tests** are available from several private laboratories. They rely on changes taking place in the shape of white blood cells when a blood sample is mixed with food extracts. Some conventional allergists accept that these type of changes can occur, but it seems that the current method of microscopic examination is far too unreliable. Cytotoxic tests produce too many false positives and negatives. *Not recommended.*

**Hair analysis** relies on detecting allergies from a sample of hair. There is no scientific evidence to back up such claims. *Not recommended.*

**Kineseology** is based on the supposition that muscle power falls when an individual is placed in close proximity to something which they are allergic to. *Not recommended.*

**Pulse testing** is amazingly simple – when an allergic individual eats a certain food the pulse will rise. *Not recommended.*

**Radionics** practitioners use a pendulum and do not require the presence of the patient. The patient and practitioner communicate by 'energy waves' which transfer all the necessary information. *Not recommended.*

**Vega testing** involves the use of electrical equipment rather like an ECG machine. It is said to be capable of diagnosing both food and chemical allergies based on the idea that there are changes in electrical resistance at acupuncture sites during illness. This particular method is regarded with extreme scepticism by conventional allergists (reference: *Medical Journal of Australia*, 1991, 155, 113–14). *Not recommended.*

## Treatment of allergies

Once an allergy or sensitivity has been found the obvious solution is to try and avoid, wherever possible, the particular allergen.

Conventional medicine treats allergies with a variety of drugs. Antihistamines, sodium cromoglycate (which covers the histamine-containing cells and prevents its release) and the powerful anti-inflammatory steroids are used according to the type and severity of symptoms. High doses of steroids are not recommended for people with ME/CFS unless really necessary for other conditions.

The only anti-allergy drug to be so far tested in a double-blind placebo-controlled trial is an antihistamine called terfenadine (reference 466). Thirty patients with ME/CFS were enrolled into a trial lasting for two months. Although initial assessment of the group confirmed an increase incidence of allergic conditions were present, treatment with terfenadine failed to produce any benefit.

Non-orthodox practitioners use a variety of different approaches to manage allergic conditions.

Two methods which are commonly used in the private allergy sector are enzyme potentiated desensitisation (EPD) and neutralisation therapy.

**Enzyme Potentiated Desensitisation (EPD)** This controversial method for treating allergies was developed by Dr Len McEwan, an allergist who originally worked at St Mary's Hospital in London. He is still the leading expert in this area and trains other doctors in how to administer EPD. Although this treatment is mainly used in the private allergy sector, there are a few allergists working in the NHS who are open minded about its possible value.

The principal use of EPD is for treating food allergies, and the technique involves a mixture of multiple diluted food allergens combined with an enzyme (beta glucuronidase) which is supposed to enhance the desensitising effect.

EPD can be given either by injection or by placing the allergen and enzyme mixture on to an area of skin.

The treatment has to be administered several times during the first year. Boosters are then given at increasing intervals depending on the response.

The cost of a full course of EPD may well run into several hundred pounds. Unfortunately, a few people have adverse reactions and cannot continue. In the absence of any published trials demonstrating clear benefits in ME/CFS, *I would not yet recommend the use of EPD.*

**Neutralisation therapy** This is another approach favoured by some doctors in the private allergy sector. A few conventional allergists feel that it may have some benefits, whereas others maintain that the investigation side produces too many false negatives and positives.

Allergies are first identified using a series of injections of food extracts which are placed just under the skin (intradermally). A series of weaker and weaker injections is given until the resulting reaction (a weal) is white, hard and raised as well as remaining the same size for 10 minutes after the test dose. This is known as the neutralising dose – a precise concentration of allergen which should be able to 'switch off' the symptoms.

Neutralisation therapy then involves taking food extracts either by drops straight under the tongue or by self-administered injections. As far as ME/CFS is concerned, this technique remains purely speculative. *I would not recommend its use at the present time.*

The subject of allergies and ME/CFS still creates heated debate between those who support the theories and others who don't see allergies as having much to do with this illness. This is undoubtedly very confusing for patients, who can't follow the scientific arguments and are baffled by what they ought to do. I've tried to present the facts as I see them. I don't believe that allergic reactions are a major part of ME/CFS, although there are some patients who have allergies (or sensitivities). Identification and correct management could help them feel a lot better.

Some useful books on allergy are listed at the end of this chapter. Details about the British Allergy Foundation can be found in Useful Addresses, page 408.

## Aloe Vera

Supplements of this product, which tend to be quite costly, contain a gel which has been extracted from the leaves of a cactus-like plant. Claims have been made that aloe vera can be useful in the treatment of a range of medical complaints, including asthma, multiple sclerosis and ME/CFS. At present, there is no reputable evidence to support such claims, particularly in relation to ME/CFS. *Not recommended.*

## Aromatherapy

Here, small quantities of plant oils are massaged into the skin, inhaled or used in the bath. Aromatherapy is undoubtedly very soothing and relaxing, especially when using an oil such as lavender in the bath. Whether these oils have more beneficial therapeutic properties (as is often claimed) remains a matter of speculation.

Occasional allergic reactions have been reported from the use of some oils (e.g. lemongrass) which are far more concentrated than their original plant form. So, do look very carefully at the label and make sure the oil is properly diluted before use.

Another concern is that some oils may be absorbed through the skin and then enter the general circulation. For this reason the International Federation of Aromatherapists have drawn up the following guidelines:

- Avoid altogether because of possible toxicity – calmus, cassia, fennel, horseradish, mugwort, mustard, pennyroyal, rue, sassafras, savin, tansy, wintergreen, wormwood, sage, aniseed, hyssop
- Avoid in pregnancy (may cause bleeding) – all the above plus basil, birch, clary sage, cypress, jasmine, juniper, marjoram, myrrh, peppermint, rosemary and thyme
- Unsuitable for anyone with raised blood pressure – hyssop, rosemary, sage and thyme. Fennel, hyssop and wormwood can also trigger epileptic attacks
- Avoid if you have sensitive skin (can cause an unpleasant irritant dermatitis) – basil, lemon, melissa, peppermint and thyme. These oils can also irritate when used in the bath. Also avoid bergamot, lemon, lime, orange and verbena in strong sunshine.

Some of the common oils which appear to be safe and may be worth trying include:

- Bergamot – calming and uplifting
- Camomile – said to reduce tension and help sleep
- Cedarwood – soothing
- Geranium – a cool calming oil useful for tension
- Lavender – supposed to help stimulate the mind
- Peppermint – said to relieve decongestion and headaches; also very cooling
- Rosemary – said to have stimulating effects
- Ylang ylang – supposed to have a sedating effect.

For more details on aromatherapy and how to find an aromatherapist see Useful Addresses, page 409. You can expect to pay around £15 to £30 for an hour-long full-body massage.

## Ayurveda

This is a traditional system of medicine which is very popular in India. It is now becoming fashionable here in the UK. The treatment involves the use of herbal medicines and massage which is said to be less 'interfering' than orthodox medicine and allegedly results in far fewer side-effects. Anyone trying ayurveda should be careful to ask questions about the use of imported herbal medicines whose safety has recently been questioned (see later in this chapter).

## Bach Flower Remedies

These were developed in the last century by a homoeopathic doctor called Edward Bach. He claimed that extracts from certain flowers could reverse what were termed 'negative mental states' which led on to various types of physical illness. Bach flower remedies are alleged to work by a process of energy transfer – something that orthodox medical opinion views with considerable scepticism. See Useful Addresses, page 409.

## Candida albicans

One aspect of ME/CFS that continues to create an enormous amount of controversy is the possible role of a yeast called candida. It's also an important reason why some doctors refuse to take ME/CFS seriously – they regard candida as yet another 'bogus illness'.

Having worked in the sexually transmitted disease clinic at London's Middlesex Hospital, I've spent more hours looking for this particular yeast under the microscope than any of the alternative practitioners advocating such a connection. I've also witnessed the whole spectrum of ill health that it can produce, ranging from vaginal discharge through to life-threatening complications in patients with severe immune deficiency. *My conclusion is that candida has no connection whatsoever with ME/CFS.*

Unfortunately, large numbers of ME/CFS sufferers do still believe that they have a significant candida problem and go to great lengths to treat it, using drugs, restrictive diets and probiotics. Some undoubtedly report improvement, in others there's no change and a third group actually feel even worse with anti-candida treatment. These results are not that dissimilar to many of the other unproven treatments.

Reading the various other self-help guide books on the subject, it's not hard to see why people become so convinced by the candida connection. The 'evidence' that more than 75 per cent of people with

ME/CFS have candida overgrowth is presented with such confidence – as though it were irrefutable. Unfortunately, it isn't – most of these 'facts' are based on supposition and pseudoscience. At the moment the case for candida leaks like a sieve. Perhaps the best way of trying to explore the arguments for and against candida is to look at how this yeast lives in our intestines, and what happens when the natural balance is upset.

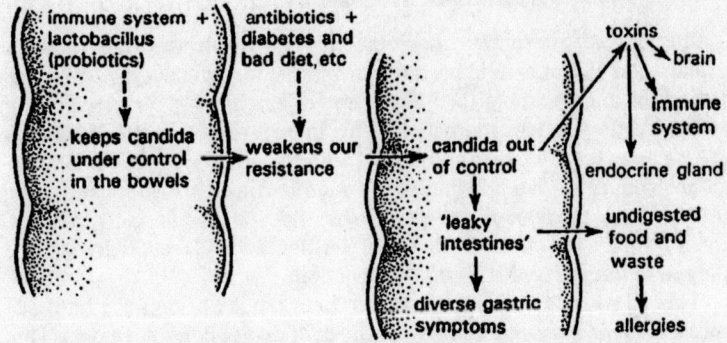

Firstly, there's no disagreement that everyone (healthy or unhealthy) has some candida living in their gut. The yeast is kept under control by the activity of 'good bacteria' (like lactobacillus) and the body's immune system. The presence of this small amount may actually be beneficial. As a result, it's not hard to grow (culture) candida in a stool sample, but this doesn't prove anything. Neither does looking for antibodies to candida – we all have this yeast as a life-long passenger, so it's not surprising that we make an immune response and produce antibodies.

From time to time certain factors allow candida to get out of control and this can lead to problems in various parts of the body. White patches in the mouth (common in babies and the elderly), vaginal discharge and skin or nail infections are all common examples; it's quite easy to confirm the presence of candida from any of these sites. People with severely disrupted immune systems (e.g. AIDS or those taking powerful steroid drugs) develop far more serious candida infections in the lung or brain. There's nothing 'bogus' about these types of candida infections. The body's natural resistance to candida overgrowth can be weakened by any of the following:

- **Antibiotics** – which kill off 'good bacteria', but the body's natural balance of gut organisms is usually quickly restored to normal after such drugs.
- **Diabetes** – which raises the level of blood sugar, the nutrient on

which candida feeds.

- **Immunosuppressive drugs** and diseases such as AIDS.
- **The contraceptive pill** is frequently cited as the fourth factor, but a review of all the current literature leads me to doubt such a connection. The contraceptive pill does not contain the type of steroids which significantly depress immune function. It does alter the body's sex hormones (oestrogen and progesterone) but whether this predisposes to candida is open to debate.

Orthodox and alternative medicine now part company. The latter's explanation is that candida turns into what is known as a hyphael form and starts to grow roots (just like a tree does) which penetrate the gut wall to produce a 'leaky intestine'. This in turn allows so-called candida 'toxins' to enter the blood and affect the brain, immune system and hormone-producing glands. Undigested food particles are supposed to be able to seep through these tiny holes and set off allergic reactions. Lastly, waste products from yeast fermentation (acetaldehyde) are alleged to interfere with blood oxygenation.

This all sounds very impressive in theory, but where is the hard scientific evidence to support the hypothesis? I do not believe it exists. This is why:

- Claims of candida overgrowth in the gullet/oesophagus and stomach could easily be verified by using a special type of X-ray (a barium swallow) or by having a look with an endoscope and taking a small sample of tissue (a biopsy). This type of oesophageal infection is a common complication of AIDS and can easily be confirmed by these sort of investigations. Nobody has, as yet, demonstrated the same findings in ME/CFS.
- There is no reputable published material to show that candida behaves in the intestine by growing penetrating roots and producing a 'leaky' gut lining.
- Claims that candida 'toxins' have adverse effects on the brain or immune system are unsubstantiated. I once asked a manufacturer of the anti-candida drug nystatin to carry out a data search for 'toxins'; they could not find a single reliable scientific reference on this connection. Incidentally, despite the enormous profit potential, manufacturers of this drug have no desire to promote it to people with ME/CFS because they, too, are totally unconvinced by any such link.
- Acetaldehyde may well be produced in the intestine but it's doubtful whether there are sufficient quantities to cause a significant lack of oxygen.
- Gastric symptoms, such as bloating and wind, along with bowel disturbances, are far more feasible, but again remain unproven. If the

gut really is 'leaking' then why don't far more serious problems arise? Why, for instance, doesn't the nystatin pass through these holes? After all, nystatin is a toxic drug which is only safe when not absorbed into the circulation.

Having examined all the arguments for and against candida, can it really do any harm embarking on a treatment regime? Possibly not, but I would still maintain that people with ME/CFS have quite enough restrictions placed on their lives without having to add limitations on diet, as well as spending money on supplements and probiotics. In addition, is it really such a good idea to be taking prolonged courses of antifungal drugs which some microbiologists feel could result in the development of resistant strains – as has occurred with antibiotics and bacteria? Although nystatin is thought to be perfectly safe inside the intestine, there are drugs such as Nizoral (ketoconazole) which can have serious toxic effects on the liver.

Finally, could it be that having some candida inside the gut is actually beneficial and forms a natural part of the environment there? My feeling is that the candida connection is another blind alley for desperate patients searching for a cure. By all means weigh up the arguments carefully, but remember that the case for candida is nowhere near as watertight as its advocates suggest.

If you want to read more about some of the research that has been published into this very controversial area, please refer to medical references 468–72.

## Treatment

Those who believe that it's essential to remove candida as part of an ME/CFS treatment regime rely on an approach which involves diet, conventional anti-fungal medication and other additional supplements.

### Diet

The theory is that to help eradicate candida, your diet will have to be free from both sugar and yeast, which denies the organism its essential nutrients. This sort of diet will involve cutting out foods such as bread (which contain yeast), sugar and honey. Even your B vitamins have to be yeast-free. Some practitioners also advocate a low carbohydrate diet to accompany this, but don't start this sort of dietary manipulation by yourself without proper supervision. One reason for the apparent success of this diet may have nothing whatsoever to do with its effect on candida. Instead, as Dr Robert Loblay, an expert on food allergies and intolerance, has explained the reason may lie in the fact that this approach eliminates a number of common foods which contain chemicals such as natural salicylates and glutamine to which many people are undoubtedly sensitive.

## Drugs

Anti-fungal medication, such as nystatin, needs to be prescribed by your general practitioner. Nystatin is the generic name, so it comes in a variety of preparations using different trade names, e.g. Nystan. It can be used as a cream or pessary for vaginal infections, drops and pastilles for thrush in the mouth, skin creams, tablets for bowel infections as well as powder. The powder form is taken between meals. The dose is gradually altered according to the individual response.

Nystatin appears to be a relatively safe drug, but like any medicine it should be used with caution during pregnancy. However, there are reports in the medical literature of occasional severe reactions occurring, including erythema multiforme and Stevens-Johnson syndrome, both of which are serious skin disorders (reference: *Archives of Dermatology*, 1991, 127, 741–2).

One anti-fungal preparation which doctors can prescribe is ketoconazole (Nizarol). This drug is potentially *very toxic* to the liver, and I don't believe it should be used by anyone with ME/CFS unless there are very strong medical indications to do so.

A variety of other anti-fungal preparations are used by practitioners who carry out this form of therapy, some of them originating abroad.

## Additional supplements

*Lactobacillus acidophilus* is a natural constituent of the bowel; its presence helps to keep candida in check. It can be killed off by taking antibiotics, but restored by eating 'live' yogurt (from health food shops), or taken in capsules known as probiotics (see later in this chapter).

Other additional supplements sometimes recommended include high doses of vitamin C, as well as other vitamins and minerals. High-dose vitamin C will produce diarrhoea and it is claimed this will aid the removal of candida.

This type of anti-candida treatment isn't scientifically proven, and enthusiasts don't claim it can cure ME/CFS. However, they do maintain that it will make a substantial number of people feel much better. There are certainly some anecdotal reports of people apparently benefiting from this approach, although others say they feel worse. Some conventional doctors are looking at the relation between yeasts and specific bowel diseases, but this research is still in its early stages and it is too soon to draw any conclusions from it.

# Cannabis

A growing number of people, including some with ME/CFS, take cannabis for purely medicinal purposes. In multiple sclerosis, cannabis is said to relieve muscle spasticity as well as improving bladder function – claims which have some support from clinical trials. Cannabis is also claimed to provide relief from pain and sickness in cancer.

Many doctors do now agree that these claims ought to be properly investigated, but this isn't going to be easy as long as cannabis use remains illegal. In some parts of the USA, the position is different – doctors there are now allowed to prescribe cannabis for a limited number of medical conditions.

The negative side to cannabis use is that it does have side-effects. In addition to producing mental relaxation and a sense of well-being, cannabis interferes with concentration, the co-ordination required to drive a car and other complex tasks. Smoking one joint is thought to be just as harmful as 20 cigarettes when it comes to increasing the risk of bronchitis and lung cancer. There's also increasing evidence to suggest that regular use can affect the immune system and levels of various body hormones. Long-term use may even trigger the onset of schizophrenia and serious mood disorders.

My own view is to support the call for more research into the medicinal uses of cannabis. Even so, *this is not the time to make it available to anyone who wants to use it until the true facts emerge*. And remember, several people with ME/CFS have ended up in court for using cannabis, even though this was purely for medicinal (pain relief) purposes.

# Carnitine

The use of this substance, which may be deficient in some cases of ME/CFS, is covered in more detail on pages 140 and 199.

# Chelation Therapy

Although orthodox medicine accepts that chelation therapy is a perfectly legitimate way of removing toxic substances such as lead and mercury from the body (following accidental poisoning), it has yet to be convinced that the process has any value in the treatment of conditions such as Alzheimer's disease, arthritis, heart disease, multiple sclerosis and ME/CFS.

Despite the lack of evidence, a number of private doctors in both the UK and USA are recommending chelation as a form of treatment for ME/CFS. A course of treatment is likely to be quite expensive and involves the antidote being infused into the body via a drip. A single treatment will take about three hours. *I am not yet convinced by the alleged benefits and cannot recommend the use of chelation therapy in ME/CFS.*

## Chemical Sensitivities

The controversial link between chemical sensitivities/allergies and ME/CFS continues to generate a great deal of publicity and is accepted without criticism by many patients. However, this is something that orthodox medical opinion, including my own, still views with considerable scepticism, because any such link is very difficult to prove. Whilst accepting that chemical sensitivity may be a problem (and occasionally a severe one) in a *small minority* of patients, I do not believe that everyone with ME/CFS needs to go to the lengths advocated by some practitioners and remove almost every form of chemical from their home environment. Equally, you should be very careful about some of the very dubious investigative procedures and treatments which are now available in the alternative health sector.

The possibility that some agricultural pesticides may be associated with an ME/CFS-like illness is discussed further on pages 110–12. See also reference 473.

## Chinese Medicine

Traditional Chinese Medicine (TCM) attaches great importance to restoring and then maintaining a person's own natural healing processes. Assessment of any health problem comes from what are called 'the four methods of diagnosis', namely observation, listening and smelling, interrogation, pulse feeling and palpitation. Following this assessment, an individual treatment programme will be devised, which could involve a combination of acupuncture, massage and the use of various herbal remedies.

Chinese herbs are classified according to their healing properties – hot, warm, cool, etc – and are prescribed to help eliminate whatever imbalance in energy channels is thought to be present inside the body.

Although there is no doubt that many of these herbs do possess genuine healing properties (especially in the case of skin conditions), there are a growing number of disturbing reports in the medical literature of dangerous side-effects occurring following their use. These include cases of severe liver and kidney damage as well as problems resulting from the presence of contaminants and toxins. *I am not yet convinced about the value of using these types of herbs in ME/CFS.* As with any other herbal remedy (see later), it's important to ask about possible adverse effects on the liver or kidney before consenting to treatment.

(For more information on TCM practitioners see Useful Addresses, page 412.)

## Co-enzyme Q10

The use of this substance, which is required as part of the cell's energy producing functions, is described on page 199.

## Dental Amalgam, (Mercury Fillings) Removal

There has been growing concern about the safety of mercury in dental fillings, especially in relation to the possibility that unsafe amounts of this potentially toxic metal could be slowly absorbed into the body from the teeth. Mercury toxicity has been linked to conditions such as Alzheimer's disease, multiple sclerosis and depression, as well as ME/CFS. And despite constant reassurance from the British Dental Association that no such connection has been scientifically proven, an increasing number of people are having their mercury fillings replaced.

Having your dental fillings removed and replaced is not a procedure that is generally available on the NHS and will probably have to be done privately at considerable expense. There is also a risk that the removal process may cause an exacerbation or relapse of your ME/CFS.

My own view is that in the current absence of any good evidence to link mercury fillings to ME/CFS, this is not a treatment option that I would recommend.

If you require further information on both sides of the debate into this controversial form of treatment for ME/CFS, then contact the British Dental Association (tel: 0171–935 0875) and the British Society for Mercury Free Dentistry (tel: 0171–486 3127).

## Detoxification Therapies

These involve various forms of 'colonic cleansing' which, in theory, help to eliminate a 'toxic load' from the large bowel. Such approaches were very popular in the early 1990s and now seem to be the subject of renewed enthusiasm amongst alternative therapists. *Orthodox medicine considers them to be wholly unscientific* and they should certainly be avoided by anyone who is already debilitated as a result of ME/CFS.

Colonic irrigation involves regular visits to a colonic therapist (about £30 a time) who uses warm water to flush out debris from the bowel wall. Although adverse effects are rare, colonic irrigation can upset the balance of electrolytes (body salts) and damage the gut lining in anyone who already suffers from any sort of bowel inflammation. More serious side-effects, including an outbreak of amoebiasis (a serious gastrointestinal infection) involving six deaths, have been reported in the medical literature (reference: *New England Journal of Medicine*, 1982, 307, 339–42). *Not recommended.*

Fasting for days, or even longer, is another method of allegedly detoxifying the body. *This is one practice which I would definitely not recommend* – it could end up doing far more harm than good (reference: *British Medical Journal*, 1992, 304, 521).

# Dietary Supplementation and Vitamins

Some practitioners advocate that people with ME/CFS need to supplement their diets with a variety of trace elements, amino acids and vitamins. This type of approach is particularly popular in America for a variety of illnesses. Once again the theories are quite attractive, although there is little evidence to back them up and win the acceptance of orthodox medicine.

The idea behind this approach is that there may be both faulty absorption of some of these essential substances, as well as an extra requirement to help in the repair process of essential cells which have been damaged by infection or immune dysfunction.

A comprehensive list of all these substances would be endless, as differing practitioners recommend their own individual treatment regimes, often using a combination of therapies. However, those amino acids and trace elements which are quite frequently advised do warrant some appraisal.

## Amino acids

These are essential building blocks which are required by the body to manufacture proteins. When food proteins, such as fish or meat, have been digested, they are quickly broken down into their constituent amino acids. These are then removed from the circulation by cells in the brain, muscle, bone, skin, etc, to build up their own proteins for either repair or growth.

Altogether there are about 20 different amino acids, of which eight are known as 'essential' because they cannot be made inside the body and have to come from our diet.

Expensive preparations containing various amino acid supplements – both essential and non-essential – are now available. *Provided your protein intake is satisfactory, there seems little advantage in using these preparations.* However, if it can be shown that there are specific amino acid deficiencies in ME/CFS, then this sort of approach could prove to be beneficial.

## Magnesium

Deficiency of this vital element has been implicated in a number of disorders including premenstrual syndrome and high blood pressure. However, researchers remain uncertain about the precise role of magnesium in the body, although it does seem to be an important factor (like carnitine) in catalysing energy production inside nerve and muscle cells.

In March 1991, *The Lancet* published a paper on the use of magnesium sulphate injections as a possible treatment for ME/CFS (reference 475). The paper created a great deal of press interest and, as a result, family doctors were inundated by requests to prescribe this new form of therapy.

The reaction from the medical profession was far more sceptical. Some doctors co-operated with requests for treatment whereas others were hostile and refused to experiment with such an unconventional approach to ME/CFS management.

The clinical trial involved patients who were selected by general practitioners and by the Centre for the Study of Complementary Medicine in Southampton. First, the concentration of magnesium inside the red blood cells was measured. (Only a very small amount of magnesium is present outside the cells, making ordinary blood tests an unreliable indicator of magnesium deficiency.) The results suggested that there was a slight deficiency in magnesium levels. Those taking part were also asked to fill in a health questionnaire so the response to magnesium could be objectively assessed.

The 32 participants were then divided into two separate groups so that a double-blind, placebo-controlled trial could be carried out. This means that neither doctor nor patient knew who was receiving active treatment (in this case injections of 1gm of 50 per cent magnesium sulphate) or a placebo dummy injection (water).

The trial continued with six weekly injections after which everyone filled in their health questionnaire once again. This covered symptoms such as energy levels, emotional reactions and sleep pattern. Out of the 15 patients receiving magnesium 12 improved, of whom seven reported a significant improvement in energy levels. In the placebo group, only three out of 17 reported any benefits.

So, although the numbers involved were very small, and the follow-up period surprisingly short (six weeks), the results were considered to be statistically significant.

But why might magnesium help people with ME/CFS? Magnesium is something that we all take in as part of a normal healthy diet. Foods such as green vegetables, cereal grains, chocolate and nuts are all good sources. So is 'hard' drinking water. About 45 per cent of this daily intake is then absorbed in the small intestine. During times of deficiency inside the body this absorption can easily rise to 80 per cent. Once inside the body, most magnesium is stored inside the bone and muscle.

The main action of magnesium is within the cells, particularly muscle and nervous tissue, where it helps with numerous enzyme systems. As far as muscle is concerned, too much magnesium can seriously interfere with the way electrical impulses are transmitted from nerves to muscles. Within the muscle, magnesium is stored in the mitochondria – the 'power house' of the cell – where it acts as a vital co-factor in energy production. So, there are some theoretical mechanisms why magnesium supplementation could be both beneficial and harmful.

According to most orthodox medical opinion, true magnesium deficiency is fairly unusual, except in some types of gastrointestinal disease (where absorption is reduced), alcoholism (which increases its removal by the kidneys, as do diuretic drugs) and some hormonal diseases (e.g. an overactive thyroid gland).

Incidentally, an underactive thyroid (hypothyroidism) can actually cause magnesium levels to rise. Whether or not magnesium deficiency is a significant factor in ME/CFS remains unproven, despite these findings from Southampton.

Publication of the trial results was followed by a number of critical letters to *The Lancet*. One of the most important concerned the actual amount of magnesium contained in these injections. According to one of the pharmaceutical companies involved, this amounted to only about 100mg, which was then released over the following few hours. Given that our average dietary intake of magnesium is about 300–400mg per day, it is difficult to see why an extra 15mg per day, on average, should produce any major benefits.

It was also pointed out that measuring the red blood cell concentration of magnesium is *not* a reliable indicator for assessing magnesium deficiency inside the body. A more objective method is to assess the concentration in either muscle or monocytes (a type of white blood cell), or to carry out what is known as an intravenous magnesium loading test. In practice though, none of these tests are easily obtainable from the NHS, so most people trying magnesium therapy will not know if they are actually deficient.

Finally, it was pointed out that the laboratory used to carry out some of the tests had been the subject of media investigations which had cast doubt on their accuracy.

It should also be noted that high doses of magnesium can cause serious side-effects, especially on the heart. So, it is a wise precaution to check that kidney function is satisfactory before these injections are given. I would not recommend that anyone with heart disease takes extra magnesium. These injections must be given into the muscle and *never* directly into a vein.

Given the way that the body absorbs and then distributes magnesium, it seems that small amounts taken by mouth are far less likely to have any beneficial effects.

The results of this small trial must be viewed with considerable caution and further independent trials are needed before any definite conclusions can be drawn. We also need to establish whether significant magnesium deficiency is indeed a part of this illness. *Magnesium is not yet a proven therapy for ME/CFS.*

## Selenium

This is another trace element which has already been advocated as a possible treatment for ME/CFS. Selenium is frequently combined in commercial preparations with vitamins A, C and E. In theory, this combination should act together to scavenge for harmful substances known as 'free radicals' which cause cell damage, ageing and possibly cancer. Selenium is also alleged to possess anti-inflammatory, antiviral and immune altering effects; concentrations are said to be reduced in some patients with rheumatoid arthritis.

Concern has been expressed in a recent editorial in the *British Medical Journal* (reference: 1997, 314, 387–8) that the normal dietary intake of selenium (from bread, cereals, fish, poultry and meat) is falling in some parts of the world. Twenty years ago, selenium intake in the UK was around 60 micrograms per day, much higher than the 34 micrograms per day found in a 1994 survey. These latter results are significantly below the government's recommended daily intake target for selenium of 75 micrograms per day for men and 60 micrograms per day for women. The editorial suggested that the fall in dietary intake could be due to a decrease in the use of selenium-rich wheat which used to be imported from America for bread-making purposes. It then went on to quote evidence supporting the view that some types of viral infection – HIV in particular – could become more virulent in people who are selenium deficient.

Although there is certainly growing evidence that selenium can affect the body's normal protective response to infection, *there is still no reliable data to show that it has any beneficial effects in ME/CFS or that blood levels are reduced.*

As with any other micronutrient, concern has been expressed about how important it is to leave a wide safety margin, and not exceed the recommended dose of any selenium supplement. Toxicity does occur, leading to hair loss, chronic eczema and damage to the sensory nerves (as with vitamin $B_6$). According to the most recent government guidelines on vitamins and minerals, a safe daily intake lies somewhere between 40 and 70 micrograms for a normal weight adult. Supplementation in excess of this should only be taken where a clear deficiency is shown to exist.

## Zinc

This trace element forms an essential part of our diet. Well over 200 enzymes are now known to require its presence to operate effectively.

At the moment there is no officially recommended daily intake of zinc in the UK, but in America it is set at 15mg per day. Most people take in about 10mg a day in their diet, which is probably quite sufficient. Meat (30 per cent) and milk (25 per cent) are major sources of dietary zinc. Fruit and vegetables contain very little. Absorption from the gut is reduced by a high intake of dietary fibre and phytic acid which is found in soya beans. Even so, vegetarians do not seem to have any problems associated with zinc deficiency.

Orthodox medicine acknowledges that severe deficiency of zinc does occasionally occur. This can result in inflamed skin lesions, increased susceptibility to infections and a general failure to thrive in children. Such deficiency is usually due to a malabsorption in the intestines, chronic alcoholism or loss during kidney dialysis.

The level of zinc in the blood is *not* thought to be an accurate indicator of zinc levels overall, as only a small amount is actually in the blood. Any chronic infection will probably reduce the level of zinc in the blood, but it seems that the total amount of zinc in the body doesn't fall significantly. So, concluding that someone has a mild zinc deficiency from a blood test isn't necessarily a logical conclusion.

Experimentally, zinc can interfere with virus multiplication, but there's no evidence that it stops the progression of the common cold (for which it's often recommended) or any other infection. Some allergists believe that people with food allergy or sensitivity have an abnormal ratio of copper to zinc status in the body and that if this is corrected there can be a considerable improvement in food-related symptoms.

Taking extra amounts of zinc may result in side-effects (e.g. stomach pains and decreased copper absorption); very high intakes can actually start to depress the immune system. Zinc also competes with iron for absorption within the gut; cases of anaemia associated with excessive supplementation have now been recorded.

*At present, many of the claims made for zinc supplementation are unfounded, but taking a little extra probably does no harm.* Nobody should take any more than 50 mg per day (Zincomed capsules contain this dose) if they decide to use this as part of their treatment. Zinc supplements should *not* be taken by anyone who has kidney problems.

## Vitamins

Vitamins, when taken in normal recommended daily doses (RDAs), are extremely safe. However, many people with ME/CFS seem to be taking ever-increasing amounts of expensive vitamin supplements. In some cases the manufacturers have been giving the prescribing practitioners a substantial commission on sales – a practice which creates a very undesirable conflict of interest.

The list of disorders that large doses of vitamins are alleged to help is becoming endless. It seems that almost any 'sick cell' in the body can be restored to normal health by these pills. This trend towards high-dose vitamin therapy is partly based on the ideas of the great vitamin C enthusiast, Linus Pauling. He argued that many psychiatric illnesses (particularly schizophrenia) were due to deficiencies in transmitter chemicals within the brain (neurotransmitters) which could be solved by dietary supplementation. The same idea has now been applied to ME/CFS – taking large quantities of vitamins and minerals should help cells in the brain, muscle and immune system to recover. This all sounds fine in theory, but any alleged benefits are based on anecdotal reports rather than hard scientific fact.

All doctors acknowledge that vitamins are essential catalysts for the correct functioning of blood and nerve cells, the immune system and hormones; in fact almost any tissue in the body. However, these requirements are in *minute amounts* which any normal healthy diet should be supplying perfectly adequately. *There is no scientific evidence that people with ME/CFS are deficient in any of the major vitamins* and it should be noted that reliable facilities for the assessment of possible vitamin deficiencies are only available in a limited number of NHS laboratories.

In the absence of any reliable proof of vitamin deficiency occurring in ME/CFS I would urge anyone with this illness to carefully consider the pros and cons of megadosing on vitamins. *I am not convinced that large doses of vitamins are either necessary or desirable in this illness.* The untoward effects of taking such large doses over a prolonged period of time are still far from certain and difficult to assess, as self-medication makes the reporting of adverse reactions very unlikely.

So, which vitamins do you need to be careful about and what are the dangers?

**Vitamin A (Retinol)** is currently being investigated as a possible anti-cancer substance; but there is no good evidence that people with ME/CFS are either deficient or would benefit from supplementation.

The medical journals now contain well over 500 case reports of people being made ill by taking too much vitamin A. In excess it can cause increased pressure in the brain and serious liver damage – deaths have even been reported. It seems that at levels as low as ten times the RDA, toxicity can occur.

A high incidence of spontaneous abortions and births that include malformations of the heart, face, thymus gland and nervous system has been observed in infants of mothers who had a high intake of vitamin A (greater than 3,000 micrograms per day) during pregnancy. Therefore, women who are, or might become, pregnant are advised not to take vitamin A supplements (including fish oil capsules) and they should also avoid eating liver or liver products, e.g. pâté, that often contain high levels of this vitamin.

**Vitamin B group** Conventional teaching on vitamins used to be that it was only the fat-soluble group (A, D, E and K) which caused harm as they could accumulate in body fat. The water-soluble vitamins (B and C) are excreted in the urine when taken in excess, so nobody thought they could also accumulate. Research has now shown that life is not quite so simple, and although vitamins $B_1$, $B_2$ and $B_{12}$ appear to be quite safe, problems are arising in connection with vitamin $B_6$ (pyridoxine) and vitamin C in high doses.

*Vitamin $B_1$ (thiamine)* Deficiency of this vitamin – essential for the way in which the body deals with dietary carbohydrates – is extremely unusual, except in alcoholics who develop heart and nerve damage as a result.

*Vitamin $B_3$ (niacin)* is required for the continuous release of energy from carbohydrates. The only people who really need to take supplements are alcoholics, those on a very poor diet and anyone having kidney dialysis. High doses of niacin (especially in the sustained release form) can cause severe liver damage and even death. *There is no rationale for exceeding the RDA in the case of ME/CFS.*

*Vitamin $B_6$ (pyridoxine)* is currently the vogue treatment for pre-menstrual tension (PMT), and it does undoubtedly seem to help some women with this condition. At doses of 150mg per day (and possibly lower) it can damage sensory nerves causing pins and needles (paraesthesiae) and lack of co-ordination. What is worrying, and still far from certain, is at what level vitamin $B_6$ actually starts to produce nerve damage in the absence of symptoms. Dr Katharina Dalton, a world expert on hormone disturbances, has noted that adverse effects reoccurred at doses of 50mg per day in patients who had previously stopped the high dosage and then resumed at this lower dose (reference 476).

In 1997, the UK Medicines Control Agency announced plans to make supplements containing a daily dose of 50mg or above available only on prescription. Only those products with a daily dose of up to 10mg would continue to remain on general sale, without the need for a pharmacist's supervision. *I can see no reason why people with ME/CFS should be taking excessive doses of this vitamin.*

*Vitamin $B_{12}$* is needed for healthy bone marrow and nerves. Deficiency leads to anaemia and nerve cell degeneration (pernicious anaemia). Deficiency occurs primarily due to lack of absorption, so it has to be given by injection. Oral preparations do no harm but their benefits are questionable.

At present there is no evidence that people with ME/CFS have problems with vitamin $B_{12}$ absorption. However, a new research study from Sweden, showing increased concentrations of an amino acid called homocysteine in the cerebrospinal fluid, does give some support to the suggestion that $B_{12}$ levels could be marginally reduced (see page 158).

A number of doctors in both America and Australia are now giving $B_{12}$ injections in an attempt to saturate the body with this vitamin. Although there are anecdotal reports of success, the only placebo-controlled trial which involved vitamin $B_{12}$ showed no significant benefits compared to a placebo (reference 479). This trial was, however, criticised because of the very short period of time (four weeks) during which the active treatment or placebo were administered.

*Vitamin C* This is probably the most common vitamin to be megadosed, due to claims that it can boost the immune system. Whether or not people with ME/CFS need their immune system boosting is a matter for debate. Even so, there is very little evidence that large doses can actually fulfil these claims in humans. If vitamin C did have these properties, it would presumably have become a standard treatment for immune-deficiency conditions such as AIDS.

What worries doctors is the increasing number of adverse reactions being reported as claims for vitamin C become more widespread. It is now known that excessive amounts can increase levels of oestrogen in the body, so converting a 'low-dose' contraceptive pill into the 'high-dose' equivalent. Vitamin C also increases the output of chemicals in the urine called oxalates, which can result in kidney stone formation. Increased intake results in the body's natural removal mechanisms speeding up, so any sudden cessation of treatment can produce a rebound scurvy – several cases of which have now appeared in the medical literature.

Another disturbing effect of vitamin C is the way it increases the absorption of iron. People with ME/CFS are *not* deficient in iron and it is undesirable to overload the system with this metal, as it can cause serious liver damage. It has also been suggested that heavy metals such as iron and aluminium may damage nerve cells and be responsible for other neurological diseases such as dementia.

*The strong possibility that excessive amounts of vitamin C intake (greater than 500mg per day) could actually be causing cell damage seem to be largely ignored whilst the benefits of large doses remain far from certain.*

*Vitamin D* helps to maintain the level of calcium in the blood. Any excess will lead to kidney stones and further muscle weakness. The best way of maintaining an adequate calcium balance is from dairy produce, and calcium supplements if necessary.

*Vitamin E* This is another fat-soluble vitamin which is enjoying considerable popularity. Many people are enthusing about vitamin E's anti-oxidant role, meaning that it can mop up free oxygen molecules circulating around the body. There is certainly a theoretical benefit here, as these molecules are capable of damaging normal healthy cells, and vitamin E has been used experimentally on premature babies whose eyes have been damaged after being given too much oxygen at birth.

On the more negative side, vitamin E raises blood fats (triglycerides), can lower thyroid gland hormones, and has been reported to cause muscle weakness along with the release of muscle enzymes (creatine kinase), suggesting that excessive amounts may actually be damaging the cells.

The benefits of this vitamin in ME/CFS remain far from clear. Higher than normal doses should be taken with care.

*Folate* This is mainly found in vegetables, fruit and some meats, but is easily destroyed during the cooking process. Well recognised deficiency occurs in people on highly restrictive diets and those with food malabsorption problems.

*Folate is the only vitamin that has ever been shown to be possibly deficient in ME/CFS* (reference 478). In this study, half of a group of 60 ME/CFS patients were found to have laboratory evidence of folate deficiency (a serum folate level below 3 micrograms/l). None were obviously suffering from folic acid anaemia. The authors – Professors Peter Behan and Leslie Borysiewicz – pointed out that adequate supplies of folate are essential for the production of genetic materials (DNA and RNA) and proteins in all body tissues, and that natural demand for extra folate occurs during both acute and chronic infections. They suggested that blood folate levels should be measured in people with ME/CFS and that, if lowered, a folate supplement of 2.5mg should be taken for two to three weeks. This advice is particularly relevant to women with ME/CFS who are contemplating pregnancy, as folate deficiency at this time is strongly associated with the development of birth defects. Anyone who is found to be folate deficient should also query the possibility of coeliac disease (see page 84) being present.

**Table 10: Vitamins and minerals: the facts**

|  | Recommended Daily Allowance* | Sources |
|---|---|---|
| Vitamin A: retinol | 1,000mcg | liver, green vegetables, carrots, oranges, eggs, cheese, milk |
| Vitamin B$_1$: thiamin | 1.4mg | potatoes, bread, milk, vegetables, cereals |
| Vitamin B$_2$: riboflavin | 1.6mg | liver, meat, milk, cheese |
| Vitamin B$_3$: niacin and nicotinic acid | 18mg | liver, meat, bread, cereals |
| Vitamin B$_6$: pyridoxine | 2mg | liver, cereals, pulses, poultry |
| Vitamin B$_{12}$: cobalamin | 3mcg | meat, milk, cheese, eggs |
| Vitamin B: biotin | 0.15mg | liver, pork, cauliflower, cereals |
| Vitamin B: folic acid | 400mcg | green vegetables and fruit |
| Vitamin C: ascorbic acid | 60mg | fruit, vegetables, potatoes, tomatoes |
| Vitamin D: calciferol | 5mcg | sunlight, margarine, fish, eggs, butter |
| Vitamin E: | 10mg | vegetable oils, nuts, eggs, butter |
| *Minerals* |  |  |
| Calcium | 800mg | milk, cheese, bread |
| Iron | 12mg | meat, liver, beans, bread, fruit, nuts |
| Zinc | 15mg | milk, liver, meat, wholegrains |

*European Community figures are quoted, which are slightly higher than the RDA here in the UK.
mcg/microgram = one millionth of a gram
mg/milligram = one thousandth of a gram

Vitamins need to be taken with the same type of caution that applies to any other medicine, especially if you're going to take more than the RDA. A daily multivitamin tablet isn't going to cause any harm and good values ones include Sanatogen Multivitamins and Boots Multivitamins. Specially formulated preparations from the health-food industry often cost more and don't offer any significant advantages. In future, I hope that alternative practitioners will give a great deal more thought (and publicity) to the possible disadvantages of high-dose vitamin therapy. Apart from the dangers I have illustrated, all this is doing is making drug companies even richer and producing some of the most expensive urine in the world, as our bodies naturally remove what we don't require.

## Electrical Devices

Over the past few years a variety of extremely dubious electronic and magnetic devices have been 'invented' by the alternative health sector. Promoters of these devices often claim that they work by 'correcting' abnormal brain wave activity – an explanation which fails to convince medical experts in this area. Unfortunately, the 1968 Medicine Act, which prohibits unsubstantiated therapeutic claims being made for drugs, doesn't apply to such devices. Consequently, some companies have gone so far as to claim that their products can successfully treat ME/CFS, depression, migraine, etc. At present, the only regulatory control comes from the Advertising Standards Authority, which can decide that promotional material is breaking their strict Code of Practice. Such rulings have been made in relation to two devices aimed at people with ME/CFS. *I do not believe that any of these expensive devices are of benefit in the treatment of ME/CFS. Don't waste your money!*

## Hair Analysis

The value of hair analysis in the assessment of nutritional status and allergies is viewed with extreme scepticism by orthodox medicine. Nevertheless, several private clinics now claim to be able to detect deficiencies in vitamins and minerals such as zinc, magnesium and chromium from a sample of hair. The problem is that hair does not necessarily reflect the concentrations of minerals found in body tissues, and there are large individual variations in these levels according to age, sex and even which part of the scalp the sample is taken from. Even more dubious is the practice of diagnosing and treating allergies from samples of hair sent by post. *I do not believe that hair analysis has any value in either the diagnosis or treatment of ME/CFS.*

## Healing

The term 'healing' covers a wide variety of different approaches, the theory being that people can be healed by 'forces' which the healer possesses.

Many healers make strong religious claims in connection with their work, assuming, rightly or wrongly, that their powers are 'God given'. In practice, the process of healing usually involves the laying on of hands or some other form of physical contact, although some healers claim to be able to transmit these healing powers by way of thought.

There seems to be an ever growing number of healers. Some of them are obviously frauds, so if you decide to embark on healing, do make careful enquiries first and try to find a genuine and respected healer. This 'mind over matter' approach can be of great value to some people, and obviously the chances of success are greatly increased if you believe in the healer and the principles of healing.

People who have strong religious beliefs (and even those who don't) may gain considerable benefit and comfort from Christian healing. Some churches now have specific 'healing services' as part of their worship – your vicar should know of any which occur locally. Part of the service usually involves the priest giving an individual blessing along with the laying on of hands for those who require healing. Relatives are very welcome to attend and to pray for recovery.

Some healers belong to the National Federation of Spiritual Healing (see Useful Addresses, page 417) but the best way of finding a healer would be by personal recommendation.

# Herbal Medicines

A recent survey in the *British Medical Journal* found that general practitioners understood less about herbal medicines than any other branch of alternative medicine. This is disquieting, because many of the drugs used by orthodox medicine are derived from plants, and some of the herbal medicines available for purchase have some disturbing side-effects if not used with care. A growing number of herbalists are now taking some form of formal training and will recommend or prepare specific herbal remedies for their patients. Many people, though, still make use of this branch of alternative medicine on a 'do-it-yourself' basis by purchasing remedies from health food stores, often without knowing a great deal about the product they're about to use. There is a vast range of herbal medicines available, and the current position with regard to licensing and control is far from satisfactory. Patients are taking substances of which the long-term effects, in some cases, have never been properly assessed. This is something that the Department of Health is currently investigating.

Although the majority of herbal remedies are probably quite safe, some herbs are known to accumulate heavy metals and pesticide residues, which can be passed on to the user. A few are known to cause cancer in animals (comfrey and sassafras) or produce severe liver damage in humans (ragwort or 'bush tea'). Ginseng, which is quite popular among people with ME/CFS, is reported to cause high blood pressure, breast development in men (it can affect hormone levels) and 'nervous irritability'. Its benefits are far from certain.

The *British Medical Journal* has reported on several cases of severe liver damage (hepatitis) caused by products containing a herb known as valerian. At the time, valerian was said to be present in over 80 different herbal medicines which were being promoted for their sedating effects – two of those mentioned by the *Journal* were Kalms and Neurelax (reference 488).

More worrying are some of the herbs used by hakims – the traditional Indian herbalists who still treat many members of the Asian community. These imported herbs have been found to contain toxic substances such as lead, mercury, arsenic and even strychnine. They should certainly be avoided. Further details on the adverse effects of herbal remedies are contained in the book *Herbal Medicines* (see page 296).

If you decide to use shop-bought herbal remedies, check to see if the product has a medicinal product licence as shown by the letters PL on the packaging. This means that the Department of Health has assessed the herb for safety and examined any medicinal claims being made. Never exceed the stated dose and always check with your doctor or pharmacist if you are taking any other medicines.

Even though many herbal remedies are of very dubious value in the management of ME/CFS, there is no doubt that others do have genuine and beneficial therapeutic effects. This is why evening primrose oil (Efamol), ginkgo biloba and St John's Wort merit serious consideration.

## Evening primrose oil

This has become an increasingly popular treatment for a whole range of conditions, ranging from pre-menstrual tension to rheumatoid arthritis, atopic eczema and multiple sclerosis.

Evening primrose oil comes from seeds of the shrub *Oenothera biennis*. It's usually combined with vitamin E, which helps to preserve the effectiveness of the oil once inside the cells. The oil is rich in two essential fatty acids. These are known as essential because our bodies can't manufacture them and we have to take them in the diet. It's thought that these fatty acids play a part in chemical pathways that eventually have an effect on the body's immune system and inflammation responses.

There's no doubt that evening primrose oil has a number of firm supporters in orthodox medicine and trials have been carried out to compare its effectiveness in relieving the pain in arthritis with traditional painkillers. The results show that it can be just as effective. There is also evidence that it can help with skin conditions like atopic eczema. For people who are experiencing joint pain, this drug might well be worth trying, especially as it doesn't have any nasty side-effects.

In 1990, the results of a properly controlled clinical trial using supplements of Efamol Marine (a mixture of gamma-linolenic acid and eicosapentaenoic acid) were published (reference 482). After 15 weeks, 84 per cent of those who received a high dose of Efamol reported improvement compared to only 22 per cent in the placebo group. Those receiving Efamol also noted a significant decrease in palpitations and heart rhythm disturbances. The authors of this study speculated that the high dose of Efamol might be reducing the production of lymphokines such as interleukin, as well as correcting any deficit in body stores of essential fatty acids resulting from a chronic viral infection. (The patients in this clinical trial took four capsules of Efamol Marine morning and evening. Each capsule contains about 35mg of GLA and 17mg of EPA.)

The oil usually comes in capsule form (250mg or 500mg). It is available from pharmacies and health food stores under a variety of trade names, and is quite expensive. EPO is available on NHS prescription, but only for the treatment of eczema and cyclical breast pain.

Although evening primrose oil appears to be perfectly safe, it can occasionally cause nausea, diarrhoea and headaches. It should be avoided by anyone with epilepsy.

## Ginkgo biloba

Extracts from the leaves of the ginkgo biloba trees have long been used by the Chinese for medicinal purposes. The principle claim is that ginkgo can improve 'cerebral insufficiency', symptoms of which include problems with memory and concentration, confusion, fatigue, depression, dizziness, tinnitus and headaches. And with several trials supporting these claims, ginkgo has now been licensed in Germany for the treatment of cerebral dysfunction (reference 484). Interestingly, the most recent placebo-controlled study from America found that it could stabilise and, in some cases, improve mental function in a group of patients with dementia (reference: *Journal of the American Medical Association*, 1997, 278, 1327–32).

Commercial supplements containing ginkgo biloba are now being promoted in the UK for the treatment of tinnitus, ME/CFS, multiple sclerosis and other neurological complaints. The dose used in most of the clinical trials has been around 120–160mg per day, taken in three divided doses. Treatment should be continued for at least four to six weeks before a decision on any possible benefits is made. Gingko should not be used by anyone with a bleeding disorder or who takes regular aspirin as it may increase the risk of a brain haemorrhage. (Lancet, 1998, 352, 36)

Whether or not ginkgo biloba can increase blood supply to the brain in ME/CFS and/or have any effect on brain symptoms remains unproven. Even so, *this is one herbal remedy which may be worth trying. The alleged benefits certainly deserve further investigation.*

## St John's Wort

The possible value of this herbal remedy in the treatment of depression is described on pages 241–2.

## Eleutherococcus Senticosus (ES)

This is a ginseng supplement which comes from Russia. There, it is claimed to promote resistance to infections, conserve stress hormones produced by the adrenal glands and even help in the treatment of cancer.

No proper clinical trials have been published using ME/CFS patients to assess both the alleged benefits and possible side-effects. Reported adverse reactions include palpitations, high blood pressure, headaches and insomnia (reference 481).

# Homoeopathy

Homoeopathy was developed by Dr Samuel Hahnemann nearly 200 years ago. It is based on the principle that 'like cures like' and involves the use of very dilute preparations, which in a healthy person would cause specific symptoms, but could cure the same symptoms in someone who was ill. For example, because scarlet fever resembles belladonna poisoning, a very dilute dose of belladonna would be used to treat scarlet fever.

Homoeopathic medicines are usually made from natural sources such as plants, minerals or animal products. The remedy is made by a process called potentisation, so that as the original solution (the 'Mother Tincture') is made more dilute, its effect is increased. Conventional medical thinking finds it difficult to understand how such a product could then be beneficial in purely scientific terms, as there's almost nothing left in the highly diluted final preparation.

Homoeopaths tend to take a holistic approach to patients and their illnesses and will adjust the treatment to each individual case. There's no one homoeopathic remedy for something like ME/CFS.

Homoeopathic treatment depends on you and your individual symptoms. It's not a do-it-yourself type of alternative therapy.

A double-blind trial involving 64 ME/CFS patients who were treated with either a single homoeopathic remedy or a placebo has been carried out in the UK (reference 489). Patients were randomly selected into either group and then made monthly visits to the same homoeopath for a period of one year. The classic method of homoeopathy was followed with each practitioner having the freedom to prescribe the most suitable homoeopathic remedy for each patient. Thirty-three per cent of those receiving a homoeopathic treatment reported a 'significant improvement', whereas 94 per cent in the placebo group remained 'largely unchanged'.

A critical review of the use of homoeopathic treatment in a wide range of medical disorders has now been published in *The Lancet* (reference 492). Other homoeopathic studies which are relevant to ME/CFS are contained in references 490 and 491.

*Homoeopathic preparations appear to be perfectly safe and free from side-effects. Many people with ME/CFS use them and I know of several instances where significant benefits have occurred.*

If homoeopathy is a type of alternative treatment that you would like to follow up, there are several consultants who are willing to see people with ME/CFS privately or on the NHS. Everyone is entitled to be referred to one of the NHS homoeopathic hospitals or clinics in Glasgow, Bristol, Liverpool, London and Tunbridge Wells, although some health authorities are becoming increasingly unwilling to fund such referrals. For further details on these clinics and a homoeopathic pharmacy in London see Useful Addresses, page 420.

## Hypnosis

Hypnosis can't and won't 'cure' ME/CFS, but it may be of help for relaxation and in coming to terms with the illness instead of fighting against it. It may also be helpful with a specific symptom such as chronic pain.

Do remember, though, that *hypnosis in the wrong hands can do a great deal of harm*, especially if it's inappropriately used for psychiatric problems like severe depression. If you are seriously considering using this approach, I'd strongly suggest discussing it with your own doctor first. Do try to consult a medically qualified hypnotist and certainly not one out of the Yellow Pages.

An increasing number of general practitioners are using hypnotherapy in their practices. One of the partners in your own practice may be interested. For a report on three case histories using hypnosis to treat ME/CFS see reference 528. ee Useful Addresses for details of medically qualified hypnotherapists, page 421.

# Iridology

Iridologists believe that by carefully examining the colour and structure of the iris (the coloured part of the eye that surrounds the pupil) they can detect ill health in almost any part of the body. They use the iris rather like a clock face in which each small segment corresponds to a particular organ or specific anatomical part of the body. Like most orthodox doctors I find these diagnostic claims to be extremely suspect.

No objective clinical trial has managed to support the theory behind iridology. *I cannot recommend it.*

# Kutapressin

This is a drug which is given by intramuscular injection several times a week. It is currently being used by some doctors in America, but I am not aware of its availability elsewhere. The active ingredients are a mixture of chemicals derived from pig's liver and amino acids. It was originally developed for the treatment of various skin disorders back in the 1940s, and came about as a by-product from the manufacture of vitamin $B_{12}$.

Doctors who use Kutapressin in the treatment of ME/CFS claim that it helps to restore imbalances in the immune system and may also have anti-viral effects. Interestingly, as far back as 1939, Kutapressin was being used as a treatment for neurasthenia – a condition which some doctors believe to be similar to ME/CFS. It is also said to be effective in treating herpes virus infections such as shingles.

Although Kutapressin is anecdotally supposed to improve fatigue and reduce muscle or joint pain (but not mental impairment), there are, as yet, no published clinical trials to back up these claims. *I would be reluctant to recommend its use until properly controlled trial data have been published.*

# Lecithin

Lecithin supplements have been promoted as a possible treatment for various neurological disorders, but no proper clinical trials have ever been carried out.

The most important ingredient of commercially available lecithin supplements is choline, a substance which is required by the body for the production of a brain chemical transmitter known as acetylcholine. Abnormalities in this particular transmitter have now been described in ME/CFS (see page 153–4) so there may be theoretical reasons why lecithin could be of benefit.

*Although lecithin supplements don't appear to have any harmful side-effects, I'm not yet convinced that they are of any real value in ME/CFS.*

# Meditation

Some people with ME/CFS gain benefit from the way meditation can relax both body and mind. Meditation can take any form you like, from the type of relaxation techniques described on pages 247–8 to Christian meditation, transcendental meditation or Zen meditation. Meditation seems particularly appropriate for anyone whose stressful life continually exerts a powerful negative effect on their body's ability to recover.

Probably the best-known meditation technique is transcendental meditation (TM), which was originally brought to wide public attention by the Maharishi Mahesh in the 1960s. TM is based on principles commonly used in India, which probably date back to well before the time of Buddha, over 2,500 years ago. It involves spending periods of about 20 minutes, twice each day, sitting in a perfectly relaxed state in a quiet room, with eyes closed, breathing easily. The aim is to use the mind to settle and slow down the body, creating 'inner stillness', using a special repetitive technique called a mantra. This can be a sound, or a repeated word or phrase, which is specially chosen to suit that individual. Once started, TM needs to be continued on a regular daily basis, as the effect is cumulative – it's not a one-off form of therapy.

There's no doubt that this form of 'mind over matter' can reduce the heart rate and blood pressure, and it's possible that these purely physical effects may in turn be producing beneficial psychological ones as well.

TM is quite an easy technique to acquire after you've been instructed by a trained teacher. This will usually involve going through a series of introductory talks, followed by individual sessions on the actual learning process. After that you can continue on your own. *TM isn't an approach that will suit everyone, but I do know of several patients who claim to have found it helpful.* (For more information on TM contact the TM National Enquiry Office on 01695 51213.)

# Naturopathy

This therapy aims to use the body's natural internal healing powers as a basis for recovery from ill health and makes little use of external treatments. Naturopaths tend to regard their role as helping people to heal themselves, so they tend to pay much more attention to the individual than the disease.

Dietary modification, with the use of fresh and unprocessed foods, is one of the most important recommendations in change of lifestyle. Herbal medicines, manipulation and massage may also be included.

Part of the process of coming to terms with and recovering from ME/CFS involves making changes in lifestyle. If a naturopath fully understand the condition, they may be able to offer some good advice. (For how to find a naturopath, see Useful Addresses, page 428.)

# Osteopathy and Chiropractic

## Osteopathy

Probably the commonest reason for patients consulting osteopaths is back pain, which is often related to problems with the bony vertebrae or structures which surround and support them – the muscles and ligaments. Osteopaths become skilled in detecting positional changes in the vertebrae and the way they move in relation to one another. Their aim is to correct these abnormalities, and hence the symptoms which occur as a result. Qualified osteopaths have to complete a comprehensive training, and then conform to professional standards.

Both osteopaths and chiropractors first carry out a careful clinical examination, and may make use of X-rays to exclude conditions which could be worsened by manipulative techniques.

Many people with ME/CFS have back pain, along with muscle spasm and pain. When this seems to be unrelieved by conventional medical approaches, these are therapies which might be worth considering, although if you have any sort of back pain, it's very advisable to discuss the use of manipulative therapy with your general practitioner before going ahead. Back pain in someone over the age of 50 could be due to osteoporosis or osteomalacia, in which case manipulation wouldn't be a good idea.

Many general practitioners now accept osteopathy as a valid form of treatment – in fact many of them use it themselves for their bad backs, and a few have even become qualified osteopaths. Osteopathy, however, is not usually available on the NHS.

The only clinical trial into the possible effectiveness of osteopathic treatment for ME/CFS has been carried out by Raymond Perrin and his colleagues from the University of Salford. Treatment consisted of a course of massage to various groups of muscles along with manipulation to parts of the spine and back. A number of patients on this trial reported a significant degree of improvement compared to a control group who received no form of manipulative therapy (reference 493).

(For details of how to find an osteopath see Useful Addresses, page 428.)

## Chiropractic

Chiropractors use a variety of manipulative techniques based on the assumption that the cause of symptoms such as back pain or referred nerve pain (e.g. sciatica down the leg) results from what they term 'misalignments' or subluxations of the spinal column. They believe that by correcting these misalignments, they can then restore the normal anatomy and so relieve symptoms, be they due to muscle spasm, bone misplacement or pressure on the nerves as they pass out of spaces between the vertebrae.

As with osteopathy, this is a form of alternative treatment that is becoming increasingly respectable amongst orthodox medical opinion; a recently published trial in the *British Medical Journal* did appear to confirm its beneficial effects.

Unfortunately, anybody can set up in practice and call themselves a chiropractor, and just like osteopathy in the wrong hands, this can have its dangers. Registered and trained chiropractors belong to a professional organisation and there are a few medically qualified ones. (For how to find a chiropractor, see Useful Addresses, page 412.)

# Oxygen Therapy

Various forms of oxygen therapy are now becoming available. The treatment is claimed to work on the idea that increased levels of oxygen in the body may help in the repair of damaged nerve tissues. In theory it all sounds very impressive – increasing the amount of vital oxygen into the tissues ought to help muscle and brain function, rejuvenate 'sick cells' and boost the immune system etc.

One form of oxygen therapy being used in the UK involves the injection of dilute amounts of hydrogen peroxide (bleach) into the muscle.

In America you can now pay out £50 a visit for 'Ozone Treatment' (three molecules of oxygen). This involves withdrawing a pint of blood, adding ozone till the blood turns bright red and then re-infusing it! In practice, playing around with the body's natural physiology is not nearly so easy or simple.

Stabilised oxygen (SO) is yet another form of oxygen treatment whereby drops are placed into drinking water to allegedly enhance body oxygen levels.

Some people with ME/CFS are now joining up with multiple sclerosis patients who use hyperbaric oxygen chambers – oxygen at very high pressures.

Despite claims that this is an effective form of treatment for a number of neurological disorders, as well as producing a beneficial effect on immune responses, a review of eight recent clinical trials (reference: *Acta Neurologica Scandanavia*, 1995, 91, 330–4) found only one trial which showed up any significant benefit from this highly controversial form of treatment. In another, deterioration actually occurred more often in those treated with hyperbaric oxygen. The remainder found no significant differences between the two groups.

Concerns have also been expressed about long-term side-effects, including serious damage to the retina at the back of the eye.

*I am not yet convinced by any of these claims about the benefits of oxygen therapies, and I suspect that most of them are of no value whatsoever.*

## Probiotics

These are concentrated cultures of 'good bacteria' (e.g. *Lactobacillus acidophilus* and species of *Bifidobacterium*) which, supposedly, help to restore the imbalance of gut organisms following anything from stress to excessively prescribed antibiotics or attacks of gastroenteritis.

This approach does have some theoretical attractions, but it is very unlikely that minute quantities of bacteria found in commercial preparations could significantly reverse any such imbalance. And there is no evidence whatsoever that people with ME/CFS have such an imbalance in their gut organisms.

The unsavoury activities of one probiotic manufacturer, who was promoting a product containing potentially harmful bacteria, led to an investigation by the Department of Health in 1989.

A recent report in *Health Which?* (reference: August 1997, 134–5) examined the bacterial contents of 17 different commercial brands. Only 8 out of 17 contained the strains of bacteria listed on the label. Many contained far less bacteria than was stated. Other products contained strains of bacteria that were not even listed! This report also queried whether capsules containing probiotics could survive a journey through the acid in the stomach before entering the intestines.

Nevertheless, many people with ME/CFS believe that they have a disturbance in their gut bacteria and regularly take expensive probiotics as part of an anti-candida regime. If used in this way, probiotics must be stored correctly in a fridge or at least in a cool dry place, away from sunlight.

*I do not believe that probiotics in this form have any useful role to play in ME/CFS and would not recommend their use.*

# Propolis

This is a resinous substance collected by bees from the bark and sticky buds of poplar and fir trees. Bees then use propolis to line the interior of their hives to protect the Queen's eggs. Propolis is said to have powerful anti-bacterial properties and has long been used as a natural treatment for various skin disorders. It is also being used by some alternative practitioners for the treatment of mouth ulcers, asthma and, not surprisingly, ME/CFS.

Commercially available tablets contain widely varying concentrations of active propolis. Those who believe that this product can be useful maintain that a minimum effective dose is around 1.5mg per day. The only side-effects appear to be occasional allergic reactions, so anyone with an allergy to bee products must take care.

*Although frequent anecdotal claims are made about propolis aiding recovery in ME/CFS, I remain unconvinced.*

# Reflexology

Reflexologists claim that by examining the soles of the feet they can detect all manner of ill health. Each part of the sole is divided into separate zones representing a particular organ or a different anatomical part of the body. For instance, the big toe is supposed to represent the head, brain and pituitary gland.

Once a diagnosis has been made, reflexologists claim that by the use of massage, blocked energy channels can be cleared in the organ or limb to restore normal health.

*The therapy itself is undoubtedly very relaxing but I cannot recommend this approach for diagnostic purposes.*

(Details of how to find a reflexologist can be found in Useful Addresses, page 430.)

# Relaxation Techniques

For anyone under stress, relaxation techniques (teaching your body how to relax) are a far wiser idea than taking tranquillisers. One of the easiest and cheapest do-it-yourself methods is to follow the instructions on tapes which are available from various organisations, including Relaxation for Living and Lifeskills (see Useful Addresses, pages 430–1).

# Royal Jelly

This is an expensive mixture of vitamins, minerals, amino acids and a 'mystery ingredient' which is alleged to have almost miraculous healing properties for an endless list of ailments including ME/CFS. Although many alternative practitioners now recommend this product, the results from the Action for ME treatment survey (see page 294) are not very impressive. The possibility of severe allergic reactions occurring after taking royal jelly products also needs to be considered. A report in the *British Medical Journal* (1995, 311, 1472) referred to the case of a 31-year-old lady who developed a life-threatening asthma attack after taking only two royal jelly capsules. Six weeks later she again took some royal jelly and within 40 minutes a similar reaction occurred. The explanation appears to lie in the fact that royal jelly products contain high levels of various bee proteins. Consequently, there is a risk of allergic reactions taking place in anyone who is predisposed to allergies, particularly when such reactions have followed bee stings.

*I cannot recommend the use of royal jelly in ME/CFS.*

# Shiatsu

This is an ancient form of oriental medicine dating back over 5,000 years. Shiatsu practitioners use their fingers and palms to press along what the Japanese refer to as meridian lines. These lines are supposed to represent 'channels of living magnetic energy' which pass through the body and connect vital organs. The aim of shiatsu is to correct any imbalance by dispersing 'vital energy' to places where it is most needed and moving it away from areas where 'congestion' is occurring. A session of shiatsu will last for about an hour, during which you are positioned on a comfortable mattress on the floor. I am not at all convinced by the theory of moving 'vital energy' around the body in this way. Even so, *shiatsu might be worth trying if you have faith in this type of approach.*

# Signalysis

This is one of the most unusual alternative therapies which have been aimed at people with ME/CFS. It involves taking a sample of blood which is then heated to a very high temperature. It is then claimed that by carefully examining the resulting crystals under a microscope an assessment can be made on the function of various parts of the body. An individual 'therapy' is then prepared for the patient based on these findings.

In 1997, the Royal Pharmaceutical Society carried out an investigation into the claims being made for Signalysis and concluded that they were nothing more than 'quackery' (reference: *British Medical Journal*, 1997, 315, 625).

*This is a process which I cannot recommend for either diagnostic or treatment purposes.*

## Yoga

This is an approach that combines spiritual, mental and physical training. The movements involve light exercises which are designed to be carried out slowly, and then the particular position is maintained for several minutes. The aim of yoga is to develop both flexibility and relaxation.

Yoga does seem to produce genuine benefits in people with back pain, anxiety, high blood pressure, asthma and PMT. I'm not sure about its value in ME/CFS, although I do know of people who have found it useful.

If you decide to try this technique do make sure that you find a teacher who fully understands ME/CFS and is able to advise on the most appropriate type of movements. The wrong type of yoga could end up doing more harm than good.

## Conclusion

As you can see, there's a bewildering choice of therapies on offer from the alternative health sector. Some seem to be of help, whereas others are nothing more than pseudoscientific nonsense and a complete waste of money. A small number (e.g. germanium) have turned out be positively dangerous, even fatal.

Alternative therapies are one area of health care where the consumer has to carefully make up their mind on the evidence that's available. If you want to find out more about a particular therapy you could contact one of the organisations listed under Alternative and Complementary Medicine in Useful Addresses.

If you're unlucky to be ripped off or harmed by an alternative form of therapy, it's worth contacting Healthwatch (see Useful Addresses, page 419) who are actively campaigning for so-called 'natural medicines' to be subjected to the same controls over efficacy and safety that apply to ordinary drugs.

## Action for ME Survey Results

In 1990, Action for ME conducted a survey into treatments which had been used by nearly 500 of its members. With kind permission, the results are reproduced below.

Perhaps one of the most interesting and disturbing points to emerge concerns cost – the average amount of money spent in the private or alternative health sector amounted to nearly £900, with one person spending over £16,000! However, only 8 per cent felt that they had wasted their money, and 53 per cent considered that it had been a combination of money well spent and wasted. The remainder did not feel strongly one way or another.

Analysing the results it seems that these therapies fall into three distinct groups. At the top of the list are those which seem to benefit the majority of users. In the middle are a much larger group where, I have to say, the results suggest a strong placebo response. Down at the bottom are a selection of treatments (e.g. steroids, tranquillisers and antibiotics) which almost everyone would agree should be avoided in ME/CFS.

Hopefully, in due course, some of these alternative therapies can be subjected to properly controlled clinical trials to see if they really are of any value.

## Table 11 Therapy

| | Useful % | No effect % | Harmful % | Trying this therapy % | No. of answers |
|---|---|---|---|---|---|
| Rest | 94.5 | 5.2 | 0.3 | 88.9 | 618 |
| Hydrotherapy (warm baths, etc.) | 79.6 | 11.1 | 9.3 | 15.5 | 108 |
| Relaxation techniques | 79.5 | 20.2 | 0.3 | 49.1 | 341 |
| Diet | 73.2 | 24.1 | 2.7 | 80.1 | 557 |
| Massage | 64.2 | 17.6 | 18.1 | 29.4 | 204 |
| Natural anti-candida treatment | 55.4 | 38.3 | 6.4 | 42.9 | 298 |
| Healing | 54.4 | 44.0 | 1.6 | 26.2 | 182 |
| Aromatherapy | 50.9 | 45.4 | 3.7 | 23.5 | 163 |
| Antidepressants | 49.4 | 22.9 | 27.7 | 48.3 | 336 |
| Vitamins and minerals | 49.2 | 48.0 | 2.8 | 87.2 | 606 |
| Colonic irrigation | 47.5 | 45.9 | 6.6 | 8.8 | 61 |
| Enemas | 47.4 | 39.5 | 13.2 | 5.5 | 38 |
| EPD allergy desensitisation | 47.0 | 42.2 | 10.8 | 11.9 | 83 |
| Anti-candida drug therapy | 46.5 | 37.9 | 15.6 | 36.8 | 256 |
| Evening primrose oil (EFAs) | 45.8 | 50.2 | 4.0 | 72.8 | 506 |
| Probiotics (acidophilus, etc.) | 43.4 | 50.0 | 6.6 | 43.5 | 302 |
| Reflexology | 43.2 | 40.9 | 15.9 | 19.0 | 132 |
| Oxygen sleep apnoea treatment | 42.9 | 57.1 | 0.0 | 1.0 | 7 |
| Homoeopathy | 42.1 | 48.1 | 9.8 | 45.4 | 316 |
| Desensitisation | 42.0 | 44.0 | 14.0 | 7.2 | 50 |

| Herbal remedies | 40.8 | 51.8 | 7.3 | 35.3 | 245 |
| Gamma globulin | 40.0 | 41.7 | 18.3 | 8.6 | 60 |
| Acupuncture/acupressure | 40.8 | 48.7 | 10.5 | 27.5 | 191 |
| Sleep treatment Charing X | 33.3 | 50.0 | 16.7 | 0.9 | 6 |
| Dental amalgam removal | 32.7 | 60.0 | 7.3 | 7.9 | 55 |
| Amino acids | 26.6 | 62.6 | 10.8 | 20.0 | 139 |
| Germanium | 18.9 | 64.9 | 16.2 | 21.3 | 148 |
| Royal Jelly | 15.3 | 73.0 | 11.7 | 44.2 | 307 |
| Graded exercise programme | 37.0 | 13.4 | 49.6 | 18.3 | 127 |
| Tranquillisers | 36.6 | 23.2 | 40.2 | 16.1 | 112 |
| Fasting | 32.9 | 22.4 | 44.7 | 12.2 | 85 |
| Steroid drugs | 14.3 | 20.4 | 65.3 | 7.1 | 49 |
| Antibiotics | 11.3 | 16.7 | 72.1 | 29.4 | 204 |

*Reproduced by kind permission of* Action for ME

# Further Reading

*The Which? Guide to Complementary Medicine* (Penguin) contains information on most of the commonly used alternative therapies as well as explaining issues such as scientific evidence, availability on the NHS and the law in relation to this type of treatment.

## Allergies

*Allergy: The facts* by R. Davies and S. Ollier (Oxford University Press) is a sound book for lay readers on a topical and controversial subject.
*The Complete Guide to Food Allergy and Intolerance* by Dr Jonathan Brostoff and Linda Gamblin (Bloomsbury) explains why certain foods cause problems and how people can identify and eliminate the common culprits. Also covers many of the more unorthodox approaches to allergy investigation and treatment.
*The Allergy Diet* by Dr John Hunter (Vermilion) is a very useful guide to the management of food allergy and intolerance.
*Allergy, Conventional and Alternative Concepts* is a highly critical report on many of the approaches to diagnosis and management referred to in this chapter. It is available from the Royal College of Physicians, 11 St Andrew's Place, London NW1 4LE.

The British Allergy Foundation (see Useful Addresses, page 408) publishes a series of useful leaflets on most aspects of allergy and also has a telephone helpline.

## Candida albicans

*Beat Candida Through Diet* by Gill Jacobs (Vermilion) supports the view that this yeast infection is involved in ME/CFS and provides detailed advice on management.

## Herbal medicines

*Herbal Medicines* by Carol Newall, Linda Anderson and David Phillipson (Pharmaceutical Press) is the most comprehensive guide available on this aspect of alternative medicine. The possible benefits of all commonly used herbs are fully discussed along with toxic side-effects. Essential reading for anyone who wishes to pursue herbal remedies.

## Homoeopathic remedies

*The Family Guide to Homoeopathy* by Dr Andrew Lockie (Hamish Hamilton) provides a comprehensive guide to the use of homoeopathic treatments.

# PART 3

# LEARNING TO LIVE WITH ME/CFS

# Three Case Histories

## Looking After a Young Child Who has ME/CFS

*by Rachel Glover's mother*

At eight years of age my daughter Rachel was an outgoing, active and very cheerful child who enjoyed ballet lessons, gymnastics and long country walks. At the crack of dawn she'd be up, singing around the house and generally driving us all to distraction with her 'get up and go'. She loved school and couldn't wait to get there each morning. She even wanted to go at weekends! Alas, I didn't realise how precious a time it was for us and I now look back on those eight short years as being Rachel's childhood. For she was then struck down, quite dramatically, with what our GP thought was glandular fever.

Rachel had swollen glands, a temperature and an ulcerated sore throat. She was racked with pain all over her body and this continued for several weeks. However, we were told to get her back to school as soon as possible.

As time went on her symptoms didn't seem to improve, so I asked for a referral to the local hospital. The consultant agreed with our GP's opinion and felt she would be fully better within three months and to continue going to school. She went back, but was too weary to take part in general activities, preferring to sit in a quiet corner. The teachers were convinced that she'd become used to being at home, and wouldn't accept my doubts and fears concerning her non-recovery.

Rachel would only be in school for a couple of days before collapsing with the return of all her previous symptoms. Even when she did manage to go she was never totally well, and this continued for two years. Daily living was never the same again for any of the family. We attempted to go on one of our favourite walks one Sunday, when she appeared to be a little brighter, but after only 300 yards she collapsed and had to be carried home.

One day, looking through the family snapshots, trying to amuse her, I was shocked to realise the drastic change which had occurred. Gone were the lovely rosy cheeks and bright eyes, only to be replaced by a deathly pallor and dark circles under the eyes. I took her back to hospital, where she had every conceivable blood test, but in the end the advice was that she should 'pull herself together', and stop thinking of herself as being an invalid.

We returned to our GP and this time asked for a second opinion at Great Ormond Street children's hospital in London. There we were told that, yes, Rachel was poorly, but they didn't know the cause. The consultant said he'd come across children like this before and that after a time they always made a recovery, but he didn't know what ailed them. He continued to see Rachel on a regular basis and fully backed us up with, for example, countless letters to the school. Most important of all, he gave us lots of moral support. However, other doctors and teachers involved with Rachel continued to maintain that there was nothing much wrong with her.

As so often happens when one has almost given up hope, I turned on the radio one evening and found myself listening to Dr Shepherd talking about ME/CFS. It hit me that this was exactly what Rachel was suffering from. I contacted the ME Association and was put in touch with another doctor who was experienced in dealing with childhood ME/CFS. After listening to our story and arranging blood tests, the diagnosis was confirmed. His advice was that there was no 'cure', but with careful management she would eventually recover. We felt a great relief that, at last, we had a diagnosis of what was wrong.

By now Rachel was starting to require a wheelchair to go any distance and by the time of her last Christmas at junior school it was necessary to push her to the local church for the carol concert.

There were times of despair and one particularly awful night she said, 'Mummy, it would be better to die than to let me suffer like this any longer.' I was shocked and so very sad for her. We had a little weep together, but I felt so angry that my child was having to suffer for so long in this way.

In the midst of all this the school decided to threaten us with prosecution for Rachel's constant non-attendance. This resulted in a meeting with the Chief Education Officer to try and sort out the mounting difficulties concerning Rachel's education, or rather the lack of it. At last we seemed to have someone who was totally on our side. Soon after the meeting a letter arrived from the school, not quite an apology, but near enough, plus a pile of kind letters from all the children in Rachel's class.

It was arranged for us to have the services of a home tutor, and the authority decided that Rachel should be 'statemented'. We'd never heard of this procedure before, so I contacted the Advisory Centre for Education (see Useful Addresses, page 411) and received a lengthy reply – all very much in favour of the statementing procedure. Statementing is basically a legal term connected with the English 1981 Education Act. It's a means of assessing the educational requirements of a sick or disabled child. It highlights the needs or support the child requires, be it a home tutor, flexible school hours, tutor support whilst in school lessons, provision of wheelchairs and ramps, etc. It outlines virtually everything the child needs within the school environment.

The process involves meetings between medical representatives, teachers and a child psychologist from the education department, along with the parents. Written evidence can also be submitted. If the parents disagree with the findings there are procedures available to have decisions changed. When it's been decided exactly what help is required, a 'statement' is prepared. When everyone is fully satisfied with this final statement it is placed with the local authority, who must carry out *all* the recommendations and make any necessary funds available. If the school doesn't comply with any of the required tasks, the authority can make it do so. In essence, it's well worth having and so far it's certainly been of great help to us.

A home tutor was provisionally allocated to Rachel for five hours a week. This was more than enough, as she was rarely well enough for more. The teacher was fully aware of the problems created by ME/CFS and on days when Rachel was well enough they'd read stories and sometimes play a board game. Unfortunately, they rarely managed to accomplish much real work as Rachel's concentration was so low. However, it was nice for Rachel to have this type of company and help – a lady who could be trusted not to push her beyond her limitations. It also gave me the first chance in many months to have an hour or so to myself.

Children with ME/CFS require a great deal of help and support when trying to return to school. Your child, like mine, may have been extremely bright and able prior to being ill, but now with concentration difficulties and muscle fatigue to contend with, they may find themselves increasingly forced into the situation where they need a statement in order to receive the requisite help.

In September, Rachel enrolled at her new secondary school, although she didn't actually make her first appearance until February. The school was our choice, even before it became obvious that she now had very specific needs. It's well known in the area for its high standards of education, coupled with a strong belief in caring for less fortunate pupils, who find the staff helpful and sympathetic to their needs. The school has ramps, a lift and other adaptations for pupils with disabilities. At present there are six children who need these aids. Disabled children are encouraged to take part in all aspects of school life wherever possible, but if, like Rachel, rest is the name of the game, they go to great lengths to make sure that they don't overdo things.

By Christmas, Rachel had been ill for four years. She hadn't yet met her classmates, but the children sent her a massive pile of beautifully written letters, jokes and stories. They said that the teacher and matron had often talked about her, so they felt they already knew Rachel, and looked forward to the day when she'd be well enough to join them. Girls had already volunteered to push her chair and be helpers. Needless to say this was all received with much joy and she started to look forward to being well enough to be able to go next term.

As her health gradually improved I left it entirely up to Rachel to decide when to start her first day. In January she proudly hung up her new school uniform on the wardrobe door, and began to collect her pens and equipment together for the big day. We had a few false starts, but by mid-February she felt well enough to go for one lesson per day. I took her to school by car, and she was pushed in her wheelchair to meet the new classmates.

After that one short visit she was exhausted and lay on the settee for the rest of the day. In the first week she only managed one lesson, but after that she gradually built things up, until she was actually staying for school lunches with her new-found friends – always the same baked beans and chips, but who cares! Suddenly she was a different girl, starting to feel a bit better day by day, and taking an interest in life again.

For me, this had been a very difficult time, having to stand back and watch her first few tentative steps, wanting to stop her from doing too much, but realising how important it was for her to learn for herself. It wasn't long before she'd actually accomplished three weeks of full-time schooling. There was nothing stopping her now. I'd hold my breath as she played in the garden with her friends, running to and fro. However, by bedtime, one evening, the results of all this new activity were beginning to show. After a restless night she awoke once again with swollen glands, feeling very low. She didn't become as unwell as I'd feared, and she didn't slip back too far. Recovering from ME/CFS is often two steps forward and one step back. Her level of activity – both physical and mental – was still obviously at a much reduced level, but a year earlier I had truly believed that my daughter had no future at all.

Her teachers have given her wonderful reports: 'Keen, willing to work and a pleasure to teach' are all music to my ears. She still has to have a home tutor for some lessons, as well as help from a welfare assistant during craft lessons. And instead of PE, she spends time with the matron doing gentle exercises.

Rachel is now 12½ years old, and remains thin and frail. She still becomes tired quite quickly and has to rely on her wheelchair at times. The local school for the handicapped have a warm pool and they've kindly agreed to let Rachel use it for half an hour each week. She just goes and lies in the water and the physiotherapist gives her some gentle exercises in the pool. She is getting better, improving slowly day by day, and one day I'm sure that all this will just be a painful memory.

I don't think that children of Rachel's age can ever come to terms with an illness of this magnitude – neither can many adults. She accepts that she has a strange illness, but she is heartily sick of it. The only time she'll put herself out to discuss the subject is if she hears of another child going through black days, and then she tries to help them feel a bit better. She no longer plans ahead; she just says she'll see how she feels on the day before deciding what to do. She used to cry a lot, but now she tries to laugh things off by saying that it's 'only the bugs' which are bothering her. Until quite recently she didn't like to talk about her future aspirations. Now, she talks about doing 'something with computers', so she's obviously feeling much more confident about the future.

The financial pressures on the family have been quite considerable during the course of Rachel's illness, especially at a time when I'd planned to return to full-time employment again. This I had to forego in order to be at home to look after Rachel. In view of her quite severe disability we applied for disability benefits. Since then, like many others, we've had to endure the full bureaucratic nightmare of the DSS system. One examining doctor wrote that she fulfilled the requirements, as the exertion required to walk exacerbated her illness. However, it then came as a shock to find that this advice had been turned down by the authorities who make the final decision. An appeal is possible, but when you're physically and mentally worn down by caring for someone, the last thing you want (or are capable of) is fighting for benefits. However, I've found a welfare rights worker, attached to the Benefits Unit of the town hall. They help prepare your case and will even attend the tribunal with you.

As for the family, Rachel's illness has taken its toll on us all. Our youngest daughter, Emma, just 11, has missed out more than anyone else on holidays, trips out, picnics, etc. Most of the time she's been uncomplaining, but just occasionally she becomes bitterly upset and jealous about the disproportionate amount of attention Rachel receives. Fortunately I'm now in a position to be able to spend more time with Emma and am trying to mend the damage. But, just like Rachel, these precious years can never be replaced. It's not been quite the same for my sons, and Ben, who's now 17, is happy with his own friends away at college.

Having to cope with this illness has taught us many things, above all to take each day as it comes. If your child can't eat, sleep or whatever, don't worry – maybe they will tomorrow. When, as undoubtedly they will, your child begins to start taking the first tentative steps back to normal life, learn to stand back, as they've now got to find their own level of activity and learn to have control over their own lives again.

Ignorance has only made Rachel's suffering worse, and I think the illness has lasted longer as a result. If only I'd known at the beginning what I know now, I think I could have handled things much more easily. Rest and a proper period of convalescence would, I believe, have significantly aided her recovery.

Believe, really believe, deep in your heart, that your child can and will get better. It happens slowly but surely – just you wait and see.

# Children and Young People with ME/CFS

## Author's note

ME/CFS is not an illness that often affects children, although an increasing number of cases are being recognised – some as young as seven. The only epidemiological survey carried out in the UK suggests a prevalence of around 7 per 10,000 children (reference 499).

As Rachel's case illustrates, children with ME/CFS present their own special problems. These include difficulties in obtaining the correct diagnosis, conflicting and sometimes harmful advice about management, and battles with education authorities over schooling.

Parents also face their own unique difficulties. Instead of receiving help and support from doctors and other caring agencies, they may have to pursue a series of battles on behalf of their sick child. They, too, can easily end up feeling isolated and bitter with the very professionals who are supposed to help.

## Symptoms

These are very similar to those seen in adults, with the onset frequently being precipitated by some form of infection. The most commonly reported symptoms involve:

- Muscle: fatigue, pain or cramp
- Nervous system: headaches, poor memory/concentration, clumsiness, writing difficulties, dizziness
- Eyes: eyestrain, pain, increased sensitivity to bright lights
- Sleep disturbances
- Digestion: poor appetite, stomach pains.

Disturbance in sleep pattern can be pronounced, with the child asleep during the day and then awake for most of the night. This sleep reversal is often accompanied by nightmares and irritability (reference 539).

Some children lose a significant amount of weight early on and occasionally this progresses on to true anorexia. After prolonged immobility in bed, there is a real danger of muscle wasting and contractures occurring.

Psychiatric and emotional problems (depression, learning difficulties) may also occur as the illness progresses. Many of these symptoms, particularly a child's energy levels and ability to carry out mental tasks, tend to fluctuate quite widely. Some may even be able to perform with relative normality for short periods, mistakenly giving doctors or teachers the impression that they're 'not really ill'.

## Diagnosis

All too often these children are misdiagnosed as being hysterical, malingering or school refusers. The result is that the child is dramatically forced back into full-time schooling and plenty of physical exercise (the 'in at the deep end' approach) which produces rapid deterioration in both physical and emotional symptoms.

Some paediatricians and child psychiatrists still maintain that ME/CFS does not exist in children, or if it does it is nothing more than a short-lived period of postviral debility. Fortunately, a growing number are now accepting that, although rare, it can present in this age group, and that for recovery to occur the doctor must take into account the physical, social and emotional factors that form a complex interrelationship in childhood ME/CFS.

In the case of children, I think it is essential that the diagnosis is confirmed by a paediatrician who understands this illness. They should then take an active role in co-ordinating all aspects of management.

Any good paediatrician will ensure that other treatable causes of chronic fatigue are ruled out. These include:

- Infections: Lyme disease, toxocara, toxoplasmosis
- Blood disorders: anaemia, leukaemia, Hodgkin's disease
- Digestive disorders: Crohn's disease, coeliac disease, giardia
- Liver, kidney and thyroid disorders
- Primary muscle diseases
- Psychiatric conditions: depression, anorexia, school phobia.

In this respect I well remember the story of a child from Devon whose case was presented to a meeting on ME/CFS at Great Ormond Street children's hospital. The boy had initially been diagnosed as having ME/CFS, then as having myasthenia gravis, before being properly assessed at this hospital. It turned out that he had a chronic infection called Lyme disease (see page 92) which was successfully treated with antibiotics.

One other advantage of having support from a paediatrician is when it comes to problems with schools or refusal of DSS benefits. Remember, if you are not happy with a specialist's opinion, or if you are told that it cannot be ME/CFS because it does not occur in children, you can ask for a second opinion from another paediatrician.

## Management

Once again, the broad principles are not that different from those with adults, taking into account the fact that children have their own emotional, practical and education problems. Striking the right balance with rest and exercise, sleep, mental activity and good nutrition are probably the most important aspects of any recovery process. It's important to remain optimistic about the chances of recovery whilst at the same time being realistic about the pace at which this will occur.

A period of bed rest may well be beneficial in the *early stages*, but following this, rest and exercise need to be carefully balanced. On the one hand there is a very real danger that prolonged immobility will result in further weakness, wasting and even contractures. On the other there is no doubt that when children do start to recover, there is a great temptation to suddenly start doing too much and precipitate a relapse. If children learn to pace themselves, both physically and mentally, they should be able to build on their progress, which in turn will have a very beneficial effect on self-confidence.

Children's appetites tend to decline rapidly when they are ill and this is especially so in ME/CFS. Although it's never a good idea to make a great issue over meals or eating habits, I would recommend that their diet contains good quality carbohydrate, protein and an adequate fluid intake. If the diet really does become very 'faddy', then a mineral and vitamin supplement is advisable.

## Drugs

These should be used as little as possible in children. However, a low dose of a tricyclic antidepressant (e.g. amitriptyline) may be helpful for sleep disturbance or severe muscle pain. True clinical depression may well require a course of antidepressants – a decision which should ideally be taken by a child psychiatrist or paediatrician. Headaches should be managed with a strictly limited amount of simple analgesics (e.g. paracetamol). Aspirin should *not* be given to any child under 12.

## Emotional and social life

For a child, any kind of unexplained illness that produces such a devastating effect on all aspects of their life is bound to be a frightening experience. So, just like adults, they need to be given some form of simple explanation about how it can sometimes take the body rather a long time to recover from an infection. They also need constant reassurance that although things may look very bleak at the moment there is a good chance that, given time, they will recover and start leading a normal life again.

The sudden loss of mobility, friendships and self-confidence can all mount up and have a severe effect on a child's emotional feelings. That's why it's important to make sure that close friends are still encouraged to keep in touch, that occasional trips outside the house are organised and that some new non-active interests are encouraged. A small pet might become a very welcome companion; some children find keeping in touch with friends by phone or letter very useful.

Occasionally, these emotional and depressive aspects of the illness end up having a very negative effect on recovery. Some children develop a clinging dependency on their parents, who in turn become over-protective and unduly cautious about altering the child's routine regarding exercise or return to school. Even though the physical side may be improving, the child becomes trapped by the psychological aspects of such a long-term illness. In this case the vicious circle needs to be broken in a firm but fair manner. If this is done correctly, the child can turn the corner and start to make a significant degree of recovery. They will require a great deal of encouragement to slowly start joining in all aspects of family life. This could involve coming downstairs for just a short period each day for a meal or to watch television, and then gradually increasing both physical and mental activity inside the home environment.

Unfortunately, at the other end of the spectrum, there are cases of very ill children in which the local authorities have decided to use a Place of Safety Order to separate the child from what they regard as 'over-involved' parents. This is then followed by compulsory admission to hospital where family visiting is deliberately limited and treatment may involve controversial forms of behaviour therapy and strenuous physio-therapy. The latter may turn out to be totally inappropriate and lead to a further deterioration in the child's condition.

Should this situation arise, I would suggest that a second opinion from a consultant with experience in ME/CFS should be requested. Secondly, legal advice from a solicitor who is well-acquainted with the law as it affects children should be sought urgently. The child may end up being made a ward of court.

## Schooling and further education

One widely publicised UK study (reference 499) suggested that ME/CFS may be the single most common cause of long-term absence from school. Although mild and recovering cases should be encouraged to stay or return to school – which will inevitably involve avoiding games, PE, tiring journeys and excessive amounts of homework – a period of absence is likely to be necessary for almost all children with ME/CFS, especially in the very early stages.

Unfortunately, many children and young people with ME/CFS are still being denied proper educational opportunities because of inflexible or unhelpful attitudes by those in authority. Children who are still too unwell to even make a small journey back to school may be denied home tuition because the authorities fear that it will encourage 'sick role behaviour' and cause a further delay in a return to school. Older children and teenagers may find that they have lost too much coursework to go back and complete exam courses, and some colleges and universities have been far from sympathetic when students have missed more than a couple of terms. Others, however, have bent over backwards to try and help by rescheduling exams and keeping a university place open for several years.

This is why it is so important to find a doctor who is prepared to fully support the child and liaise on their behalf with the school or college. There should then be no difficulties with medical officers over suspected school refusal and they may well be able to persuade a college to hold open a place for a further year.

Planning a return to school can be one of the most difficult aspects of management. Ideally, this should involve the family doctor, the education welfare officer, the teachers and possibly a child psychologist if there has been a prolonged absence. Careful advance planning needs to include transport arrangements, avoidance of exam pressures and, initially, being very flexible about the actual amount of time spent in lessons. A sudden return to full-time education is likely to be unrealistic.

Where the child still has significant physical disabilities (e.g. uses a wheelchair), the statementing procedure (a statement of special educational needs) described in Rachel's story, may be very helpful.

If you are having problems with the educational authorities, it is well worth contacting an educational welfare officer (EWO). If this fails, write to the Chair of the Education Authority, sending a copy to your MP.

If home tuition is refused, you can write to the civil servant responsible for home tuition at the Department of Education and Employment in London.

Sadly, disputes with local authorities over home tuition have sometimes only been resolved by parents taking the matter to court in an attempt to obtain even a few hours of education per week. The results of such action have not always been successful, and this type of action obviously requires expert legal advice.

Difficulties in obtaining home tuition for children with ME/CFS may well increase in view of an extremely unhelpful conclusion contained in the Royal Colleges' report: 'As far as possible we discourage home tuition . . . Tuition at home should be reserved only for the most severely affected and should be for as short a time as possible, and always in close liaison with the school' (para 10.12).

## Benefits and practical support

A number of DSS sickness and disability benefits are available to children and teenagers. Relevant ones include the severe disablement allowance (16 years or older), disability living allowance (no lower age limit for the care component; five years or older for the mobility component), a vaccine damage payment (if severely disabled following vaccine-triggered ME/CFS) and income support (16 years or older if severely disabled).

Extra financial help might be available to help with education or adaptions to the home. Chapter 19: Additional Help and Benefits contains further information, as does the *Disability Rights Handbook* (see Useful Addresses). You may also find it helpful to ask your social services department to carry out a formal assessment of your caring needs in regard to the Carers Act (see pages 327–8).

## Outcome

Very few studies have looked at the long-term outlook for children with ME/CFS. Those which have included children indicate that the chances of recovery are significantly better than those of adults – provided the child receives good management advice early on, along with appropriate help and support with their educational needs. Recovery may well take a considerable period of time and you're likely to receive a considerable amount of conflicting advice along the way, but never give up hope.

The ME Association runs a separate section – the Young People's Group – to look after the needs of children and teenager with ME/CFS.

For details of organisations which can provide further advice and information on issues relating to health, legal problems and the education of sick children, see Useful Addresses under 'Children'.

Medical papers which have been published on the subject of ME/CFS in children can be found on pages 475–77. Unfortunately, many of them have been written by doctors who see ME/CFS in childhood as being more of a behavioural problem than a medical illness.

# Further Reading

The 1998 National Task Force report on ME/CFS and Young People, which deals with diagnosis, management and education issues, is available from Westcare (see Useful Addresses, page 403).

Information on the education of children and young people is contained in the ME Association's booklet *Guidelines for parents and children with ME.*

Dr Alan Franklin, a consultant paediatrician, has written aan excellent medical paper which reviews the practical management of children with ME/CFS (reference 543).

# Pregnancy and ME/CFS

*by Frances H. Woodward*

I had suffered ME/CFS for two and a half years before we decided to have a baby. It was a very difficult decision to make because, at that time, my 'vertical hours' averaged only about five or six a day. My best time was, and still is, in the mornings. I would get up and potter around doing small jobs but by early afternoon I would start to fade away. For the rest of the time I was in bed. My daily routine was not exactly congenial to having a baby.

One factor which encouraged us was that my condition was gradually improving. I'd had quite a dramatic start to my illness with an attack of viral meningitis. I was in hospital for a week and then in bed at home for several weeks. During the following months I suffered extreme fatigue; sometimes brushing my teeth was all I could manage before having to go back to bed. My doctor said that it was a slow recovery from meningitis, but I knew there was something else wrong with me. I was experiencing more and more symptoms: muscle pain, back and neck pains, head pressure, difficulty in walking and extreme fatigue. After almost a year I was eventually sent to a neurologist who diagnosed benign myalgic encephalomyelitis. I couldn't believe there was an illness with such a long name and thought I would never remember it! I was, in fact, greatly relieved that what I was feeling had a name.

I immediately joined the ME Association and discovered the importance of rest and sleep. Instead of trying to push myself to do things, I established a new daily routine. I would get up in the mornings, at first for only one or two hours and then return to bed. Gradually, over the next year or so, I increased those vertical hours to five or six.

My husband and I had always wanted children and were anxious that this debilitating disease might prevent it. My GP and specialist had suggested it would not be a good idea. However, we asked the advice of Dr David Smith, who was then the ME Association's Medical Advisor. His advice was what we wanted to hear. If we really wanted children, then life without them may make us unhappy and discontent. It was better to go ahead, being fully aware of the problems and with the provision of plenty of help.

When my pregnancy was confirmed, I really became very anxious about whether our decision had been wise. I wrote to Dr Smith for reassurance and also to another lady with ME/CFS who had had a baby. Her letter boosted my morale as she was coping well and was, in fact, expecting her second child.

My first visit to the hospital was interesting because, at that time, little was known about ME/CFS. The nurses and midwives were all interested to know how the disease affected me, were sympathetic in their manner and admired our decision to battle against the odds and have a baby. The gynaecologist had little experience of the illness but suspected that I would cope all right with the first stage of labour but might have a problem in the second stage and be incapable of pushing. As I was 37 he recommended an amniocentesis which I had at 16 weeks. My stomach was sore and uncomfortable for a week afterwards and I found it difficult to stand upright. Presumably this was because the muscles were particularly tender and took longer to recover. Anyway, three weeks later the results came through as clear, so all was well.

I think having ME/CFS prepared me quite well for the aches and pains of pregnancy. I was used to resting and pacing myself – other people have to learn to do that while pregnant. Gradually, over nine months, my symptoms all seemed to ease. The acute pains I suffered in my neck, head, back and arms became less severe, but the major relief I had was the fading of that awful 'ill' feeling. My head cleared, although I still had pressure in it, and that mental numbness which was constantly with me disappeared. I felt almost part of the real world, a real person instead of a zombie.

I must explain here that all through my pregnancy I was having acupuncture. I started a course of treatment about three months before I became pregnant, in an anxious attempt to do something positive to help myself. It is difficult to judge which made me feel better – pregnancy or acupuncture – but I am inclined to attribute the growing feeling of well-being to pregnancy and the more specific relief of things such as heart palpitations and nerve pains to acupuncture.

During the later weeks of pregnancy we discussed with the consultant the possibility of a Caesarean if labour became too much for me. General anaesthetic can worsen ME/CFS symptoms, so it was decided that an epidural Caesarean would be our best option.

I thoroughly enjoyed my pregnancy. Not only was I relieved of some of my symptoms but I developed a sense of purpose. Previously I had felt worthless, now I had something to live for.

In August, our daughter Anna was born. As the consultant predicted, I could cope with the first stage of labour, but by the second stage I was completely exhausted. I had no urge to push and no strength to push either. It was decided to use forceps. Anna was very solid (8½ lb) and needed tremendous tugging to get her into the world – an experience I would not want to endure again!

The nurses on the ward were marvellous. I had been in labour for 17 hours and was totally exhausted. I could not walk for about 24 hours and during that time they brought me bed pans and gave me bed baths. When Anna cried a nurse would give her to me to feed and then return her to her cot to save me the effort. My arms were too weak to hold her so I fed her lying down. At night the babies were taken to the nursery and mothers were woken to go and feed their babies there. I did not have to do that. A nurse would bring Anna to me, return to change sides and then return again to take her back to the nursery. This was such a help to me, and whenever I expressed my appreciation they merely said that's what they were there for. I was touched by their kindness and regard for my problems. One sister even stayed on duty late one night in order to show my husband how to change a nappy and bath the baby. She had realised that he would be doing much of the caring when we got home, and took it upon herself to teach him. We really appreciated her concern.

I stayed in hospital for six days after the birth before I felt strong enough to go home. My husband took the first week off work and then my mother came for a week so it was a little while before I had to cope on my own.

We had decided that my limited energy should be concentrated on Anna and looking after her. We employed a cleaner to do the housework and a child minder to have Anna for two afternoons or whenever I needed a rest. We installed such labour-saving devices as a microwave, a tumble drier and a dishwasher. I used disposable nappies to save time and effort. I could not have coped with carrying a nappy bucket, let alone washing and drying them. I find hanging clothes on the line difficult and still only put them out if it's a perfect day. There's nothing worse than having the effort of bringing clothes in, because of rain, before your arms have recovered from putting them out. If I am having a bad day or there is a hint of rain I use the tumble drier.

I found breast feeding worked well for me. Those who prefer to bottle feed have the advantage that other people can help – especially at night. However, I enjoyed breast feeding and found it relaxing. My arms were weak and my back prone to spasm, so I lay down to feed Anna, which was restful for me and cosy and comfortable for us both.

To save my arms I would lift Anna and then sit down so her weight was supported on my lap. I bought a second-hand carry cot which was left permanently in the car, so that I only had Anna to carry in and out – not a carry cot as well. To save my back and leg muscles I had two sets of changing equipment, one upstairs and one downstairs, with the mat at table height to save bending. I only ever tried to do one task a day, apart from caring for Anna. I would see a friend, or do a little shopping, or go to the clinic, all on different days.

My husband helped with the more strenuous daily tasks. He would empty the nappy bucket (used for disposables), put out or bring in washing, do ironing, empty the dishwasher, push the shopping trolley and often cook the meal. His main daily task was bathing Anna. I found it impossible to bend forward and hold her, so bath time was his time.

Motherhood would have been virtually impossible without a sensitive and willing partner. My husband has been indispensable in caring for Anna. As well as all the daily tasks he helps with, every Saturday and Sunday afternoon he takes over completely while I go and rest.

Although having a baby is hard work and often very tiring, the rewards far outweigh the difficulties. Anna has brought joy to our lives. She has given me an aim in life and stopped me focusing attention on myself. When I'm in pain or feeling down, her smile uplifts me and a cuddle makes it all worthwhile.

We are so glad that we risked the consequences of having a baby. Not everyone with ME/CFS experiences a relief of symptoms during pregnancy, but I'm sure they will all agree that life with a baby is a reward to be treasured.

## Author's note

I now know of several women, like Frances, who have decided to start a family during the course of their illness. However, this is a decision which must never be taken without a great deal of thought and careful advance planning.

For many women, the onset or continuation of ME/CFS into their thirties means that they face the inevitable problem of steadily decreasing fertility. In purely practical terms they may soon lose the option of ever becoming pregnant. Even so, I would not advise anyone with ME/CFS to contemplate pregnancy until their condition has significantly improved or remained stable for at least a year. If time is on your side then it is far better to wait till you are well on the road to recovery.

Ideally, any pregnancy should also be planned to avoid giving birth during the late autumn and winter months when infections are far more common, and the cold weather is making you feel less well.

Good nutrition is extremely important, especially if you've been avoiding certain foods before becoming pregnant. Do make sure that your intake of folic acid is adequate, as this particular vitamin has been shown to be deficient in some people with ME/CFS (see pages 278–9) and low body levels have been linked to spinal cord disorders in babies.

For anyone who does decide to go ahead and become pregnant, two important questions will inevitably pass through your mind.

First, what effect does pregnancy have on ME/CFS? In my experience about 75 per cent of women notice an improvement in their general health, sometimes quite significantly. This type of improvement also occurs in several other conditions, including rheumatoid arthritis, where there is an immune component. The precise reasons are uncertain but are probably connected with changes in the levels of various sex hormones, as well as the partial suppression of the immune system which helps to prevent the foetus being rejected. However, I must emphasise that a significant minority of women will find that pregnancy causes an actual *deterioration* in their condition, so it should never be viewed as a way of trying to get better.

The real practical problems tend to arise at the end of the nine months and during labour. So, you must inform the doctors and midwives about the practical effects of your illness (even though they are unlikely to know much about ME/CFS) because labour is likely to be very exhausting and you may require additional help.

One of the main concerns for anyone with ME/CFS who decides to have a baby is whether they're going to have enough energy to cope with labour. Fortunately, uterine contractions are extremely strong and should continue to dilate the cervix (opening of the womb) regardless of your general state of health.

If you become really exhausted during the first stages of labour, then it may be necessary to have some form of assisted delivery, either by using forceps or a ventouse (which involves attaching a soft plastic suction cap over the baby's head). This type of assistance should allow you and the obstetric team to work together and achieve a successful delivery.

If you're concerned about problems with pain relief during labour, then you should ask about having an epidural anaesthetic. This will allow a relatively painless dilation of the cervix to occur and gives you the opportunity to conserve some energy, and even have a short sleep, so you're prepared for the time when you need to start pushing.

Once you are back home again, looking after a newborn baby will become very demanding – both physically and mentally. Arranging family and social support to help you cope must be planned well in advance. It's also important to remember that otherwise healthy women commonly experience fatigue and emotional changes during this period, which are once again related to changes in the hormone levels. These problems may be even more pronounced in someone with ME/CFS, especially if they have had any form of depressive illness in the past.

As far as the baby is concerned, breast feeding has many advantages, including the fact that it's an excellent way of transferring vital antibodies. On the other hand, bottle feeding will provide your partner with the opportunity to become actively involved as well as taking some of the strain away from night-time feeding.

The second important question is whether a mother's ME/CFS presents any risks to the unborn child. As far as miscarriage is concerned, we know that 10–20 per cent of all pregnancies end this way, but there is no published evidence to suggest that this is any higher in ME/CFS. There is, however, a *small theoretical possibility* that a persisting viral infection could be passed across the placenta to the foetus. Even so, I know of plenty of women with ME/CFS who, like Frances, have gone on to produce perfectly healthy babies. I am only aware of a couple of cases where the baby has failed to thrive and no obvious cause has been found. Here, the possibility of transmission of a virus during early development cannot be discounted. This is obviously an area where accurate data needs to be collected from women who became pregnant during the course of having ME/CFS.

Any final decision on pregnancy is bound to be influenced by a number of factors – your social circumstances, your age and above all, your current state of health. Before going ahead with such a major decision I would strongly advise discussing this with your family doctor, as well as someone else, like Frances, who has been through pregnancy and knows all the benefits and problems at first hand.

Parentability, a group which forms part of the National Childbirth Trust, provides information and support for parents with disabilities (see Useful Addresses, page 412).

# ME/CFS and the Single Person

*by 'Sue'*

Perhaps the first thing to say is that coping with ME/CFS, whatever your circumstances – alone, with a partner, with children or other dependants – is made a good deal easier once a correct diagnosis has been made, especially if one's nearest and dearest can then understand what is happening and are able to be supportive. No more feeling 'I should be able to do this so easily. Why can't I? and no more pushing beyond personal limits. One can then take account of the illness in practical planning from day to day. So much of the secret of dealing with ME/CFS is illness management – but first you have to know the beast you're dealing with.

I write as someone who has had the syndrome for the best part of 25 years. It started in my teens and I am 40 now. I have only known what is wrong with me for three of those years. My illness has followed a chronic relapse/remitting course, with about five prolonged, major relapses and never quite feeling 'well' in between. For years, I've alternated between saying to myself, 'Oh, this is just how I am. Not much stamina. Always tired. Often ill,' and asking, 'Do other people ever feel like this, and so often? Surely there must be something fundamentally wrong with me?' Now I know!

For part of my 25 'ME/CFS years' I was married. So, in writing about coping as a person who lives on her own, I can also look back and compare lifestyles. Such comparisons are difficult because the major difference between then and now is not between being married and being single, but between not knowing and knowing what is wrong. Coping with this illness has its good and bad, its difficult and easier bits, irrespective of your personal situation. The great divide lies between before and after diagnosis.

The next hurdle is acceptance and learning to live within your limitations. Glibly said. At first, and perhaps for some time, there will be trial and error. You have to find out what you can do, and when to stop, to prevent a relapse. One way in which living alone can be a real boon is that it's so much easier to leave tasks half-done, to be flexible and alter a set routine, if you don't have a family to look after, or anyone else to take account of. Conversely, of course, there is no one there to help either. Shopping, cooking, cleaning, washing and all the other household chores have to be managed, spaced out between periods of rest. Forward planning has to be done with military precision.

For someone with ME/CFS who lives alone, there are several things that make life a bit easier. First, friends can be persuaded to form a rota to do basic tasks. If that is difficult to organise, or if a sufferer prefers to seek out voluntary help on a less personal basis, then most towns have a Council for Voluntary Service, and some have a school or university where students may have formed a 'caring group'. Or use your local church if you have one.

The key is not to be afraid to ask for help, not to be deterred by apparent rebuffs, and to keep on asking until you succeed.

For shopping, be on the look-out for firms that will deliver, and large stores that operate special bus services, often door to door. Ask around, and don't hesitate to make your special needs clear. You may find that other customers are having similar problems, and just one query can trigger the start of a delivery service.

Find out if your area operates a dial-a-ride system for the disabled. Contact the Disability Unit of the council, the Passenger Transport Authority and/or social services. If the answer is no, then ask for one!

To take the best advantage of bulk shopping, a small freezer is invaluable for single people. It's also useful for bulk cooking. I always make sure that I have plenty of convenience foods and a range of items that are easy to prepare. Then I'm ready for the bad days, because I know that however careful I am, there will be relapses.

If, like me, you have a lot of muscle problems or arthritis, don't hesitate to apply for a home help. I have one who just does the vacuum-cleaning. The rest I can manage without too much distress. In other words, choose carefully what you can do without ill effect and follow up all channels of possible help for what you can't do. Contact with the home help section of your nearest social service office is likely to produce an initial visit from a social worker, along with the home help organiser. This can be a helpful contact to have in reserve for when the going gets really rough and extra help (meals on wheels, household aids and so on) is needed.

Once your basic routine and regular sources of help are all sorted out, it's a good idea to plan, *in advance*, ways of coping in a crisis. If you can, organise an emergency 'back-up' team, using the kinds of resources and techniques described above: friends, volunteers, home help, social services. Make it clear in advance what your requirements will be if you do have a long period of relapse: meals cooked, washing done, all the shopping and so on. Divide out the tasks, so that people are prepared to take on whatever they can best cope with. Get it all sorted out when you are having a reasonably good patch, and have your 'emergency services' at the ready for when you are most decidedly not. Just the knowledge that you have such a team of people to call on can be a great security blanket.

If you feel too ill to remain at home during a relapse, a referral from your GP to a local consultant and hospital admission for the short term can be invaluable. If that can't be achieved, another possibility to consider is going on a 'retreat', if necessary using the Ambulance Service to get there and back! Some religious orders offer board and lodging irrespective of one's beliefs or denomination. It can be a good way of obtaining rest and being looked after, if friends or relations can't produce a short-term place to stay, and there's no hospital bed in time of crisis. Ideally, however, a good back-up team will make it possible to remain at home even during the worst of a relapse.

For anyone living alone, the worst problems can occur when both the routine mechanics of life and crisis management have been sorted out. All too often the illness leaves one with just enough energy to cope with basic survival, and no more. But what of work, social life and hobbies?

My current relapse has been the worst ever, though I am now slowly starting to recover. I have had to stop work and am now reconciled to not being able to do my old job again. It is too hectic, too physically, emotionally and mentally demanding. Work has always been a major part of my life and a large chunk of my identity. Not being able to continue has been a considerable loss. And yet, changing my perspective in this regard, looking at new ways in which I can value myself, without such a work-centred existence has been very productive.

Those of us who live on our own are perhaps even more likely to put a lot into our work. However, if stopped in our tracks, there can be advantages because there's now an opportunity to try to reorientate ourselves without the added worry of letting our families down. After a period of adjustment, we can start to enjoy a more balanced lifestyle. Perhaps, eventually, we can find a less demanding job.

I am not saying that giving up on work is an easy habit. But it can be a process that offers its own rewards – and professional help is obtainable if necessary to assist in making the adjustment.

If one can continue at work, then it is essential to be quite up-front about what is going on. If people know about the restrictions, many will understand, make allowances and be supportive. Job-sharing, going temporarily part-time and working from home can all be discussed as possible solutions.

And what of the rest of life? For those of us who have the illness badly, that has to be very restricted too. The person who is less ill, and so able to carry on working, may be too exhausted to do anything else. There may be no energy left for friends, going out, and all the things that are normally taken for granted and that make it good to be alive. All too easily, friendships fall away, people lose touch, and the person living on their own becomes increasingly isolated. Once again, it helps to be well-organised and not backward in announcing one's needs. I try to take the initiative in organising visits to and from friends, and other social events, so that I have control of when I do things, and can plan surrounding time accordingly.

Despite all the problems, this illness can have a positive effect on social life. It doesn't just illustrate who friends really are, but also forces one to reassess the basis of friendships – what one values friends for and vice versa.

For anyone on their own it may be particularly difficult to share the various facets of the illness with others, because so few people see us at our worst. Most, therefore, will not know what the whole syndrome is really like. So, for anyone alone, perhaps the best people to turn to to discuss the illness are others in similar circumstances. The 'Singles' Group run by those members of the ME Association who are living alone can be of particular help here.

Useful though friends and acquaintances can be, the bedrock of being able to deal with this illness successfully has to lie inside yourself. Try to develop a sense of self-value and enjoyment of your own company, of small details, the daily minutiae of life, that can be savoured on your own: having a few plants and watching them grow, a beautiful picture to look at, a tree outside, and so on.

What also keeps me going is 'breaking out' occasionally. A person alone lacks people to sound-off to about the illness. A lot of the time they simply have to keep going because there is no one else there to take over. Occasionally, having a good cry does wonders for pent-up frustration, grief, anger and failure to make any real progress on the road to recovery.

Likewise, giving yourself a treat can help – even if this is detrimental in the short term and causes a temporary flare-up of symptoms. Sometimes it is good simply to 'live' and take the consequences of any flare-up that comes after. In such ways it is possible to overcome some of the feelings of loss, sadness and frustration caused by ME/CFS.

So far I have talked of loss in conjunction with not being able to work and not being able to pursue an active social life. There is one other important area to look at: the effect ME/CFS has on a person's ability to sustain a close sexual relationship.

Some of us 'aloners' may have a sexual relationship with a partner, although we may not actually share a house. The amount of energy and effort needed if two people are to sustain a close, loving sexual relationship whilst living apart can become at worst prohibitive and at best a great source of stress, if one partner develops ME/CFS. And for those who are prevented from developing any close sexual relationship at all because of the restrictions of the illness, or whose relationship has ended because of it, there is another whole area of grief, loss and loneliness to come to terms with. I feel the only way to do this is again to try to use the experience of illness to re-evaluate both one's own sense of self, and the range of ways in which one is able to relate to and value other people. Our society tends to emphasise the importance, above all else, of having a sexual relationship, but in reality, there are lots of ways of loving other people that can be equally satisfying. If one can accept this, then one opens oneself to what is on offer, rather than using up energy in hankering after the unobtainable. Obviously this is easier said than done, and there will still be moments of acute sadness, not to mention sexual frustration, but these can at least be tempered, by masturbation on the purely physical level, and by the quality of life that can come from being completely open and responsive to all kinds of relationships with other people, and all kinds of experiences.

But what if none of this is possible? What if your illness is so bad that you simply cannot manage to live alone at all, never mind about such luxuries as work or relationships? What happens then?

Any solution to this will mean giving up a measure of independence, which is difficult for anyone accustomed to living alone. If your parents are fit, and able to care for you, you can then return 'home'. Alternatively, other relatives or friends may offer somewhere to live. In such situations a 'granny flat' can be a good compromise, offering carers and sufferers alike a measure of freedom, privacy and independence, whilst also affording regular care and mutual company/privacy for all. In such circumstances, maximum use still needs to be made of additional outside help to ensure that neither carers nor sufferers are over-burdened, the former by practical tasks and resentments, the latter by guilt and claustrophobia.

Another solution for anyone able to look after themselves is some form of sheltered accommodation. This, however, is difficult to come by. Supply is vastly outstripped by demand. It is only those of us who have the illness very badly who are likely to qualify for a place, either in a council-run complex, a Housing Association development or in accommodation provided by one of several voluntary organisations working in this field.

Most of us do get better, even if the illness lasts a long time; most of us do have good periods in among the relapses. In this hard-pressed world of cut-backs, such fluctuations often place people with conditions such as ME/CFS at the end of a very long queue when it comes to obtaining sheltered housing. However, there may come a time when a fight needs to be made to obtain an adequate placement, with help from the local housing manager, GP, consultant or social worker.

As a final point, it should be stressed that, even with quite bad illness, by enlisting the type of help described above, it should be possible for anyone with ME/CFS not just to manage on their own, but still obtain real enjoyment out of life.

# Relationships

One of the most distressing aspects of ME/CFS is the way it interferes with all aspects of one's personal and social life. It can be very difficult maintaining friendships, but don't ever lose the ones who are kind and understanding. You're bound to find that existing friends will take varying attitudes towards you and your illness. But the more they understand about the condition and the way it affects you, the more likely it is that they'll remain the sort of friends you still want to see. There will be others who just can't comprehend what you're going through, and will probably end up making insensitive remarks or passing on inappropriate advice on what you might do to try and get better. It may be better to let these sort of friendships dwindle.

Most people with ME/CFS find that a whole range of sporting and social activities, which previously made life so enjoyable, now have to be abandoned or curtailed. This inability to participate in any form of social activity is a severe blow, as outside work, sports and hobbies are an important way of meeting people and maintaining friendships. Some try to maintain their involvement by becoming spectators instead. It may also be possible to keep in touch by performing some sort of administrative function for a club or organisation.

This reduction of interests and social life is something which partners and carers also find difficult, and for their sake it helps to try and maintain a 'non-active' social life which you can both enjoy and participate in. This could be a trip to the cinema or a quiet meal out at a restaurant. If you really can't face the thought of going out, why not make an event out of an evening at home, perhaps by hiring a video and arranging a take-away meal?

Don't ever forget about those people who are closest to you – your partner, your children and your best friends. Such relationships are going to come under great strain from time to time, but these are the sort of people you're going to rely on for a great deal of support.

## Caring for Someone Who Has ME/CFS

The person who is closest to someone with ME/CFS – be it spouse, parent or child – has a very difficult job.

Suddenly, the carer finds that their family member is not the person they once were. They cannot cope physically as they once did, and there may be psychological problems as well, including loss of confidence and self-esteem, exaggerated mood swings and depression. And just as the person who's ill is coming to terms with their problems, so those with a caring role may be about to experience similar difficulties in learning how to cope.

Caring isn't just providing physical help, but involves a great deal of emotional support as well.

Neither of you can predict the eventual outcome of this illness – something which makes forward planning so very difficult. It's all too easy to give up hope when someone with ME/CFS has been ill for several years and become convinced that they're never going to recover. Even so, many people do start to improve, sometimes after quite a long period of ill health, and gradually return to leading a normal way of life. A key part of the carer's role is not only to understand what their partner is putting up with, but also to give hope and encouragement that recovery will take place.

One aspect of this type of positive approach is to encourage the person with ME/CFS to look after their personal appearance, to maintain their friendships and social contacts, and pursue their work, hobbies and interests – provided they are not exceeding their capabilities.

It helps to talk about the illness. Join the ME Association, where at a local group meeting you'll be able to meet other people who are close to someone who's living with ME/CFS.

Anyone with this illness will have differing physical and emotional needs when it comes to receiving help from other people. Many will be the sort of individuals who haven't been used to asking for assistance in the past, so it's not easy to be specific about what to do for them. Here are some guidelines which need to be followed with a wide degree of flexibility, according to each individual's needs and personality.

# A Four-Point Plan to Help Carers and Relatives

## 1. Find out all you can about ME/CFS

One of the first practical steps that any relative or carer must take is to find out as much as possible about this illness and the way it's affecting their partner or child.

Above all, this means listening and learning. It may also involve encouraging the person concerned to express feelings about both physical and emotional problems – something which many people find hard to do, especially if this hasn't been the case in the past.

It's a good idea for both of you to go along together, on at least one occasion, to a consultation with the general practitioner or consultant – any reasonable doctor shouldn't object to this. It's quite likely that there are questions which the sufferer may not want to ask – here the doctor may be willing to see the carer separately, but some would regard it as unethical to talk about a patient's illness without their permission. Do find out all you can about how the doctor feels the individual illness should best be managed, any drugs that are being prescribed, and whether there is any reason for referral to a specialist who has expert knowledge about how to manage ME/CFS.

It's a completely natural reaction for some relatives, when an illness like this has been diagnosed, to start spending vast amounts of money and time chasing an elusive 'cure'. They write to experts all over the world and request second opinions from anyone involved with the condition. Others take a completely opposite view and almost deny that any problem exists, or that it will go away if ignored. Some are so successful in this approach that they don't realise they're doing it! If someone with ME/CFS wants to try out an unusual form of treatment or change their diet, don't denigrate such an approach. It may help and many people undoubtedly feel better simply because they are taking some of their own management decisions.

Read all you can about the illness; it's not hard to find up-to-date medical information. The ME Association can help if you're having difficulties. Once the basic facts are straight in your head, it should be a lot easier for both of you to start making the sort of essential changes in lifestyle without which progressive recovery is unlikely.

## 2. Involve the whole family

Where someone with ME/CFS is part of a family group, it's often a good idea to arrange a meeting so that everyone can appreciate how the illness is going to affect all aspects of family life. It's an opportunity for everyone to make their feelings – positive and negative – known about any particular difficulties or anxieties, as well as reallocating some of the household and family duties. Hopefully, everyone can be flexible and decide on practical ways of getting around any current problems. This is far better than individual family members grumbling away and no practical solutions being found.

Getting children to understand the effects of ME/CFS on one of their parents can be a particularly difficult task. Try to explain the illness to them as honestly as possible, so they understand why mum or dad can't do the sort of activities with, or for them, that other parents do.

Children often find it very difficult to cope with a parent who has ME/CFS. Some will be extremely supportive and even start to take on an adult role in the way they help about the house. Others will be the

exact opposite, being completely unhelpful and even isolating themselves from their mum or dad.

At the age of five or six many children will want to know why mum or
dad doesn't go out to work like other 'normal' adults, and why he or she
can't come out and help with a game of football or go on a weekend
camping trip. Some children even make up fictitious occupations for you
in order to avoid teasing and embarrassment at school – children can be
very cruel to each other at times.

There aren't easy solutions to problems with children, but talking to
other families in a similar situation might be helpful and give you some
ideas as to how your own problems might be tackled.

## 3. Get organised – find out about help that's available

Find out about all the extra sources of help and advice which are available and might be appropriate to your particular needs and circumstances. Practical help for the disabled and advice on social security
benefits (e.g. the invalid care allowance) are covered in Chapter 19:
Additional Help and Benefits.

Don't forget that neighbours may be only too willing to help – if
asked. If you're receiving assistance from people not closely associated
with you, it's a great help to them if you carefully explain the nature of
the illness and how it affects the person involved. People tend to be
afraid of illnesses (and people with illnesses) which they don't understand, so it's important that you or your partner puts them in the picture.
They may be quite happy to offer a bit of practical help, such as regular
shopping each week. You or your partner might then be able to do something for them in return, such as looking after a pet when they go on holiday.

With the loss of mobility that ME/CFS imposes, many people find
that new friendships now come from neighbours and others living close
to them, when previously they may have only known one or two people
who lived in the same street.

There is an umbrella organisation, the Carers National Association
(see Useful Addresses, page 410) which is there for people who are caring or helping to look after people with disability. It acts as a source of
further information on a whole range of practical problems that anyone
acting as a carer may face. It also organises local groups where you could
meet other people who are having to cope with similar feelings and
experiences. It's not the sort of help that everyone requires, but it's there
should you need it.

The Carers section in Useful Addresses lists a number of other organisations which might be worth contacting for advice and information.

## 4. Self-help for the carer

It's all too easy, when caring for somebody else, to start putting your own interests and life into second place. After all, you're trying to perform a balancing act between your own needs, the rest of the family and caring for your partner. It's all too easy to start neglecting your own health, both physical and emotional, and there's no point in falling ill as well when you've become the central pillar to family life. If you find yourself becoming depressed, then do seek help from your general practitioner. And if you've any physical symptoms, don't neglect them – make sure they're attended to.

You'll also have a lot of personal feelings about the way ME/CFS is affecting both your lives; some will be positive, but many will be negative and upsetting. You'll probably start to feel fed up at times about the numerous restrictions being placed on your own way of life. You may start to feel despondent when your partner doesn't seem to be making any real progress, or some new treatment isn't having any effect.

These are all very natural reactions. There aren't any *easy* solutions, but whatever feelings you have about either your partner or their illness, try not to bottle them up. If you don't find it easy to discuss them with your partner, it can help to talk to a close friend or relative, or the partner of someone else that you may have met at a local group meeting. A third party may even be able to intervene and help defuse a family crisis by tactfully putting your point of view about a particular issue.

There may be times when a relationship comes under great stress, even crisis. If you find it difficult dealing with frustrations or putting your feelings into words, try writing them down. It's something of a last resort, but just occasionally it can be an effective way of relieving an impasse.

A variety of worries often build up: health, personal and financial. It may then be helpful to talk things over with someone completely detached from the family. This might be a social worker, a sympathetic general practitioner or even a professional or volunteer counsellor. (The British Association for Counselling trains such people – see Useful Addresses, page 413).

Although you may find that for much of the time you're having to put your interests, and even your work, into second place, it's terribly important not to abandon them altogether. Most people with ME/CFS don't actually require full-time physical help throughout the day, so giving up work for that reason isn't usually necessary. However, when a wife with small children develops ME/CFS (especially if they're of pre-school age), the husband may well have to make some major decisions regarding employment, especially if he spends a large amount of time away from home. Alternatively, if a breadwinner has to give up work due to

ME/CFS, it may be the carer who now has to consider going out to work.

Making the correct decisions in such circumstances isn't easy, so do try and talk to other people who've had to make similar decisions before finally making up your mind.

If you're already working and happy in what you're doing, and there are no practical problems at home, there are good reasons for you to continue. It gives you respite from each other, and the opportunity to keep up with outside friendships and social life. And try not to give up hobbies and interests, even though there may be practical difficulties, or activities which you can no longer do together any more.

Don't feel guilty about going out on your own once or twice a week to an evening class, or a game of sport with some friends, even though your partner isn't well enough to come. At the same time it's important to try and develop new interests and hobbies which you can do together. These could include swimming, gentle walks in the countryside, or a trip out for a meal or the cinema.

# Additional Help for Carers

## *Respite care*

Although the importance of caring for carers is gradually being recognised, most still experience enormous difficulty when it comes to having a break from looking after a severely ill partner or child.

One advantage of admitting someone who is severely ill to hospital for a while is that a careful review of the current situation can be carried out at the same time, but few NHS hospitals are willing or able to use their beds for this purpose. Even if a place can be found, it may not turn out to be a happy experience for the person involved.

The Community Care Act states that 'A key responsibility of statutory service providers should be to do all they can to assist and support carers.' It may therefore be advisable to contact a social worker (see page 369–70) to find out if there are any local residential facilities which are suitable for someone with ME/CFS. You could also contact the various carers organisations listed in Useful Addresses for further help with obtaining respite care.

## *Care Attendant Schemes*

These are being increasingly organised by both local authorities and voluntary organisations. They provide paid helpers who help disabled people with a wide range of tasks on a fairly flexible basis. The type of care provided can be on a personal basis, e.g. helping with washing or dressing, or more general tasks in the home. Such help is generally only available for those who are quite severely disabled and either living alone or being looked after by a carer who also isn't in the best of health. This sort of service doesn't occur everywhere, but your local social services department or citizens' advice bureau will know if it does.

## Crossroads Care Attendant Schemes

These aim to relieve some of the stresses which inevitably result from looking after a disabled person in their own home. They have been set up to complement, but not replace, existing statutory services and to work closely with them in the home. One particular area where Crossroads tries to offer practical help is when a carer also falls ill and there is a danger that the whole system of care will break down necessitating admission to hospital or residential care. Crossroads Care Schemes are now operating in well over 100 different towns in the UK. They are all locally administered but form part of the national organisation. For further details on your nearest Crossroads branch contact their headquarters (see Useful Addresses, page 410).

# The Carers (Recognition and Services) Act 1995

This Act, which came into effect in April 1996, is now regarded as one of the most significant developments in legislation affecting those who care for sick or disabled people.

The two main results of this Act are that:

- Carers now have a right to ask for a formal assessment of their ability to care for someone else.
- Local authorities have a duty to take this assessment into account when looking at the kind of support which needs to be provided for either the carer or the person being cared for.

The Act covers adults who care for other adults as well as those who care for ill or disabled children under the age of 18. Carers must be providing a *regular and substantial degree of care* in order to be eligible for an assessment. But carers don't have to be living with the person they look after, nor do they have to be the sole provider of care in order to request an assessment.

The important thing is to ask for an assessment as soon as you realise that your partner/child is starting to require an amount of care that takes up a considerable degree of your time and energy. Don't wait till you've almost reached the point where you can no longer cope with the demands of caring.

To obtain an assessment, you need to contact your local social services department, who will then make an appointment for an assessor to visit you at home. For further details phone the Carers National Association on 0171–490 8898 and ask for their leaflet *How to get my carer's assessment.*

A social services representative will then arrange a home visit in order to fully examine your circumstances and decide what sort of additional help and/or services might be appropriate. This could include meals on wheels or additional help in the home. Other assistance might include day or night sitting services to provide a regular weekly break for the carer or some respite care.

Following an assessment, you should then be sent a full written report on the results. In a recent survey carried out by the Carers National Association, 55 per cent of carers had their services increased following an assessment, so do take advantage of the Act. Unfortunately, local authorities are under tremendous pressure to keep social services expenditure under control. This means that at the same time as the Carers Act is starting to have an effect, those who provide the bulk of the services may well be trying to reduce (or charge for) the help that is currently available to facilitate care in the community.

## Sexual Relationships and ME/CFS

Sexual feelings are a natural and essential part of any caring relationship, especially in the age group affected by ME/CFS. In fact, sex may be one of the few pleasurable physical activities that people still feel they can enjoy!

It's hardly surprising that many people with ME/CFS experience sexual problems at some time during their illness, with both physical and emotional factors interacting. Those who are going through a bad patch may withdraw emotionally from those around them. When this happens, the partner will inevitably feel rejected, so they may lose interest in sexual activity as well. Others develop a negative body image, no longer seeing themselves attractive to their partner. In such cases experienced psychosexual counselling can be very helpful.

People who have become anxious or depressed because of the illness, especially when they are taking prescribed drugs, may find that this causes a further dampening down of sexual feelings. Normal sexual arousal stimulates nerves which open up tiny blood vessels in the penis to allow an erection to take place. Any anxiety will dampen down this nervous activity, and if the male partner fails on one occasion to achieve an erection, subsequent anxiety about a repetition may prevent him achieving an erection on the next occasion. Male impotence isn't a part of the physical disease process in ME/CFS. When it does occur, emotional factors are probably much more significant. I've also become aware that some men with ME/CFS go on to develop a variety of other sexual problems, particularly in maintaining an erection. If your GP seems unable to help, I would recommend asking for a referral to a specialist who is interested in this type of sexual problem.

For some people, the physical problems associated with ME/CFS may make sex no longer an appealing activity. Pain in the muscles and joints can severely limit capabilities, and sexual intercourse involves the expenditure of a large amount of energy in a very short space of time!

Intimacy doesn't have to end in intercourse, so foreplay, caressing and touching can be equally satisfying as an alternative to 'active' sex, if the energy just isn't there! Remember, too, that sex doesn't have to necessarily take place at night when you or your partner are feeling tired and ready to go to sleep.

If pain in the muscles, joints or back is a significant factor in reducing sexual pleasure, try taking a warm bath before going to bed and consider taking an aspirin or other anti-inflammatory drug a couple of hours before. Back pain can be eased by placing a pillow under the lower back of the partner in the passive position. Don't be afraid to explore new positions which you may find more comfortable. Get a 'guide book' if you're not quite sure what to do! A man with ME/CFS will use much less energy if he lies underneath. Alternatively, lying side-by-side may be more comfortable.

Sex can also be therapeutic. Arthritis sufferers sometimes report pain relief following orgasm. This is thought to be due to the release from the brain of chemicals known as endorphins, which are like the body's self-produced morphine.

If you are experiencing sexual difficulties, do ask for help. Some GPs are excellent, but others don't have a clue when it comes to sexual problems and are just as embarrassed as their patients. If your GP doesn't seem the right person to approach, then the local family planning clinic or marriage guidance council will point you in the right direction. The British Association for Counselling has counsellors available and SPOD (Sexual and Personal Relationships of People with a Disability) can also provide advice (see Useful Addresses, page 430).

As far as contraception is concerned, having ME/CFS is *not* a contra-indication to either using the standard contraceptive pill or the progesterone only pill. In fact, for many women with ME/CFS, using the most reliable form of contraceptive is extremely important because pregnancy is not something that I would recommend in the early stages of the illness; (see page 310–15).

Equally, dealing with the problems of an unwanted pregnancy may well cause a further relapse. One method of female contraception that I would not normally recommend is the intra-uterine contraceptive device (IUCD) because of its associated risk of infection. If you've completed your family, then the ideal method of contraception may be for your partner to have a vasectomy – something which can be done quickly and easily using a local anaesthetic. However, it should be noted that concerns have been expressed as to whether vasectomy could be a factor in the development of a small number of cases of ME/CFS.

## Further Reading

The Carers National Association (see Useful Addresses, page 410) produces a large number of publications on all aspects of caring. Among the most useful are:

Information booklets on emotional aspects (e.g. *When caring becomes a crisis*), services (e.g. *Getting the most from your primary health care team*) and employment problems (e.g. *Juggling your job and caring?*)
*Signposts through the maze* by Glenys Ruan and Luke Clements is a useful guide to community care law as it relates to carers.

# ME/CFS and your Job

One of the most urgent problems facing many people with ME/CFS is trying to adjust financially to the limitations imposed by this illness.

Where someone has been the main breadwinner, and is also quite young, with rapidly rising financial and promotional expectations from work, the loss of income can be abrupt and severe. A large mortgage might have been taken out on a new house, or other costly financial planning entered into, and now these commitments may be impossible to keep going. Even the most fortunate individuals are unlikely to receive more than six months' full sick pay and an equal period of half pay. After that, the total family income may rapidly diminish to a combination of state sickness benefit and whatever other members of the family are bringing in. And where a wife is at home looking after small children, this may mean no other source of earned income.

A financial crisis may then ensue, forcing sudden decisions to cut back on spending. It's far preferable to try and avoid this by talking to one's bank manager or building society before such a crisis occurs, both to put them into the picture and hopefully make some arrangements to ease the burden in the short term.

This chapter is designed to give practical help and advice on the sorts of problem which occur, and the options to consider in trying to solve them.

## Returning to Work

For those who have been diagnosed early on, a period of sick leave and rest, followed by *proper convalescence* is the aim.

If all goes well, a return to work should then be considered, taking into account the following sensible advice:

*'Care should be taken to match the proposed duties in employment to the subject's capabilities. Strenuous physical work, long working hours, rapidly changing shift patterns, work requiring sustained high levels of attention and concentration and work likely to place sustained high pressure on the employee are inadvisable or at least require careful monitoring until it is clear that recovery is complete and sustained.*

*A further concern arises where there is the possibility of exposure to agents in the working environment which may themselves give rise to symptoms which may resemble those of CFS because of the potential for confusion concerning the cause of any exacerbation of symptoms. For this reason work which may involve potential significant exposure to substances such as heavy metals or solvents is probably inadvisable for those with persisting CFS symptoms.'*

Reference: *Occupational Medicine*, 1997, 47, 217–27.

Those who are diagnosed much later, when the condition may have stabilised, inevitably have much more difficult decisions to take. The choice may have to be between making a major readjustment in working routines or leaving the current type of occupation, if the physical and mental stresses are too much.

Unfortunately, the financial and psychological consequences of giving up work may produce their own negative effects on recovery – unemployment can also damage your health. So, like all other routes to recovery, it's a question of trying to strike the right balance between the advantages and disadvantages, and at the same time keeping within your limitations.

It may not be easy to find such a person to talk to, but I believe it can be of immense help in these circumstances to listen to someone else in the same occupation as yourself and find out how they managed to cope. The ME Association might be able to put you in touch with a suitable colleague.

Here is a quote from an article in the *Journal of the Society for Occupational Medicine*, by Dr Mike Peel, who was an occupational physician with British Airways. It's an account of the problems in returning to work which some of their employees have faced. It is to be recommended to any other occupational health physicians.

*'The most important impression is that they are all very active, fit and dedicated workers: the last ones likely to exaggerate symptoms. Managers have expressed relief that a trusted colleague is genuinely ill and not hysterical. It is probable that the attitude of fighting on despite illness is a critical factor, in that they continued working long hours and taking regular exercise long after their bodies told them to stop.'*

*J. Soc. Occup. Med.*, 1988, 38, 44–5.

## Problems at Work

In the early stages of ME/CFS, often before a firm diagnosis has been made, employers tend to be fairly sympathetic about sick leave. This approach tends to rapidly evaporate as the months pass by and your absence becomes a steadily increasing inconvenience. There comes a time when the employer begins to wonder if you're ever going to return to work. Just how long can this ill health continue? Unfortunately, neither you nor your doctor can provide them with the answers, and their impatience may steadily grow worse.

You may attempt to go back to work, even though you know you're almost certainly not well enough to do so. When the attempt fails, you end up feeling even more demoralised. The employer then decides it's looking extremely unlikely that you're going to return in the near future and the next thing you hear is that somebody else has been promoted into your position: there's no job to go back to even if you are well!

It's a popular misconception that you can't lose your job due to ill health – unfortunately this isn't so. After a prolonged period away from work your employer may be able to argue that this is a valid reason for dismissal.

The first important step, if you feel you're about to enter this situation, is to contact your trade union or professional body and talk to one of their industrial relations advisors. It's essential to take expert advice here, as the law is complicated. These advisors should be fully up-to-date with employment legislation, and be able to refer you on for appropriate legal advice if necessary. If you don't belong to such organisations, the local citizens' advice bureau should be able to help.

Secondly, do keep in touch with work (probably the personnel officer) and let them know what's happening about your progress, or lack of it – they may even be able to help financially. Admittedly, some employers are excellent when it comes to problems related to ill health, but others just don't want to know and hope you'll quietly go away.

It's also worthwhile making an appointment with the company doctor, if you have an occupational health service, to keep them informed. Doctors who are interested and sympathetic towards ME/CFS may be able to offer help in the future. This is obviously important if it comes to taking early retirement on the grounds of ill health.

If you are claiming sick pay under an occupational sick pay scheme, dismissals shouldn't be a way of stopping such benefits. Again, check the law with your trade union.

## Dismissal on Grounds of Ill Health – Going to Law

If it comes to the point of actually being dismissed because you have ME/CFS, there may be an internal company appeal procedure to which you or your trade union could present your case. Your employer may argue that your contract of employment has been terminated, because in the legal jargon, it has been 'frustrated'. (This means that your employer now considers that you are unable to perform your contractual duties due to continuing ill health.)

If you are dismissed, and all appeals to the company have failed, you may still have a case which could be taken to an industrial tribunal – but you *must* do this within a certain time limit of being dismissed. The industrial tribunal will have to decide if your employer was acting in a 'fair and reasonable manner' when they decided to terminate employment. You may think that it's very unfair to be dismissed through no actual fault of your own, and a tribunal may agree with you if you can successfully argue points such as:

- You were never in any way consulted about your illness and possible return to work by the employers.
- The employer never went to the bother of obtaining relevant medical reports on your state of health from either your doctor or their own occupational health physician.

The tribunal also has to take into account the fact that your ill health could be endangering other employees, and in the case of ME/CFS, this could well be relevant when operating dangerous machinery or driving public transport.

The law regarding employment and dismissal on grounds of ill health is extremely complex, so do obtain expert legal advice before making any irretrievable decisions. You may also find that parts of the new Disability Discrimination Act (see later) relating to employment are relevant to your circumstances.

Two useful legal precedents involving failure of an employer to adequately consult with an employee and their doctor are Polkey v A E Dayton Services Ltd [1987] 3WLR 1153 HL and Wright v Eclipse Blinds Ltd [1990] 411 1RL1B 11 EAT.

# Problems with Personal Health Insurance (PHI) Policies

Disputes over eligibility for payments from personal health insurance policies have become increasingly common for people with ME/CFS. To start with here are some general guidelines on how to proceed if your PHI payments are abruptly terminated or refused:

- All correspondence with the insurer should be typed, clearly set out and kept to the point. If you are unable to type out your letters, try and find someone who can.
- Important letters should be sent by Recorded Delivery. This makes

certain that the insurer cannot claim that 'your correspondence was never received'. It also helps to emphasise that you are taking the matter seriously.

- Always keep copies of your letters and any important documents (e.g. medical notes) which are included.
- Obtain a copy of your policy if you are covered by a company scheme, as many employees are. The best person to ask is the personnel officer.

The most important point in any dispute involving an insurance company is to establish the principal reason(s) for the decision to stop payments. This means finding out whether there is a dispute over diagnosis, level of disability or prognosis (outcome) in your particular case. If the dispute centres on the issue of whether or not ME/CFS is a mental or physical disorder, refer to the fact that ME is now classified by the World Health Organisation as being a 'Disease of the Nervous System' (ICD10, 10, G93.3). You could also point out that the 1996 Royal Colleges' report on CFS stated that 'CFS cannot be considered either "physical" or "psychological" – both need to be considered simultaneously to understand the syndrome.' If the insurer still requires more evidence to support a physical basis, refer to the research findings described earlier in this book.

If the dispute concerns prognosis/outcome and the often quoted but inaccurate assumption that almost everyone recovers from ME/CFS within two to three years, then you will need to provide evidence from published studies which show that this is definitely not the case. Further information and references relating to outcome/prognosis are contained on pages 118 to 121.

If the response to your initial correspondence is unsatisfactory, it's a good idea to write to the insurer's Chief Medical Officer. A further unsatisfactory response then means enquiring if there is some form of internal appeal/complaints procedure to which you can present medical evidence to support your case. Ideally, this ought to include:

- A written report from your GP.
- Details of any state sickness or disability benefits being claimed (e.g. incapacity benefit), along with dates and findings of recent DSS medical examinations carried out by Benefit Agency medical advisers.
- An up-to-date report from your consultant. This is particularly important. If you don't have a consultant, try to arrange an appointment with a reputable (preferably NHS) doctor who has acknowledged expertise in the management of ME/CFS. You may end up having to do this on a private fee-paying basis, but if you still belong to a trade union or professional organisation they may help with the cost.

(A private consultation and report is likely to cost around £250).

If your internal appeal fails, you have three other options:

## Legal advice

In the first instance this is very desirable and an initial consultation shouldn't be too expensive. It can even be free. If you are on a low income or welfare benefits, you can seek advice and assistance via the Green Form scheme. If you decide to go ahead and take legal action, then it's possible that you may be eligible for legal aid (this can also help to pay for any further medical reports). Legal aid is means tested and granted on a sliding scale related to your income and other financial circumstances. Do make sure that you see a solicitor who is well used to dealing with this type of case – a citizens' advice bureau or the Law Society should be able to supply a list of suitable local names. Always take a copy of your PHI policy and any relevant medical reports plus correspondence with the insurer. The very fact that the insurer knows you are considering legal action may be enough to force a change in mind and bring about an amicable settlement.

## Personal Insurance Arbitration Service (PIAS)

This service is free and can be used, provided the insurer is a member of the PIAS scheme. The arbitrator will examine papers from both sides and can then ask for an informal hearing (so can you or the insurer). The claimant is entitled to reject any PIAS decision and then proceed to use the courts, but the decision is binding on the insurer. For more details see Useful Addresses, page 421.

## Insurance Ombudsman

Again, this is a free service and any decision will be binding on the insurer up to the sum of £100,000. If you are unhappy with the result, you can reject the decision and go to court. The Insurance Ombudsman may request further medical reports or expert advice before trying to settle the dispute by giving suitable advice. If this fails, then a formal decision will be made. People with ME/CFS who have taken their dispute to the Insurance Ombudsman seem to be generally satisfied with the way it has been handled. For further details see Useful Addresses, page 421.

It's worth noting that under the 1988 Access to Medical Reports Act you have a right to see medical reports prepared for employment or insurance purposes which have been written by your own GP or specialist. If you ask for access to the report, the doctor must allow 21 days for the report to be seen. This gives you the opportunity to correct any misunderstandings or factual inaccuracies. See also pages 176–7.

If the insurance company indicates that they would like you to see a specialist of their choosing for an up-to-date report, it's not being unreasonable to insist that you would like to see someone who has some recognised expertise in dealing with people who have ME/CFS. Unlike medical reports prepared by your own doctors, you don't have any right to see those prepared for the benefit of the insurer. The company may, however, be quite happy to let you see a copy of such a report if it confirms their view that you are fit to return to work again!

While any dispute is in progress over a PHI policy it's important to be extremely careful what you do outside the house. Insurers are now employing private detectives to snoop on claimants whom they believe may be acting fraudulently. This can involve video surveillance and even people pretending to be visitors to your home. Whilst having no sympathy with anyone who commits fraud, this sort of undercover 'evidence' can easily be misused against perfectly genuine claimants. Insurance companies do, however, have to be extremely careful when employing such tactics. In November 1997, a woman with ME/CFS was awarded £116,000 in the High Court after being secretly filmed in the hope that her claim could be discredited.

# Retirement on the Grounds of Ill Health

If you're in a company pension scheme and decide to apply for early retirement on the grounds of ill health, then some form of pension may now be payable.

The qualifying criteria will vary considerably, but most schemes stipulate that in order to obtain a pension, the claimant must be able to show (with varying degrees of certainty) that they have a 'permanent' inability to undertake their employment duties. The Local Government Pension Scheme Regulations (1995), state that an employee must be 'incapable of discharging efficiently the duties of that employment by reason of permanent ill health or infirmity of mind or body' (D71b). The NHS pension scheme and several private schemes apply similar criteria. The key word is, of course, 'permanent', which implies that the disability will continue till normal retirement age. For someone in their mid-thirties this could mean assessing the likely prognosis for the next 30 years – not an easy task to predict. Other pension schemes have criteria which aren't quite so strict and include phrases such as 'incapacity which is likely to be permanent' or 'incapacity sufficiently serious to prevent the applicant from following his or her employment for the foreseeable future', i.e. the next few years. Some pension schemes, however, have criteria which are very strict indeed, e.g. 'permanent incapacity which is likely to prevent any form of gainful employment'. So you can

see how important it is to check through the small print in the agreement
before sending in an application.

A small number of pension schemes are rather more flexible and
agree to grant a pension subject to ongoing review. In practice, this
means that it may be easier to obtain a pension initially, but it could then
be withdrawn if medical evidence suggests that a significant degree of
recovery has taken place when your situation is reviewed.

There are a number of important variables which most pension
schemes are likely to take into account when a claim for early retirement
is being assessed.

- First is your age. The older you are, the more likely that such a
  request is going to be considered sympathetically. For anyone over
  the age of 50, and not too far from normal retirement age, then this
  factor ought to count in your favour.
- Second is the severity and course of your illness. If your condition is
  steadily improving, then permanent disablement is far less likely,
  even if progress is rather slow or erratic. It obviously helps to have a
  medical report from a reputable consultant to back up your case. If
  you can't obtain one on the NHS, it may be worth arranging a private
  appointment.
- Third is how long you've been ill – probably the most crucial factor.
  Anything less than two years' duration is extremely unlikely to be
  regarded as being permanent. Between two and four years falls into
  a rather grey area when it comes to predicting outcome; experience
  suggests that most pension providers would be reluctant to regard
  ME/CFS as causing permanent disability until three or four years'
  chronic ill health has elapsed. Once you have remained unwell for
  more than four years, and no significant degree of recovery has taken
  place, the possibility of permanent disablement must be taken very
  seriously. *My own view is that it would be very unfair not to grant a
  pension at this stage.*
- Fourth is the type of occupation you normally do and whether there
  is any possibility that you could return to some form of lighter or
  more flexible duties in the future. It may be useful to obtain a copy of
  the agreement to see what the small print states.
- Fifth is the question of how your ME/CFS is being managed by both
  you and your doctor. Although there is clearly no effective drug treatment at present, you may well be asked for details of how you are
  managing your lifestyle and whether or not you have participated in
  either a graded exercise programme or a course of cognitive
  behaviour therapy (CBT) – two approaches to management which
  are currently viewed by some doctors as being the most effective way

of treating ME/CFS. Failure to have tried out such treatments could provide the pension provider with another excuse for deferring acceptance of your claim.

- Sixth is the unfortunate fact that some doctors who advise pension providers on eligibility for ill health retirement are misinformed about many aspects of ME/CFS. If this is the case, you may have to provide information on outcome, quality of life, etc (see pages 114–122), along with references to published medical papers which demonstrate that this illness can cause permanent and severe levels of disablement.

If you do decide to go ahead and apply for a pension, it is always a good idea to first discuss this with your trade union or professional body. They should be able to guide you through any legal technicalities as well as acting on your behalf when necessary. If a dispute arises, find out whether there is any form of internal appeal procedure that can be set in motion. Failing that, do consider taking legal advice from a solicitor who's used to dealing with this type of dispute (it's worth pointing out that the new Disability Discrimination Act covers certain aspects of pension entitlement). Disputes involving pensions can also be referred to the Occupational Pensions Advisory Service or the Pensions Ombudsman. The latter adjudicator is unlikely to intervene unless all reasonable steps have already been taken to solve the dispute. (See Useful Addresses, page 421, if you want to contact either organisation.)

## Occupations Commonly Affected by ME/CFS

Although ME/CFS undoubtedly affects people across the entire social spectrum and in all types of occupation, there does seem to be a bias towards those who are employed in healthcare professions and teaching. I believe that there are a number of factors which may help to explain this curious vulnerability. The most important lies in the fact that both groups are working in an atmosphere of above-average physical and mental stress; they also face considerable pressure not to go 'off sick' when ill because it's often extremely difficult finding colleagues who are willing to cover their absence. In addition, teachers and health workers are frequently in close contact with other people's infections.

As far as medical and nursing professions are concerned, there is now a possibility that permanent disablement with ME/CFS will be regarded as a work-related illness – provided there is reliable evidence that the triggering infection was contracted from a patient (or in the case of vaccination, been given for an occupational hazard such as hepatitis B).

A survey carried out by the ME Association suggested that the situation was nowhere near as satisfactory for teachers. The average age at which they first became ill was 41 and of those off work nearly 45 per cent did not expect to return to classroom duties. This is not only a tremendous loss to the country in terms of professional experience, but there is also a very large economic cost in terms of pensions and sickness benefits.

Stress in the classroom was frequently cited as a major factor, not only in precipitating ME/CFS but also in perpetuating their ill health. The lack of part-time or flexible working opportunities appeared to be a major obstacle in planning a graded return to work.

The National Union of Teachers has campaigned on behalf of a number of members who have been forced into unwise decisions over their contracts without taking competent professional advice. Others, under pressure, have just opted out and resigned. If you are a teacher in this position, do consult with the NUT and also try to speak to another colleague who has had to make similar decisions, preferably one who has been employed by a sympathetic local authority.

The high incidence of ME/CFS in the teaching profession has also been confirmed in a survey by Dr Darrel Ho-Yen into the occupation of 275 patients in Scotland (reference 17). Teachers and students accounted for 22 per cent of the total; 16 per cent were retired; 13 per cent were housewives; 11 per cent worked in various service industries; 9 per cent were clerical staff; 9 per cent were skilled workers; 8 per cent unskilled; 7 per cent worked in hospitals, and the remaining 5 per cent were in various professions (lawyers, civil servants, etc). These figures should finally dispel the myth that ME/CFS is almost solely confined to middle-class *Observer*-reading professionals!

Other occupational groups who appear to be unduly susceptible include staff in mental subnormality institutions, and water and sewage workers – all of whom are exposed to an above-average incidence of infective illnesses.

## Self-Employment and ME/CFS

One further possibility worth exploring is that of becoming self-employed and carrying on some form of work from home. This certainly has attractions, as it can be flexible, carried out at times when you're fit enough and temporarily abandoned when you're unwell.

Obviously, this is only an option for those who feel able and want to continue with some form of work. I fully accept that for many people with ME/CFS, this option isn't possible now, but it may be later on when you start to make progress. It's also important to appreciate that if you continue to claim incapacity benefit, there may come a time when the DSS will review your position. If they feel that despite being unable to perform your normal occupation, there is some 'suitable alternative work' you could do, this could be used as a reason to stop benefit.

## Some Other Options with Employment

You may feel that if you've had to give up your job, there's nothing else you can now do, but it is important to explore other possibilities.

It may be possible to arrange some part-time work in your previous type of occupation, or do some 'flexitime' to fit in with times of day when you seem to function most productively. Another employer might be able to offer you a similar type of job, but at a less demanding pace, and probably at a less demanding salary! However, for many people these options simply don't exist, and there's no other choice but to rely on financial support from the various state sickness benefits.

Being at home all day, no longer making decisions and missing out on the social life and friendships that are all part of 'being at work' is a very demoralising aspect of ME/CFS, which often exacerbates feelings of isolation and loss of self-esteem. In this situation it may be worth considering making an application to the Open University. They are particularly keen to encourage students with disabilities on to their courses, and have a special tutor who can give further advice (see Useful Addresses, page 422). Specific areas where the Open University can help disabled students include tutorials by phone; home visits by tutors; flexibility about the necessity to attend summer schools; exams being taken at home and allowances for problems with memory/concentration. It may also be possible to obtain assistance with fees or computer charges, depending on your financial circumstances.

It obviously depends on how unwell you are, what stage the illness is at, and how variable the symptoms are, but giving up work for good is one of the most difficult decisions to make in ME/CFS, so *do* look at the other possibilities – state of health permitting. It may also be worth making contact with an organisation called Opportunities for People with Disabilities (see Useful Addresses, page 416) who liaise with employees who are sympathetic to the needs of disabled employees.

Whatever you decide to do about work, try not to make any hasty decisions – take time to consider all the options available and take account of what other members of the family feel is right. Don't ever resign from your job because of ME/CFS till you've first taken expert advice – you may end up disqualifying yourself from financial assistance.

There are no simple answers to the very common question: 'What do

I do about my job?' It very much depends on the stage of your illness, what you do for a living, and the attitude of your employers and possibly the company doctor.

# Help from the Government

There are a number of different sources of advice, information and financial support available for disabled people who wish to remain in work or intend to return after a period of ill health.

## Jobcentre services

Jobcentre staff are now supposed to be trained in providing information and advice on suitable vacancies and employment services which may be applicable to disabled people. If your disability is more severe, then you may be referred to a Disability Employment Adviser (DEA) in the Placement, Assessment and Counselling Team – known as the PACT. Your DEA will be able to provide a great deal of practical information regarding disability issues and employment. DEAs also help with introductions to the various special schemes outlined below, which are designed to assist disabled people return to work.

*Registering as disabled* Since the introduction of the Disability Discrimination Act, it is no longer necessary to register your disability with the Employment Service. You can, however, still register yourself as being disabled with the local Social Services Department (see page 368).

*Job Introduction Scheme* This is available to any disabled person who, in the opinion of a DEA, requires a period of suitable reintroduction to work to allow them to demonstrate their abilities to a new employer. The Employment Service pays £45 per week (1998/9) to the employer who agrees to take on a disabled person for a six-week trial period.

*Access to work* This programme is run by the Employment Service to help cover the costs of providing extra support in the workplace for a disabled employee. The type of assistance on offer includes:

- Support workers for anyone who requires practical help at work or in travelling to work
- Special equipment or adaptations to existing equipment
- Alterations to premises or workplace environment so a disabled employee can work there
- Help with travel costs, including adaptations to a car, or taxi fares for someone who cannot use public transport.

The amount and type of support available under this scheme is supposed to be extremely flexible and so fit in with individual needs. Grants are made for up to three years, but you can then make a further application. For more details contact your local PACT.

*Rehabilitation* The Employment Service helps with numerous aspects of employment rehabilitation. Initial assessment of your needs is usually arranged by PACT. During rehabilitation you might be entitled to a Rehabilitation Allowance and other necessary expenses.

*Government sponsored training* This is the responsibility of the Department of Education and Employment. Disabled people who have special training needs may find the Training for Work (TFW) scheme worth enquiring about. TFW is delivered by Training and Enterprise Councils (TECs) in England and Wales, and Local Enterprise Companies (LECs) in Scotland. These two bodies work closely with local employers, training and disability organisations to promote employment prospects for disabled people.

## Benefits and training allowances

- The disability working allowance (see pages 387–8) is designed to supplement the income of disabled people on low wages who are working 16 or more hours per week.
- The disability living allowance mobility component will not be affected if you receive a training allowance, but the care component could be.
- Anyone receiving incapacity benefit or severe disablement allowance will have to stop claiming if they join a training course.

*Employment rights* It is important to remember that anyone with a disability has exactly the same legal rights as able-bodied employees when it comes to protection against unfair dismissal, redundancy, maternity pay and time off for public duties. Disabled people also have additional rights under the new Disability Discrimination Act (see later). For more information on employment rights, obtain a copy of an information pack by RADAR (see Useful Addresses, page 416) called *Employment Rights: A Guide for Disabled People*. Trade unions, professional organisations and local law centres will provide additional advice and information on legal disputes.

*VAT concessions* may also be available – see leaflet 701/7/94, *VAT Reliefs for People with Disabilities*, available from your local VAT enquiries office (look in the phone book under Customs and Excise).

# The Disability Discrimination Act (DDA)

The DDA, which came into force in 1996, makes it unlawful to discriminate against disabled people in relation to employment, the provision of goods and services, or the sale/management of property. Despite the Act's many good intentions, the Disability Alliance has criticised the way in which employers with fewer than 20 employees are exempt from employment legislation and the lack of any Commission with enforcement powers to pursue individual cases.

*Defining disability* This is defined as 'a physical or mental impairment which has a substantial and long-term adverse effect on [your] ability to carry out normal day-to-day activities'.

'Long-term' means effects which have lasted for at least 12 months, or are likely to last at least 12 months, or are likely to last for the rest of your life. The definition also includes a disability from the past, even if you have now recovered.

'Day-to-day' activities involve: moving from place to place, manual dexterity, physical co-ordination, ability to carry or move objects, memory and concentration.

The DDA does not define a list of specific illnesses which are automatically covered by legislation. In practice, your disability starts from the date on which you first develop symptoms that affect your ability to carry out normal day-to-day activities. One exception is the way the Act automatically covers anyone registered as disabled under the Disabled Persons (Employment) Act on both 12 January 1995 and 2 December 1996 for a period of three years from 2 December 1996.

*Employment rights* The DDA makes it unlawful for an employer to treat you less favourably than someone else because of your disability – unless they can show such action is 'justified'. The DDA applies to temporary staff and contract workers as well, and covers all areas of employment, including recruitment, training, pension rights, promotion and dismissal. In addition, the DDA requires employers to make 'reasonable' changes to employment arrangements which might be needed to help an employee. These could include widening a doorway for wheelchair access, changing working hours, purchasing special equipment or allowing time off for medical appointments. As a disability is not always obvious, employers are now expected to take *reasonable steps* to find out whether job applicants or employees have disabilities – ignorance is no longer bliss! Equally, employees with disabilities now have a duty to keep their employer or occupational health doctor informed about any difficulties which are occurring at work.

*Access to goods and services* The provision of various types of services to disabled people are covered by another part of the Act. Examples of such services include shops, hotels, banks, cinemas, restaurants, as well as hospitals, libraries and leisure centres. Size doesn't matter, neither does whether you have to pay for the service. Insurance companies are also covered, but special rules apply to some of their services. Discrimination in the supply of a service could include giving you a lower standard of service or charging some form of supplement. However, where a health and safety risk can be proven, there may be grounds for treating a disabled person less favourably.

*Housing* The DDA makes it unlawful for anyone who lets or sells property to discriminate against disabled people.

*Schools* The Act states that schools in England and Wales must now include details of admission for disabled pupils and facilities which are available in their annual reports. Unfortunately, the Act contains no real powers to substantially improve access to schools for children with disabilities.

*Transport* The Public Transport Vehicles section covers taxis, buses, coaches and trains. Transport terminals (e.g. airports and bus or rail stations) are covered under the Access to Goods and Services section. In theory, this means that all new public transport vehicles should become much more accessible to disabled people, as should places where you catch buses, trains and planes.

*Making a complaint* If you feel that some form of clear discrimination has taken place at work you can take your case to an industrial tribunal. In addition to employers with fewer than 20 employees, there are a number of groups of workers who are *not* protected by the DDA (e.g. prison and police officers). Disputes under other parts of the Act are enforceable through a local County Court (or a Sheriff's Court in Scotland). If the tribunal or court finds in your favour, you may then be awarded damages for loss of income and/or hurt feelings.

For expert legal advice contact the Disability Law Service (see Useful Addresses, page 422) or your local law centre. A solicitor may be willing to take on your case on a no win, no fee basis. It's also worth contacting your trade union or professional body for advice and possible help with legal costs.

To obtain a DDA Information Pack (DL50) contact the DDA Information Line on 0345 622 633. A range of booklets are also available covering all the different aspects of the Act.

## ME/CFS and the DDA

The first industrial tribunal case involving the DDA and someone with ME/CFS was heard in Reading in April 1997. Here, a clerical worker claimed that she had been unfairly dismissed from her job in the previous December after posting a sick note which stated that she was suffering from ME/CFS. Her employers claimed that the sick note had never been received and she was subsequently dismissed for a breach of contract. The case was lost at the tribunal, not on the grounds of disability resulting from ME/CFS, but on her failure to establish that a sick note had been sent in.

Below are some of the principal conclusions reached by the industrial tribunal. They have important implications for anyone with ME/CFS who may wish to make use of this legislation to protect their rights to employment.

'We consider that ME/CFS most certainly can be a disability for the purposes of the Act.

On the evidence before us we have no hesitation in stating that the applicant was suffering from a disability within the ambit of the Act. We are clear that the applicant was suffering from an impairment which affected her ability to carry out normal day-to-day activities because she was affected by a number of matters referred to in paragraph 4 (1) of Schedule 1 of the Act.

In conclusion, we find that the applicant suffered a disability for the purposes of the Act, but she was not dismissed because she had a disability or discriminated against because of her disability.'

In a second case, involving a health visitor who was dismissed by an NHS Trust in 1997, settlement was reached days before the case was due to be heard by a tribunal. The settlement here involved a payment of £16,000 compensation to cover loss of earnings and injury to feelings.

The lady in question had hoped to make a gradual return to work duties after a 10-month period of sick leave due to ME/CFS, but after a series of meetings with Trust managers she was dismissed only three days after the employment provisions of the DDA came into force. The result of this particular case should have important implications for many NHS staff with ME/CFS who are currently in the position of being too ill to work, but not considered sick enough to be retired on the grounds of ill health.

# The Economic Cost of ME/CFS

Although very little work has been carried out on assessing the economic cost of ME/CFS, a survey published in Australia in 1992 (reference 519) estimated the direct costs (those incurred in both the diagnosis and management) to be around $1,950 per case per year (approximately $2,500 at present). After inclusion of indirect costs (those relating to lost productivity) the total cost was estimated to be around $9,500 per case per year (current estimate $12,200). Based on a very conservative estimate of two cases per 10,000 of the Australian population, these figures imply a minimum total cost to the Australian economy of $416 million per year.

An unpublished study carried out by the ME Association and ME Action, from details on 3,000 of their members, concluded that the economic cost of ME/CFS to the UK economy was at least £641 million and possibly as much as £2.1 billion per year.

# 17

# Running your Home

The disabling physical symptoms of ME/CFS mean that many people share the same sort of practical difficulties that other chronically disabled groups have in trying to lead a normal life. These may range from the pure physical inability to summon up sufficient strength to carry out a routine task like mowing the lawn to difficulties with gripping or manipulating everyday objects used in the kitchen.

The combination of muscular fatigue and unsteadiness often produces great difficulty in coping with tasks that involve prolonged standing and concentrating. This not only prevents many people following their normal occupation but also makes many of the domestic tasks involved in running a home equally difficult.

To make life easier there are a number of practical aids available either free, on loan, or to buy, which can help to make physical and manipulative tasks less fatiguing. There are also various professionals and agencies who can give invaluable help when it comes to learning to cope with disability. It's perfectly natural to feel reluctant to label yourself as being 'disabled'. You don't have to use the term if you don't want to, but if difficulties are occurring, then do make use of the resources which are available.

Before approaching anyone for help it's a good idea to make a comprehensive written list of the sort of practical problems with which you require help. These might range from something as simple as opening tight tops on the marmalade jar to obtaining expert assistance and financial help in making major adaptations in the home for someone who is becoming more severely disabled. Don't be afraid to go round asking questions.

Organisations that are involved in helping people with the practical aspects of disability are only too willing to provide the necessary information and advice. In the meantime, here are some suggestions that could help to make life a bit easier:

## In the Home

### Kitchens

- Keep commonly used foods and kitchen utensils together in an easily accessible place – preferably at chest height, to avoid repeated reaching up and bending down.

- Use level work surfaces for heavy objects – they can be pushed around instead of lifted.
- Raise the washing-up bowl in the sink so you're not stooping over, and let the washing-up dry by itself.
- If you can afford it, consider purchasing a dishwasher.
- Again, if you can afford it, consider other types of electrical apparatus which can make life easier: a microwave, a freezer to store some essential foods in, or an electric tin opener.
- There are numerous aids which make a whole range of domestic duties and cooking much easier, e.g. specially adapted cutlery and cooking utensils, electric plugs with small handles so they're easier to pull out of the socket, etc. Visit one of the disabled living centres (see Useful Addresses, page 414–5) and see what's on display that might help you.
- With modern adjustable ironing boards it's easy to iron while seated, and with coat hangers to hand, plus an airer to put all the ready ironed items on to, you need not move from start to finish. Obviously, try to keep ironing to a minimum, and train the rest of the family in how to do this vital task! You may even be able to find someone who charges a small fee to do the weekly ironing for you. Check out the notice boards in your local shops.
- When cooking, consider preparing double quantities and then freeze the remainder for a later date.

## Living rooms

- If you have difficulty getting out of a low chair or sofa due to weakness in the hip muscles, consider buying a comfortable high chair, or one with a raised seat.
- A sofa bed may be a very useful additional piece of furniture if you're frequently confined to bed for 'relapses' and don't like spending your time upstairs confined to the bedroom.
- A remote control for the television set.

## Stairs

- These can be a major problem for anyone who has been severely weakened by ME/CFS and may mean being confined to either the downstairs or upstairs for long periods. Chair lifts, although expensive, are a very useful device in such circumstances, but do take expert advice before spending large amounts of money – visit a

disabled living centre for further practical help.
- If you do tend to live downstairs during a relapse, and sleep down there, it may be worth considering installing a downstairs toilet and shower.

## Bathroom

- A hand rail, fixed to the wall by the bath, will help getting in and out.
- Buy a non-slip bath mat.
- Sitting in a shower can be less tiring than taking a bath. Use a special board across the bath top to sit on, but make sure it's stable and won't slip. (The Red Cross may loan you one.)
- Washing hair in the bath is a lot easier than bending over the sink.
- If your 'carer' is often having to lift you in and out of the bath, consider installing some form of hoist device.

## Bedrooms

- Cut down on bed-making by making use of fitted sheets and duvets. The amount of warmth provided by a duvet is shown by its tog value. In a well-heated house a 10.5–12-tog duvet should be fine for all-year use. If you feel particularly cold, an extra-warm tog 13.5 might be better. If you really cannot tolerate the cold winter months, it's now possible to purchase 15-tog duvets!
- Remember that all the household bedding doesn't necessarily have to be changed on the same day.
- Keep a comfy upright chair in the bedroom for use when you're recovering from a period of bed rest.
- A lightweight vacuum cleaner saves lifting a heavy one up the stairs each time. If you use an extra long flex you can do an entire floor from just one plug.
- An extra telephone socket or a portable phone can be a great help, especially when you're not well and there's nobody else at home.

The most useful source of information on all forms of practical aids for disabled people is an occupational therapist, who can also give useful advice regarding more major adaptations within the home. If you think that an occupational therapist might be able to help then contact your GP or local social services department.

# Housing Grants

A variety of grants to help with repairs, improvements and/or adaptations to your home are available from local authorities. Don't be put off from claiming because you're not sure about eligibility. The rules covering these sort of grants can be quite complex, but as long as honest information is provided about your circumstances it can't do any harm.

## Disabled facilities grant

This is designed to help meet the costs of adapting a property for the needs of a disabled person. Grants can be given to owner occupiers, private tenants, local authority tenants or housing association tenants. To qualify for a grant you will need to satisfy *one* of the following disability criteria:

- have a mental disorder or impairment of any kind
- be substantially disabled (physically) by illness
- be registered disabled with the Social Services Department.

Mandatory grants are available to assist with:

- improving access to a disabled person's house
- making a house safer for a disabled person
- improving access inside the house to rooms such as the bedroom, bathroom, kitchen and principal living room
- improving facilities used for bathing, cooking, going to the toilet, washing, etc
- improving the heating system.

Discretionary grants can also be made to help with other types of adaptions aimed at making a home more suitable for someone with a disability.

As with all types of housing grant, a financial assessment of your resources will be undertaken. For those under the age of 18 this assessment will apply to the parent(s) who has main responsibility for care. Any application will have to be supported by a certificate stating that the disabled person will live in the property for at least five years after any work has been completed. Shorter periods are sometimes allowed in exceptional circumstances.

Applications should be made to the local authority, who may well request that the Social Services Department carries out an occupational therapy assessment of your disability and resulting needs.

## Home energy efficiency scheme

This provides grants to home owners and tenants who are in receipt of a relevant state benefit, including disability living allowance, disability working allowance or an attendance allowance. Under the scheme you could qualify for up to £315 (1998/9) worth of draught proofing, insulation and energy advice. For further details contact the Energy Action Grants Agency on freephone 0800 072 0150.

You might also be eligible for a decrease in council tax under the disability reduction scheme (see pages 392–3).

All these housing grants are described in more detail in the *Disability Rights Handbook* (see Useful Addresses, page 414).

# Out and About – Shopping

*Here are some ideas for making shopping easier:*

- Local voluntary groups may be able to provide an able-bodied volunteer to help with a weekly shop or a driver to take you there. Some schools also have volunteer sections.
- Find out about any local dial-a-ride services or other schemes to improve mobility. Shopmobility schemes now operate in over 150 towns throughout the UK – see Useful Addresses, page 427.

  The schemes provide battery operated scooters and wheelchairs to help people who have limited mobility to use all the shopping facilities in a city centre. Shopmobility is particularly helpful if car access is very restricted and where large shops are grouped together in pedestrianised zones. Anyone with mobility problems can make use of this facility – you don't have to be registered as disabled or possess an orange parking badge to qualify. Neither do you have to be resident in that particular town. Although there is no charge made for using the scheme a small deposit will be required. Shopmobility is usually open from 9.30 a.m. to 5 p.m. from Monday to Saturday. It's a good idea to book in advance, and car parking spaces are sometimes provided. Staff are also available to demonstrate the use of wheelchairs and scooters. Remember, you will need some form of identification such as a driving licence.
- Consider alternatives to going out to the shops. Shopping from home can be done via mail order; some shops will still deliver groceries; and the milkman now carries an increasingly diverse range of produce.
- Ask a friend or neighbour to buy certain goods on a regular basis when they go to the supermarket.
- Find out about supermarkets and department stores which have special shopping hours reserved for the disabled; some also have priority parking facilities. An increasing number of shops are also willing to provide extra help for their disabled customers.
- Ask able-bodied members of the family (or friends) to buy certain

items in bulk, as long as you have the storage space.
- Make sure that you always have a stock of essential items of food, so that in a relapse when you can't get out for several days, there is something to eat.

## Telephone services

Anyone who is housebound ought to consider making use of the increasing range of services being offered over the phone:

- Banking services are available from most of the leading banks and some building societies. First Direct, a division of the Midland Bank, offers a complete range of financial services including share dealing and insurance. Ask around to find the best service to suit your needs.
- Clothes, household and electrical goods are now available from home shopping catalogues. Orders can be taken over the phone but there may be a small charge. Catalogue shops such as Argos also operate home delivery services if you live within a reasonable distance of the nearest store.
- Supermarkets are introducing home-shopping schemes which allow you to order by phone or fax and then either collect the goods or have them delivered for a small extra fee. Stores to contact include Sainsbury's, Safeway and Tesco. So far, this type of service is largely confined to London and other cities. If successful, it will inevitably spread to the rest of the country.
- British Telecom has a free guide for people who are disabled which outlines the products and services provided to make communication easier. For a copy, telephone 0800 444 122 or write to: BT, Action for Disabled Customers, FREEPOST, Bristol BS1 2BR.

## Further Reading

The first four publications are available from the Disability Information Trust (see Useful Addresses, page 414).

*Communication and Access to Computer Technology* All kinds of advice and information on ways in which disabled people can make use of computer technology.
*Furniture* Describes a wide range of items which might be needed for the home and office.
*Hoists, Lifts and Transfers* Information on equipment designed for lifting and moving more severely disabled people.

*Home Management and Housing* Information on equipment and devices designed to make everyday tasks around the home easier (e.g. wheelchair-accessible kitchens, building design and all kinds of gadgets).

*Everyday Aids and Appliances* Articles from the *British Medical Journal* with 16 different chapters dealing with practical aids for all manner of disabilities. Available from BMJ Publishing, PO Box 295, London WC1H 9TE (tel: 0171 383 6185).

*More Everyday Aids and Appliances* Acts as a companion to the first book, and concentrates on aids which enable people to manage in the home and those which improve indoor/outdoor mobility. Available from BMJ Publishing.

*Shopmobility Directory* Contains details of all the individual schemes currently operating in the UK. Also has details on suppliers of projects and services for disabled people. Available from Shopmobility (see Useful Addresses, page 427).

# 18

# Increasing your Mobility

Problems with mobility are a major cause of social isolation for the disabled, as well as creating extra difficulties when it comes to obtaining employment, so do take advantage of any help that's available and appropriate to your individual needs.

Financial assistance may be forthcoming from the DSS with a mobility component from the disability living allowance. The Department of Employment can help with fares to work. Other types of financial assistance are described later in this chapter.

## Walking Aids

A walking stick will help to provide extra support, relieve muscle and joint pains, and increase mobility.

Make sure the stick you buy is the correct length for your body – you shouldn't end up leaning towards the stick (too short) or away from it (too long). If the stick has a metal or wooden tip it can easily slip in wet weather. A soft rubber tip is the best way to increase friction and grip, and just like the tyres on a car, these rubber tips need to be changed when worn. Pyramid sticks have either three or four legs and may be helpful if you require a considerable amount of support. If you're out and about quite a bit, it might be worth buying a shooting stick which has a fold-up seat on the top.

For those who are severely disabled, the Zimmer type of walking frame may be necessary – a physiotherapist or occupational therapist will provide appropriate advice.

## Wheelchairs

A small but significant minority of people with ME/CFS eventually find that they have to make use of a wheelchair. This may only be on a temporary basis to aid mobility during an arduous day's activities such as passing through an airport or a full day away from home. Sometimes, though, a wheelchair becomes a much more permanent necessity.

Wheelchairs can be obtained from a variety of sources:

*From the NHS* Wheelchairs (including powered wheelchairs) are supplied and maintained free of charge to disabled people who have a genuine and fairly permanent need for such assistance. Any wheelchair on the market can be supplied by an NHS Wheelchair Service Centre, depending on the circumstances of the individual concerned and the resources which are available.

Powered indoor/outdoor wheelchairs can be provided by the NHS for severely disabled people, provided you are unable to manage an ordinary wheelchair.

Attendant controlled wheelchairs can be issued where it would be difficult for the disabled person to be pushed out of doors, e.g. due to being overweight or living in a very hilly environment.

Each health authority currently makes its own eligibility criteria, but this has to be within broad national guidelines.

New legislation also permits NHS trusts to supply, at the request of a user, a wheelchair which is more expensive than is clinically necessary. In these cases, the cost difference is then recovered by the NHS from the user.

At present, a new voucher scheme is being phased in which provides financial aid from the NHS if you decide to purchase a wheelchair from the private sector. A voucher enables you to pay the difference between a wheelchair prescribed by the NHS and a more expensive model of your choice. Vouchers are not yet available for powered indoor/outdoor models.

You can also consider using the Motability scheme (see later in this chapter) to purchase an electric wheelchair on hire purchase.

If you feel that you might benefit from making use of a wheelchair, ask your GP/physiotherapist/occupational therapist to refer you to a local Wheelchair Service Centre for further assessment of your precise needs. Centres are listed in the phone book or contact the Health Information Service free on 0800 665544.

*Purchased privately* There are perfectly reputable private suppliers of wheelchairs, but do take expert advice before spending large sums of money. The British Association of Wheelchair Distributors (see Useful Addresses) can supply a full list of companies.

*The British Red Cross* can make a short-term loan to anyone who just requires extra help for a short period, e.g. when going away on holiday. Most large airports offer this kind of temporary assistance in the arrival/departure areas.

The exact type of wheelchair you eventually choose will depend on a number of factors. Are you going to use it indoors and out? Do you want to self-propel it or be pushed? Do you want to spend a lot of money on a powered wheelchair? Most people will require a chair that's suitable for both indoor and outdoor use, which will fold up to fit in a car, and which is comfortable.

Features which will increase the comfort and ride include pneumatic tyres (which, along with the brakes, need regular checking), a good cushion and a reliable base. You can also add various accessories such as trays and cushioned backrests.

You may decide to purchase an electric wheelchair, but there are certain disadvantages – they're heavy, can't be folded up, require quite a lot of space and are much more expensive.

Local authority housing departments may be able to help with ramps and widening of doorways to your home, but you might have to ask for support from your GP, occupational therapist and local councillor.

If you decide that a wheelchair might help to increase your mobility, either temporarily or permanently, do go and talk to other users about their experiences and opinions on the models which are available, and seek help from professional organisations such as RADAR who can offer expert advice.

Useful publications on wheelchairs are listed at the end of this chapter.

## Powered Vehicles

Besides electric wheelchairs, there are a variety of different types of electric scooters and powerchairs available. These vary in size from small three-wheeled scooters up to the much larger four-wheeled vehicles which generally travel longer distances (as they have much larger batteries). The three-wheeled vehicles tend to be more manoeuvrable, but many disabled people feel safer in a four-wheeled model. Smaller vehicles perform well indoors and on flat ground, but aren't always so useful at negotiating kerbs and other outside obstacles.

If you are considering purchasing one of these vehicles, then it's a good idea to go through a check list of your most important requirements. Where are you going to keep it when not in use? (These vehicles have to be stored under cover.) Will you need to take the vehicle inside a car? How far will it need to travel on most single journeys? (All kinds of factors, including your weight, the local environment and size of vehicle will be relevant here.) How much can you afford to pay? (Remember, you'll also need to pay for replacement batteries, maintenance and insurance cover.)

The next stage is to check out all the various models and manufacturers and send off for some brochures. There are several useful leaflets and books available (see Further Reading at the end of this chapter) on choosing a wheelchair or powered vehicle. You could also contact a local Disabled Living Centre (see Useful Addresses) for advice. Before visiting a Centre, phone to check that they have the sort of models you want to try out.

The final stage is trying out different models from the same range and possibly from a number of manufacturers to see which one suits your particular needs best. Some manufacturers are willing to arrange home demonstrations; this is particularly helpful as you can properly assess the pros and cons of the vehicle in the environment where it's going to be used. Otherwise, you'll have to visit a showroom. Make sure you have a friend or relative with you when you go for a demonstration or test drive.

A number of distributors also sell second-hand models, but do take care when purchasing one through a newspaper advert. And don't forget to check whether financial assistance could be provided by the Motability scheme (see later in this chapter) or the NHS Wheelchair Service.

Further information on powered vehicles and assessments is available from the Banstead Mobility Centre (see Useful Addresses, page 426). Insurance cover can be arranged through: Bradstock Yarrow Young Ltd (tel: 0181–863 5577); M. J. Fish & Company (tel: 01772 724442) or Chartwell Insurance (tel: 0181–958 0901).

# You and your Car

## *Help from motoring organisations*

For those who continue to drive there are two motoring organisations specialising in the problems faced by disabled drivers – the Disabled Drivers' Association and the Disabled Drivers' Motor Club (see Useful Addresses, page 426). Membership may provide financial concessions on car ferries, motor insurance and RAC membership.

The AA has a special telephone information line for disabled motorists. This service provides help and advice on all aspects of motoring for the disabled. The AA helpline is on freephone 0800 262050. A special AA breakdown service for disabled drivers – Mobility Assistance Membership – is available to anyone who has been granted an orange badge. The RAC operates a similar scheme, known as Response, which is again restricted to orange badge holders. Phone 0800 550550 for more details.

## *Insurance and the Driving and Vehicle Licensing Agency (DVLA)*

Anyone with ME/CFS who continues to drive a car should consider informing the DVLA about the current state of their health, especially if such driving involves a commercial or passenger service vehicle. This may then involve a medical assessment on your current 'fitness to drive' or a medical report from your GP. Whether or not you should still be driving very much depends on how muscle fatigue and problems with concentration are affecting your ability to control a car and make quick decisions when necessary. My view is that there are a significant number of people with ME/CFS who continue to drive when they are not really fit to do so.

Insurance companies usually want to know about any physical or mental condition which could 'in any way impair your ability to drive', so do check the small print on your policy, otherwise you could be invalidating the insurance cover. If in doubt, most insurance companies have a medical officer to whom you could write for further guidance.

## *Mobility Advice and Vehicle Information Service (MAVIS)*

This is an organisation set up by the Department of Transport to help disabled drivers choose a suitable car and any adaptions which are appropriate to their needs. A range of vehicles is available for test driving on a private road system, each equipped with hand controls showing different driving systems and adaptions. Information is free but a charge may be made for other kinds of help (see Useful Addresses, page 427).

## *Mobility Information Service*

This is a voluntary organisation offering a wide range of information on cars and adaptions. It also produces leaflets on choosing, buying and converting a car. Personal assessment can be arranged within a 100-mile radius of Shrewsbury (see Useful Addresses, page 427).

## *Motability*

This is a voluntary organisation, sponsored by the government, which aims to help disabled drivers use their higher rate mobility component of a disability living allowance (DLA) to obtain a car or powered wheelchair. New cars can be obtained on either a contract hire basis or on hire purchase. Servicing, maintenance, AA membership and loss-of-use insurance cover are included.

For the hire purchase scheme, special discounts have been negotiated with a range of car manufacturers (e.g. Ford, Renault, Volvo) but virtually any make of car can be purchased over a two to five year period. There are also hire purchase schemes for used cars and powered wheelchairs. Motability schemes operate when the disabled person agrees to the DSS paying their DLA supplement to Motability Finance Ltd for the period of the agreement. (For more information see Useful Addresses, page 427.)

## Orange Badge parking scheme

This scheme, which is designed to help people with severe mobility problems, currently applies throughout England, Wales and Scotland with the exception of four areas in central London (the City, Westminster, Kensington and Chelsea, and part of Camden). These areas have severe parking problems and so run their own schemes – contact the Greater London Association for Disabled People at 336 Brixton Road, London SW9 7AA (tel: 0171–346 5813) for more details.

In order to qualify for an orange badge you need to be over the age of two and meet one of the following disability criteria:

- be in receipt of a higher rate mobility component of the disability living allowance
- have a grant towards running your car
- have a severe disability in both arms so you cannot turn a steering wheel by hand
- have a 'permanent and substantial disability which causes inability to walk or very considerable difficulty in walking'.

Orange badge holders can park free and without time limit at on-street parking meters, 'pay and display' parking locations and in time-limited parking zones. You can also park on double or single yellow lines in certain circumstances. However, the orange badge is not a licence to park anywhere you wish to. Although you shouldn't be wheel-clamped, your car will be removed if it causes an obstruction.

An application form and explanatory leaflet can be obtained from your local Social Services Department or Regional/Island Council in Scotland. Some local authorities request a medical report from your GP to confirm that you have a real need for an orange badge. A few authorities employ physiotherapists to make these assessments.

There is no formal right of appeal if an application is refused, but you could try contacting your local councillor to see if they are willing to help.

Orange badge holders who visit certain overseas countries can take full advantage of similar concessions. Full details can be obtained from the Department of Transport (see Useful Addresses, page 417). The Orange Badge Network (see Useful Addresses, page 427) represents the rights and needs of Orange Badge holders.

## Special adaptions

Various types of adaption to a car can make life much easier for both disabled drivers and disabled passengers. For example, a rotating car seat, which swings around and outwards, will help with getting in and out. This type of device can be supplied by Elap Engineering, Fort Street, Accrington, Lancashire BB5 1QG (tel: 01254 871599). Advice on other types of adaptions can be obtained from organisations already listed in this section.

## Vehicle excise duty (road tax) exemption

This is an extremely useful item of financial assistance for anyone who is receiving a higher rate mobility component of the disability living allowance. Technically, the vehicle is only exempt whilst being used by or for the purposes of a disabled person, but what this means in practice has never been satisfactorily defined. Clearly, regular use for purposes not connected with a disabled person would be highly illegal. However, where a car is principally being used or the proper purpose, there shouldn't be anything to worry about.

Anyone who receives a higher rate mobility component of DLA should be automatically sent a VED exemption form by the DSS. If not, contact the Disability Benefits Unit on 0345 123456.

You can also nominate another person's vehicle for this exemption, provided it is still being used 'by or for the purpose of' the disabled person.

There is no formal appeal procedure in operation if an application is refused. Further information on VED exemption can be found in the *Disability Rights Handbook* (see Useful Addresses, page 414).

# Public Transport

For many people with ME/CFS who've had to stop driving, or never even driven, increasing reliance on public transport becomes a necessity. Fortunately, the administrators of public transport are becoming much more aware of the needs of their disabled passengers – British Rail and the airports in particular. The situation is likely to improve still further with the implementation of the Disability Discrimination Act, which has specific sections on public transport.

Genuine financial help is available with fares on public transport and taxi rides, but the level of disability required to qualify tends to vary between local authorities.

Local voluntary organisations are now producing a range of access guides to toilets, shops and public buildings (see Further Reading at the end of this chapter). RADAR (see Useful Addresses, page 416) has a scheme involving specially designed toilets for the disabled. For a small fee you can have a key which provides automatic access to these conveniences.

## Train Travel

Train operators charge a small fee for their disabled person's railcard which gives a third off fares for both the holder and a companion. Anyone who receives a middle or higher rate care component or higher rate mobility component of a disability living allowance, or a severe disablement allowance should qualify.

If you are severely disabled, particular if you have to use a wheelchair, and require extra help at stations and during the journey, do let the correct train operator know (in good time) as staff can be extremely helpful. A special seat/wheelchair space can be reserved on many InterCity connections and other reservable trains. There is a comprehensive leaflet, *Rail Travel for Disabled Passengers*, which provides information on all the ways in which they are able to help, and whom to contact for particular services. RADAR also produces a book providing information on accessibility to over 500 stations (see Further Reading at the end of this chapter).

## Bus travel

Many local authorities provide financial assistance by issuing concessionary fare tokens to people who are registered as disabled. Check with your local council for eligibility criteria.

## 'Dial-a-ride' schemes

Some towns operate dial-a-ride schemes for disabled people who are unable to make proper use of public transport. These can be of immense value for shopping trips or just being able to leave the house for a while. The service usually operates on a door-to-door basis. Your local citizens' advice bureau should know if there's a service operating in your area.

In London, this scheme is operated by London DART (Dial-a-ride and Taxicard). Tel: 0171–482 2325 for further details.

## London Transport

Runs a specific Unit for Disabled Passengers (see Useful Addresses, page 426) which is aimed at making public transport more accessible to people with disabilities. Among the services provided are:

- **Stationlink** – for across London train connections
- **Airbus** – for travel between the centre and Heathrow
- **Mobility Bus** – wheelchair accessible buses now operate on several

different routes linking residential areas to the main shopping centres.

For leaflets giving details of these services tel: 0171–918 3312.

*Shopmobility*

This organisation provides a range of battery operated wheelchairs and scooters on loan for the day in shopping centres of most large towns (see page 427).

# Taking a Holiday

Just like everyone else, people with ME/CFS, along with their carers and relatives, need to enjoy a good holiday from time to time. However, the effort involved in the process can be extremely tiring. But once you've safely arrived, a pleasant holiday in the right climate with good-quality accommodation and food can provide a considerable degree of improvement.

The first step is to plan well ahead and discuss with the whole family exactly what sort of holiday seems most suitable – home or abroad. Obviously, a holiday in the UK may be much easier if you're planning to travel by car and you have to help with the driving. Alternatively, many parts of France can easily be reached by using the ferries or channel tunnel, although this may mean the frustrations of having to depart at odd hours and climbing awkward stairs to and from the car decks. If you can't cope with stairs, contact the ferry operator well in advance; they should make arrangements for you to use a lift. Some ferry operators offer financial concessions to disabled drivers, but they may only be available to those who belong to one of the disabled drivers' associations already mentioned.

Some families have invested in a caravan – obviously with this there needs to be a very fit member of the party, but this is an option worth considering.

Most of the large tour companies are perfectly willing to accept travellers with disabilities. In fact, it's now very difficult to do otherwise, thanks to the Disability Discrimination Act. Most of them advise people to contact their client services department well before booking to find out if the hotel, resort or country you intend to visit will be suitable.

If you're severely disabled and have to use a wheelchair, there are many hotels which have specially adapted rooms with good access and washing facilities. If you have special dietary needs, these should be made known well in advance.

The National Trust has specially adapted cottages which can be rented. For information on these, as well as details of other self-catering holiday accommodation, see Further Reading at the end of this chapter.

Some people with ME/CFS mistakenly believe that the hot sun will automatically improve their condition. Unfortunately, this is rarely the case because excessive heat makes many symptoms worse. I personally find a warm, but not hot, rural part of France, with clean air and good food, to be the ideal place for the family's summer holiday.

If you are going abroad, do make sure that you have adequate health insurance and check the policy to make sure about exclusion clauses relating to 'pre-existing medical conditions'. There are still plenty of insurers who will readily provide cover for someone with ME/CFS at no extra cost, but you may have to shop around for the best deal. Going abroad should be fine, providing you don't travel 'against your doctor's advice'. And don't forget to fill in form E111 (available at a post office) for you and your family if the holiday is going to be taken in the European Community. This form acts as a passport to the use of state health facilities whilst abroad.

Compulsory vaccinations are seldom required for most of the popular European holiday destinations, and the chances of picking up serious infections are fairly remote, provided you stick to simple rules of hygiene. For further advice on vaccinations see pages 219–20.

If you suffer from travel sickness, then cinnarizine (Stugeron) is a useful drug to try. If you're going abroad, it's worth taking a list of any important drugs which you use translated into the relevant foreign language, just in case you lose any of them. The same applies to details of other important medical conditions which may require treatment. The chances of finding a doctor who knows anything about ME/CFS is, however, rather remote!

If you want further information on health aspects of foreign travel, I can thoroughly recommend Dr Richard Dawson's book *Traveller's Health* (Oxford University Press).

## Specialist advice on holidays

A number of organisations provide advice and information on all aspects of holidays/travel abroad for people with disabilities:

- **RADAR** (see Useful Addresses, page 416) produces a series of useful books (see Further Reading) and has a list of organisations that provide escorts.
- **The Holiday Care Service** (see Useful Addresses, page 410) provides information and support for anyone with special needs. It is the accommodation specialist for disabled people.
- **Tripscope** is a transport specialist which runs a telephone-based (on

0181–994 9294) information service for people with mobility problems.

## Travelling by Air

Aeroplanes can be an exhausting experience, with crowded departure lounges, long walks with luggage to the plane and the almost inevitable delays. If you use a wheelchair, or have special dietary requirements, let the flight operator know in good time as they can be immensely helpful. One friend of mine – an occasional wheelchair user – always uses his (or borrows one) for transit through an airport. Your travel agent should be able to give you some idea about conditions in foreign airports if you're considering travelling abroad. A great deal of useful information on facilities for disabled people at major UK airports is contained in the AA's *Guide for the Disabled Traveller* (see Further Reading).

If your disability is more severe, it may be necessary for you and your doctor to fill in an incapacitated passengers handling form (an INCAD) stating the nature of your disability and confirming that you are fit to travel. For anyone who travels quite frequently by air it can be worthwhile obtaining a frequent traveller's medical card (FREMEC card). This is issued free to disabled travellers who can satisfy the airline's medical officer that their condition is significant and stable. The card is accepted by most major airlines and provides a useful passport to extra assistance. *Care in the Air*, produced by the Air Transport Users Committee, is a useful leaflet (see Further Reading).

If you're flying early in the morning, it's often a good idea to go to the airport the day before and stay at a hotel for the night.

Whatever sort of holiday or travel you're planning to undertake, always try and do as much of the packing and attend to anything else that needs doing in the home several days before departure. Ideally, this should then leave you with a 48-hour gap before you leave, in which you can rest as much as possible.

Finally, don't forget about the needs of your partner or the rest of the family. If they're having to do most of the packing and organisation, why not suggest an overnight break on the journey? After all, this is likely to be a very stressful few days for them as well.

# Further Reading

Below are some of the most useful publications relating to mobility issues. Those marked with an asterisk* are available through RADAR (see Useful Addresses, page 416).

## Access and mobility

*AA Guide for the Disabled Traveller* Contains details about disabled facilities in hotels, motorway service areas and tourist attractions in the UK. Also has comprehensive information for anyone intending to travel abroad by car (including the channel tunnel), ferry or plane.

*A Guide to British Rail\** Information on the accessibility of over 500 British Rail stations including details of toilet and parking facilities.

*Access in London\** A guidebook to London for disabled people.

*Access to the Underground: A Guide for Elderly and Disabled People* Available free from ticket offices and the Unit for Disabled Passengers, London Regional Transport, 55 Broadway, London SW1H 0BD.

*Adaptation of Car Controls for Disabled People* Guidelines intended to help garages and individuals who are asked to convert vehicles to suit the needs of a disabled person. Available from: Maria Clark, Institute of Mechanical Engineers, 1 Birdcage Walk, London SW1H 9JJ (tel: 0171–222 7899).

*Care in the Air* A useful booklet for anyone with disabilities who intends to travel by plane. Available from: The Secretary, Air Transport Users Council, 5th Floor, Kingsway House, 103 Kingsway, London WC2B 6QX (tel: 0171–242 3882).

*Door to Door* A guide to transport for disabled people, published by the Department of Transport and available from their Disabled Unit at Room F10/21, Department of Transport, Marsham Street, London SW1P 3EB.

*RADAR Mobility Factsheets\** (1–10) include *Motoring with a Wheelchair, Insurance, Motoring Accessories and Car Control Manufacturers, Suppliers and Fitters.*

*The Disabled Motorist\** A guide to all aspects of motoring, including chapters on choosing a car, aids and adaptations, and insurance.

## Holidays and leisure

*Country Parks\** An access guide giving information to disabled people on facilities in parks, such as parking, toilets and catering.

*Holidays and Travel Abroad\** An annual guide which provides basic holiday details on around 100 countries and advice on the best organisations to contact for more details.

*Holidays in the British Isles* An annual guide which includes chapters on planning and booking a holiday, and the voluntary organisations and commercial companies involved in holiday provision for disabled people.

*Nothing Ventured* (Harrup Columbus) is one of the best guides for disabled people intending to travel to more remote destinations.

*RADAR Holiday Factsheets\** (1–13) include *Holiday Transport, Equipment for Hire* and *Holiday Accommodation with Nursing Care.*

*Spectator Sports\** A guide to facilities and access for disabled people at sporting venues.

*Stay on a Farm: A Guide to Farm and Country Holidays* includes details of establishments suitable for disabled people. Available through bookshops or Tourist Information Centres.

*The World Wheelchair Traveller* (AA Publications) is produced by the Spinal Injuries Association for disabled people who need to use a wheelchair.

## Walking aids, wheelchairs and powered vehicles

Disabled Living Foundation Fact Sheets are available on *Choosing an Electric Wheelchair* and *Choosing a Scooter or Buggie* (both cost £2.50). (See Useful Addresses, page 414.)

*How to Choose a Powered Vehicle* This contains a check list of requirements and brief descriptions of all the various models from different manufacturers. Available from the Banstead Mobility Centre (see Useful Addresses, page 426).

*The Ins and Outs of Buying a Mobility Vehicle* Available from Mobility Matters, Freepost, Kettering, NN16 8BR (tel: 0990 134131).

*Walking and Standing Aids* Available from the Disability Information Trust. Information on a wide range of walking and standing aids.

# Additional Help and Benefits Available in Britain

## Registering as Disabled

One of the first things you can consider doing to obtain further help is registering yourself as being disabled with a local authority, provided your disability would be regarded as 'substantial and permanent'. If you want to register, contact the area office of your local Social Services Department. Registration will then involve an appointment with either a social worker or occupational therapist, who will assess your level of disability. This can be done in your home if you wish.

Registering is quite voluntary, but it can help you obtain certain benefits which the local authority administers. It also gives your local authority some idea of the number of disabled people in their locality, what their needs are and to what extent they're meeting those needs. The actual benefits aren't great, but the more people who register, the more pressure 'the disabled' as a group can put on both central and local government to take notice of their problems. So, by registering, you're not only helping yourself.

## Service Providers

### Local authorities

These can help with advice (and sometimes finance) on adaptations to the home. They are also responsible for administering housing benefit (see later) and rebates connected with the Council Tax.

Financial help for alterations is limited, but anyone who is a tenant in council property should qualify if they have a good cause for, say, a wheelchair ramp. If you are disabled and assessed as needing one of the services listed in Section 2 of the Chronically Sick and Disabled Persons Act, your local authority has a duty to make the necessary arrangements.

Social workers know about all the services that a local authority can and should provide; if you're not happy with the response from the council's officials, phone the local Social Services Department and ask to speak to the relevant social worker.

You can approach your local councillor or citizens' advice bureau if you're not satisfied by their response.

Local authorities also administer home helps, meals on wheels, transport concessions and orange parking badges.

*Home helps* are very sought after, but often not available! The home help organiser at your local social services office will be able to give you further information. If you are able to obtain this help, you'll probably have to pay part of the cost, unless you're on a very low income. Due to demand often exceeding supply you'll probably only qualify for local authority help if you're living alone (or with a relative who isn't very fit) and have considerable difficulty in carrying out most household tasks. A doctor's letter may well be of help. Any duties carried out by a home help should be suited to your own particular needs, but can include help with cooking, cleaning and shopping.

If you can't obtain help from the local authority you could always try to find someone by advertising in the local shop or newspaper, or ask around to see if a neighbour has a home help who might be prepared to work a few extra hours each week.

*Meals on wheels* This service operates in most parts of the country, but again tends to be overstretched, so has to be limited to those in real need, who aren't well enough to be up and about to shop and cook a hot meal every day. The service operates on weekdays only, and a small charge is made. The quality of the food is usually very good. Contact your local social services for further information.

If you have a freezer, and are living alone, check out the ready prepared meals for one, which can be kept in store.

## Social workers

These offer a wide variety of practical help and advice. They don't just spend their time dealing with problems, and can put you in touch with an appropriate agency or help you steer the correct path through the minefield of DSS benefits.

Many social workers are experienced in listening to people who have a multitude of difficulties -- financial, social, emotional, medical, etc -- and don't see any way out of their predicament. If you feel you've reached this stage, it's often useful to sit down and talk about your anxieties with someone such as a social worker, who's detached from the situation, yet has helped many others in similar circumstances. They should know all about local authority services which are available, and may possible 'negotiate' with the relevant department on your behalf. They also tend to have good contacts with local community and volunteer groups.

Some social workers are now attached on a part-time basis to general

practitioner health centres, but the best way to contact one is to phone
the local Social Services Department and ask for an appointment, or a
home visit if necessary.

## District nurses

These are nurses (sometimes with non-qualified helpers) who undertake extra training to become expert in the problems of nursing patients
at home. For someone with ME/CFS who is spending long periods in
bed they can offer practical advice to the carer on how to lift correctly, as
well as assisting with bathing and dressing if there's nobody else to help.
They are able to advise on what other sources of help may be locally
available, and provide aids such as sheepskin mattresses to help prevent
bed sores, hoists for the bathroom, bath seats, etc. The best way to make
contact is via your general practitioner.

## Health visitors

These provide information and advice on local services and will liaise
with the Social Services Department on your behalf. Contact with a
health visitor can normally be made via your GP or surgery staff.

## Physiotherapists

These don't just work in hospitals; they also care for patients out in the
community. Intensive physiotherapy isn't usually part of ME/CFS treatment and may well be harmful, but treatment from a physiotherapist
who understands about this illness can be helpful in some selected
cases.

If you're on prolonged bed rest, a physiotherapist could come in and
show you how to carry out passive exercises on the arm and limb
muscles, to stop them becoming too weak. Physiotherapists also provide
advice on wheelchairs, and what sort of walking aids may be available,
e.g. Zimmer frames.

Ask your general practitioner if there is a community physiotherapist
available. For information on how to obtain private physiotherapy
services see Useful Addresses, page 429.

## Occupational therapists

These therapists work in both hospitals and out in the community,
where they're employed by the local authority. You can contact your
local occupational therapist directly (without a doctor's letter) at the
local Social Services Department. One will probably come and visit you
at home to assess and advise on ways in which your daily living can be
made easier. Occupational therapists are quite used to advising people
about aids to help with washing, bathing, dressing, etc, as well as equip-

ment for the kitchen and the possibility of making more major alterations to the home.

If you're going to start making life easier in the way your home is run, you'll have to accept that a whole range of domestic duties aren't going to be carried out as often, or perhaps as efficiently, as they used to be. If you find standing and carrying out tasks particularly difficult, try to sit down whenever possible. It's obviously not so easy to do the cooking, washing up or ironing from a seated position, but it may be the only practical way to complete the task. Here, an occupational therapist can help with advice on lowering of work surfaces and suitable high seating.

## Home visits

Such visits can be made by a chiropodist, dentist and optician. Your local Family Health Services Authority (FHSA) should know if this is possible. A citizens' advice bureau worker will try to visit you at home if you are housebound when it's not possible to give advice over the phone or by letter. Some local authority libraries make arrangements for home visiting as well.

## Prescription charges

ME/CFS is not an illness which entitles you to exemption from NHS prescription charges. If you regularly need two or more items every month it may be worth buying a four-monthly or yearly 'season ticket' which gives you unlimited free prescriptions for a set charge. Apply on form FP95 (EC95 in Scotland) which is available from a chemist, post office or DSS office.

Free prescriptions are available to anyone who is:

- under 16 or under 19 if in full-time education
- aged 60 or over
- pregnant or is looking after a child under one year old
- claiming income support, income-based job seekers allowance, disability working allowance, family credit or living on a very low income
- also suffering from diabetes, myxoedema, hypoparathyroidism, Addison's disease, myasthenia gravis, epilepsy or who has a permanent colostomy or ileostomy

Forms FP29A (EC29A in Scotland) explain about prescription exemptions.

## Public services

British Gas, British Telecom and the Electricity Boards have all become much more aware of the needs of disabled customers, and may be able to help with special adaptations to their equipment (e.g. easier knobs on a gas cooker) or, in the case of British Gas, offer free safety checks if you are registered as disabled. If you cannot manage to handle a large printed phonebook, register for free use of Directory Enquiries by calling 195 for an application form from British Telecom.

# Further Sources of Practical Help

*The Disabled Living Foundation* This is probably the most important, and now has around 40 disabled living centres throughout the country. (Full list on pages 414–5.)

The Foundation has well over 10,000 different technical aids for the disabled on its database, and many of these can be seen on display at the living centres. Potential users, carers and healthcare professionals can find out what's available, and where they can buy or hire such equipment. The centres don't actually sell anything on display. Occupational therapists and physiotherapists are on hand to give advice on aids for any individual problem. This can be for any aspect of daily living, indoors or outdoors, ranging from those designed to help with bathing and dressing to highly sophisticated electronic aids for the severely disabled. There's no charge made to visit the centre, and they're usually open weekdays from 9.30 to 5.00.

You don't require a doctor's referral, although staff do like you to phone or write beforehand to arrange a fixed appointment, so they can give individual attention. If you have a severe disability, it's useful to obtain a letter from your doctor as well, giving some information on your current state of health.

*Disablement Information and Advice Line (DIAL)* provides locally based information on how to obtain aids. There are numerous local centres, listed in the phone book.

*The British Red Cross* Local branches (see phone book) can make short-term loans of aids such as wheelchairs and commodes.

*The Centre for Accessible Environments* will provide advice if you are considering extending or making some major alterations to the home. They are in contact with the sort of architects who are interested and experienced in this type of work. (See Useful Addresses, page 413.)

*Department of Health* publish a booklet HB6: *A Practical Guide for Disabled People: Where to find Information, Services and Equipment.*

*Disability Information Trust* provides a series of illustrated booklets on a wide range of disability problems, and act as a reference source for aids and equipment. (See pages 353–4 and Useful Addresses, page 414.)

*The Royal Association for Disability and Rehabilitation* (RADAR) offer advice on a whole range of issues affecting the disabled, and publish a number of useful books. (See Useful Addresses, page 416.)

*Volunteer Bureaux* exist in many areas and aim to put disabled people in touch with willing, able-bodied helpers, who are prepared to assist with a wide variety of tasks. Your citizens' advice bureau will know if there are local groups in operation, and they sometimes have a list of volunteers available and jobs to be done printed in the local paper. If you have a specific task which needs attending to, e.g. some gardening or decorating, or require help with transport, contact your local bureau organiser (see Useful Addresses, page 432).

## The DSS: Sickness and Other Benefits Available

You may find that you now need to make use of the wide range of state social security benefits. You contribute taxes and National Insurance contributions throughout your lifetime, so there shouldn't be any feeling of guilt in claiming such benefits at a time of need.

Over the past few years there has been a significant change in the way that the DSS views ME/CFS as an illness and the disability it causes. Claims for benefits are generally being considered in a far more thoughtful and sympathetic manner, and it is quite acceptable for doctors to write ME or CFS on a sick note. In February 1997, the Chief Medical Officer at the Department of Health wrote to all doctors in the UK to make it perfectly clear that ME/CFS 'is a potentially debilitating and distressing condition which may affect thousands of people and their families' (reference: *CMO Update 13*, Department of Health).

The different benefits, and rules governing eligibility, are often confusing and complex. They're sometimes even misunderstood by the very people who are supposed to administer them. If you're in any doubt about eligibility, do make a claim and see what happens – it can't do any harm, providing you're not being dishonest in the information you provide. If the application is refused, don't give up and make an appeal if this is possible – after all, you're not only fighting for yourself, but for other people with ME/CFS in the same position.

If it becomes necessary to appeal against a DSS decision, some lawyers aren't very well informed or helpful when it comes to benefit issues. It may be better to 'do it yourself' with help from one of the various disability rights organisations, local citizens' advice bureau and welfare rights centres set up by local authorities. Many of these organisations publish extremely useful reference books on benefit issues (e.g. the *Disability Rights Handbook*).

## Table 12: Benefit Help

Phone Lines Providing Help and Advice on Benefits
**Benefit Enquiry Line (BEL):** 0800 882200 (in Northern Ireland 0800 220674)
This service specialises in benefit information for both claimants and their carers. BEL will only provide general advice as the operators have no access to personal files at the DSS.

**Disability Living Allowance Central Telephone Answering Unit:** 0345 123456
Available to answer queries about a disability living allowance claim or general enquiries about disability benefits.

**Disability Working Allowance Central Telephone Answering Unit:** 01772 883300
Available for queries relating to disability working allowance claims.

**Family Credit Helpline:** 01253 500050
Advice and information on applications for family credit.

**Forms Completion Service:** 0800 441144
Provides help over the phone on the filling in of disability benefit claim forms.

**Senior Line:** 0800 650065
General advice on a range of benefits and information for older people. Organised by Help the Aged.

Other Sources of Advice and Information from the DSS
**Disability Benefits Unit**
Warbreck House, Warbreck Hill Road, Blackpool, Lancashire FY2 0YE
Tel: 0345 123456
Handles all disability living allowance and attendance allowance claims.

**Independent Tribunal Service, Office of the**
Whittington House, 19–30 Alfred Place, London WC1E 9LW
Tel: 0171–957 9200.

Deals with disability appeal tribunals, social security appeal tribunals, medical appeal tribunals and vaccine damage tribunals.

**Invalid Care Allowance Unit**
Palatine House, Lancaster Road, Preston, Lancashire PR1 1NS
Tel: 01253 856123
Deals with all invalid care allowance claims.

Other Useful Contacts
**Benefits Agency, Chief Executive's Office**
Room 4CO6, Quarry House, Quarry Hill, Leeds LS2 7UA
Tel: 0113 2324000

**Social Security and Child Support Commissioners for England and Wales**
5th Floor, Newspaper House, 8–16 Great New Street, London EC4A 4DH
Tel: 0171–353 5145

**Social Security and Child Support Commissioners for Northern Ireland**
Lancashire House, 5 Linenhall Street, Belfast BT2 8AA
Tel: 01232 332344

**Social Security and Child Support Commissioners for Scotland**
23 Melville Street, Edinburgh EH3 7PW
Tel: 0131–225 2201

## Some practical advice on dealing with the DSS (and other parts of officialdom)

- Always try to find out who you are talking to, either on the phone or at an interview.
- Preferably do things by letter and *always keep your own, dated copy of any correspondence.* If you're sending important documents, keep a photocopy of them in case they get lost, and post them by recorded delivery. If you deal with the office by phone, always make a note in your diary about what was said, and by whom.
- If you want to discuss something at the office, phone to make an appointment, and if you're not happy about tackling officials by yourself, take a friend or relative along as well. There shouldn't be any objection if you explain your disability.
- Make a written note of what you want to ask before you go. Make a full written note of the response.
- If you're not happy with the answers, ask to speak to a supervisor of the relevant department, or write a letter to the manager.
- If you're getting nowhere with a claim, a letter to your MP (at the House of Commons, London SW1) will be passed on to the local DSS office with a request for a swift reply. As a last resort write to the Minister for Social Security at The Adelphi, 1–11 John Adam Street, London WC2N 6HT.

If this doesn't work a letter to Her Majesty the Queen can be extremely effective in making officialdom move!

## Guide to individual benefits

DSS benefits for the sick and disabled fall into three broad categories:

1. Those which help replace income for anyone who is no longer able to work:
   Statutory Sick Pay
   Incapacity Benefit
   Severe Disablement Allowance – if you've no national insurance contributions.
2. Benefits providing extra help for the severely disabled, including:
   Disability Living Allowance
   Disability Working Allowance
   Attendance Allowance
   Invalid Care Allowance
   Home Responsibilities Protection
   Independent Living Fund
3. Benefits to help people on a low income:
   Income Support
   Family Credit
   Housing Benefit
   Council Tax Benefit
   Council Tax: The Disability Reduction Scheme
   Social Fund
4. Other types of benefits and payments:
   Vaccine Damage Payments
   VAT Concessions

## Statutory Sick Pay

At the onset of any illness, providing you're in work, you should be eligible for Statutory Sick Pay (SSP) from your employer, which will then be 'topped up' to a percentage of normal pay, depending on how long you've been employed. SSP does not depend on National Insurance contributions and can be paid for up to 28 weeks in any period of sick leave.

## Incapacity Benefit (ICB)

*What is it?* A benefit paid to people who are unable to work due to sickness or disability. To qualify you must have contributed a sufficient amount of National Insurance contributions during previous periods of employment. ICB is not means tested, so is unaffected by your income or savings. Additional payments may be made for your partner and/or any dependent children.

*Incapacity for work* During the first 28 weeks, this is generally assessed by what the DSS call an 'own occupation' test. This considers whether you are fit enough to carry on working in your normal occupation. Eligibility for benefit at this stage is based on medical certificates signed by your GP. In some circumstances you may have to be assessed using the 'all work' test at this stage. There are, however, a number of situations (e.g. already having a higher rate DLA care component or being assessed as 80% disabled for an SDA claim) which will provide exemption. After 28 weeks' incapacity from work, the 'all work' test applies to everyone.

*Incapacity for work questionnaire (form IB50)* This relates to the 'all work' test and involves filling in a lengthy questionnaire which asks about the practical effects of your physical disabilities. Various aspects of mental health are also covered – some of these questions may be particularly relevant to the memory and concentration problems commonly associated with ME/CFS.

The questions deal with your ability to undertake 14 specific activities. These include walking, climbing stairs, getting up from a chair, standing, bending and kneeling, lifting and carrying, reaching out with your arms. There are also several questions about disabilities (e.g. fits) which are not really relevant to ME/CFS. Under the title of each activity there are a series of statements (called 'descriptors') from which you are asked to choose the most appropriate one to describe your current state of disability. Each of these descriptors has a score (although the numbers are not given on the form) which ranges from an upper threshold (at or above which you would be regarded as being unfit for work and so automatically pass the test) to a lower threshold (above which the DSS accepts that there is a problem which is going to have some affect on your ability to work).

For example, there are seven different descriptors regarding the ability to walk on level ground. These range from 'cannot walk at all' (score = 15 points) through to 'no walking problem' (score = 0 points). If you are unable to walk more than 50 metres (score = 15 points) you will still be above the upper threshold and so pass the test. If you cannot walk more than 800 metres (score = 0 points), this is below the lower threshold and so judged by the DSS to have no practical effect on your ability to work. When walking ability lies somewhere between the two (e.g. you cannot walk more than 400 metres = score of 3 points), this will still give you some points which can then be combined with those obtained elsewhere in the questionnaire.

You need to score a total of 15 points on the questionnaire to qualify for ICB. There's no requirement to score points in every single activity, and you can, of course, pass the test by obtaining a full score in just one activity.

*Filling in the questionnaire* Before attempting to fill in this extremely lengthy form it's well worth taking some time to carefully plan out in rough the various answers you intend to give, along with any other written information which may be relevant to your claim. Here are some of the key issues relating to ME/CFS which need to be considered when filling in the form.

- Think about the way in which the various activities would relate to your ability to carry out meaningful employment. If you feel that you could not perform a particular activity *reliably, safely or at a reasonable speed*, then do make this clear in writing.
- Symptoms such as pain, fatigue or unsteadiness/dizziness are all going to have an effect on your ability to carry out work-related tasks. Once again, make this clear if it is relevant to your particular case.
- If you feel that *repeating* one of the activities (e.g. walking up and down stairs) would be so tiring that you would not be able to do so repetitively, then this is almost the same in practice as not being able to do it at all. You could also point out, if appropriate, that the process of travelling to work is likely to have a significant adverse effect on your ability to then carry out work-related tasks with a reasonable degree of efficiency.
- If your symptoms show a considerable degree of *variability* on a day-to-day basis – as frequently happens in ME/CFS – then you should make this point clear. The DSS accepts that this test is not intended as a snapshot of your ability to carry out various tasks on one particular day. It is designed to show what is happening to you over a period of time.
- If you regularly take any *prescribed medicine*, or suffer from drug-induced side-effects which can affect your ability to perform any of the activities, do describe this problem in the area provided.
- The main questionnaire only deals with physical health problems. A separate mental health questionnaire lists additional activities relating to mental functioning (e.g. sleep problems interfering with daytime activities = 1 point). It may even be possible to score some extra points here as a number of these questions are relevant to people with ME/CFS who have difficulties with memory or concentration, or who suffer from depression as well.

If you're not sure about precisely what to write down contact your local citizens' advice bureau, welfare rights advice centre, DIAL, or the ME Association for help. The ME Association publishes an extremely useful booklet to guide you through filling in the whole of this questionnaire.

*Returning the questionnaire* This must be sent back to the DSS within six weeks along with a medical statement (Med. 4) from your doctor. The Med. 4 provides details of your diagnosis, resulting level of disability and an opinion on your ability to return to work. Your GP will not be given access to the answers on your questionnaire.

The questionnaire is then assessed by a DSS doctor (from BAMS, the Benefits Agency Medical Service) before being passed to a DSS Adjudicating Officer (AO) to make a decision on eligibility. If the AO feels unable to grant ICB then you will be offered a medical examination.

*Medical examination* You should be given a full seven days notice that this has been arranged. At the examination centre you'll be asked a series of questions about everyday activities and then given a full medical examination. All this takes about 30 minutes. You might also be given a 'mental health assessment', if it seems appropriate. As with the information you provide on the questionnaire, the purpose of the examination is to build up a picture of how you are being affected by ME/CFS *over a period of time*, not how you are feeling on that particular day. Make sure you explain how specific symptoms (e.g. pain, fatigue, problems with balance or concentration) affect you and the way in which the variability of the condition is likely to cause difficulties in relation to employment.

It's worth making a note of the name of the doctor who carries out the examination. If you feel that you are not being treated correctly, try to stay calm and polite. Afterwards, if you consider that the attitude of the doctor was inappropriate, it's worth making a written complaint to the DSS Office.

*Appeal procedures* If the DSS turns down your application for ICB and states that you are capable of working, you can appeal against the decision. Along with the refusal you'll be sent a copy of the Adjudicating Officer's assessment, which will describe those activities where it is agreed that you do have some limitations. You will also be told how many points the DSS have scored as a result of their assessment.

To appeal against the decision you need to obtain form NI246, which can be obtained from your local DSS office or Jobcentre. Any such appeal must be made within three months of the decision being notified.

I believe it's well worth appealing if you feel you have a good case because around 45% of all ICB appeals are successful. Whilst making an appeal, you can still sign on for a jobseekers' allowance. Doing so will not prejudice your chances at the appeal and it also protects your right to National Insurance credits.

Finally, in order to increase your chance of success at an appeal there are several important aspects of preparation which may need to be undertaken:

- Obtain a copy of the DSS doctor's medical report. There may be statements/comments in it which you need to dispute or misunderstandings requiring correction.
- Obtain advice from a citizens' advice bureau, welfare rights advice centre or the ME Association.
- Carefully reconsider how your various symptoms and practical disabilities affect your ability to carry out work-related activities. You may need to emphasise the difficulties that ME/CFS creates in relation to reliability, safety, accuracy and speed when performing physical and/or mental tasks. Remember that with walking problems, any distance you are able to walk after the onset of 'severe discomfort' should be ignored.
- Obtain as much written medical evidence to support you as you can. This may mean asking your GP, consultant, physiotherapist or occupational therapist for a written report. Try to make sure that their comments relate to your ability to perform the sort of tasks quoted on the questionnaire.
- As far as pain, fatigue and variability of symptoms are concerned, it may be necessary to refer the tribunal to case law (CSIB/17/96, CSIB/12/96 and CIB/14587/96) and DSS guidance. Check with a welfare rights advice centre about any recent case law decisions which could be relevant to your circumstances.
- If a medical point needs clarifying at the actual appeal, ask the chairperson to consult with the doctor. If you consider that more medical evidence is required from your own doctor(s), then ask for the tribunal to be adjourned.

Finally, if the Social Security Appeal Tribunal (SSAT) refuses your appeal, you may be able to make a further appeal to the Social Security Commissioner. Unfortunately, this has to be done on a point of law, so you will almost certainly have to obtain expert advice in such circumstances.

*Therapeutic work and ICB* You can still claim ICB and carry out a limited amount of work, provided it helps to 'improve, or prevent or delay deterioration in, the disease or bodily or mental disablement which causes [your] incapacity to work'. Any such employment must only be carried out with the full approval of your GP and you should not earn more than £48 per week (1998/9), after any reasonable deductions.

## Severe Disablement Allowance (SDA)

This is a weekly cash benefit for anyone who has been incapable of work for at least 28 weeks but doesn't have sufficient National Insurance contributions to qualify for incapacity benefit. SDA is neither means tested nor taxable and may include additional payments for dependent children and your partner.

To claim SDA you must first:

- have been incapable of work for a continuous period of 196 days before the first day any payment is made; and
- be at least 16 (or 19 if in full-time education) and under 65.

Most people who claim SDA will have to show that they suffer from 'loss of physical or mental faculty such that the extent of the resulting disablement amounts to not less than 80%'. However, it is possible to be automatically passported to SDA if you have been:

- found to be incapable of work on or before your 20th birthday
- assessed as 75–80% disabled for the purpose of an industrial injuries scheme
- claiming a disability living allowance (DLA) care component at the higher rate.

Once a claim has been made the DSS will arrange for you to be examined by an Adjudicating Medical Practitioner (AMP) to assess your level of physical and mental disability. In the case of ME/CFS the disabilities which are particularly relevant are:

- limited energy, which affects your ability to walk or carry out physical tasks
- brain malfunction, affecting memory and concentration.

It's important to have these facts clear in your mind before attending the medical examination. You can then present them to the examining doctor when questions arise about how ME/CFS affects your ability to carry out normal day-to-day activities.

The AMP may request a medical report from your GP or consultant, but there's nothing to stop you obtaining one, provided you think such information will help your claim. If the medical issues are complex, particularly if you have other conditions besides ME/CFS, then you may be referred to a medical board for a further opinion.

If the AMP or medical board decided that you are 74% or less disabled, you still have a right of appeal to a Medical Appeal Tribunal. This has to be done within three months of the decision to refuse SDA. My feedback from people with ME/CFS who have been refused on the first attempt is that it is well worth making an appeal. This is because different doctors are inevitably going to make different assessments of percentage disability in something as complex as ME/CFS.

Claims for SDA should be made using a claim pack SDA1 from the DSS or post office. It's also possible to carry out a limited amount of therapeutic work whilst claiming SDA. You can find out more about the 80% test in the *Disability Rights Handbook* and the *Severe Disablement Allowance Handbook for Adjudicating Medical Officers* (£13, available from the Stationary Office.)

## Disability Living Allowance (DLA)

This is a benefit for adults and children who require a considerable degree of help in looking after themselves and/or have difficulties with walking. You can claim even if you live by yourself. What counts above all is your actual *need* for help, not whether there is anyone currently providing it.

DLA is tax free, not means tested and not related to any National Insurance contributions made in the past. It can be paid on top of any earnings or income you already have coming in, including most social security benefits. It consists of three rates of care component and two rates of mobility component. Eligibility depends on the amount of personal care required and how severe your problems with mobility are in practice.

*Age limits* The care component has no lower age limit. However, there is an additional test for children under the age of 16 and the 'cooking test' (see later) is not applicable till the age of 16. To qualify for the mobility component a child has to be five or older. All children have to pass an additional test of disability to qualify for the lower rate mobility component. Although DLA can be granted for life, only those who apply before their 65th birthday can continue to receive DLA.

*Care component* To qualify, your care needs must relate to a significant degree of disability – physical, mental, or both. The key qualifying criteria are severe mental and/or physical disability such that you require:

**During the day**
1. Frequent (meaning several times, not just once or twice) attention in connection with your bodily functions (these refer to activities such as eating, drinking, walking, sitting, getting out of bed, dressing, going to the toilet, washing, etc).
or
2. Continued supervision in order to prevent you accidentally harming

yourself or others (i.e. someone needs to keep an eye on you for most of the time).

or

**At night**

3. Prolonged (at least 20 minutes) or repeated (at least twice) attention in connection with bodily functions.

or

4. The need for another person to be awake for a prolonged (at least 20 minutes) period or at frequent intervals (at least two or three times) to avoid you accidentally harming yourself or others.

or

**Part-time day care**

5. You need attention from someone else for a significant part of the day (one hour or more in total) in connection with bodily functions.

or

6. You cannot plan, prepare and cook a main meal for yourself – the 'cooking test'. This test doesn't depend on what sort of equipment is available in your kitchen, it simply questions *whether you are capable of preparing the main meal.*

Qualifying criteria for the three different rates are as follows:

- higher rate – either or both 1 and 2 of the daytime tests *and* either or both 3 and 4 of the night-time tests
- middle rate – either or both 1 and 2 of the daytime tests *or* either or both of 3 and 4 night-time tests
- lower rate – either or both of 5 and 6 part-time day-care tests.

Children under 16 have to satisfy any of the tests numbered 1 to 5, as well as demonstrating that they require a substantial degree of care or supervision.

*Mobility component* To qualify for the *higher rate* you must be 'suffering from a physical disablement'. Problems with mobility resulting from psychiatric illnesses (e.g. severe depression) are excluded, and this is an important issue where the presumed cause of ME/CFS can have a negative effect on benefit entitlement if the Adjudicating Officer takes the view that your particular situation is psychiatric in nature. Your physical state of health must be such that you are either:

- completely unable to walk (means what it says)
- virtually unable to walk (this can be severely limited in regard to distance, speed or resulting pain from exertion)
- so disabled that the 'exertion required to walk would constitute a danger to [your] life or would be likely to lead to a serious deterioration

in [your] health'.

To qualify for the *lower rate*, your walking problems can be due to physical or mental disabilities. The lower rate is designed to help people who can actually walk but are unable to make use of that ability when outdoors unless they have someone to guide or supervise them. Children under 16 must show that they require substantially more guidance or supervision.

In practice, the success rate for people with ME/CFS who claim the higher rate mobility component tends to be rather disappointing, and disputes over whether this is a physical or psychiatric disorder certainly account for some claims being refused. By contrast, the success rate for obtaining the lower rate is often quite good, provided you satisfy the criteria.

*Making a claim* You can order a DLA claim pack by calling the Benefit Enquiry Line (BEL) on freephone 0800 882200. Filling out the form can, however, take a great deal of time, so don't try to do it all in one go. To start with, write out all your answers in rough and make sure you don't underestimate how much practical care you require along with the various difficulties you have with mobility. If you're not sure about precisely what to write down, contact a local welfare rights advice centre, DIAL or the ME Association. The ME Association produces an extremely useful booklet to guide you through filling in every single page of the DLA claim form.

If you fail to provide the DSS with an adequate amount of detail, or your answers don't really provide them with a clear picture of your level of disability, they may send a visiting officer to go through the questions with you. Alternatively, a report may be requested from your doctor or a medical examination arranged.

*Processing the claim* DLA eligibility is decided by a DSS Adjudicating Officer (AO), not by a doctor. To help the AO make a decision they will probably refer to a guidebook produced by the Disability Living Allowance Advisory Board (DLAAB). This lists in some detail how the DSS and DLAAB view the various personal care and mobility needs associated with a range of common chronic illnesses, including ME/CFS. The relevant sections for ME/CFS, which were thoroughly revised in 1996 after complaints from the ME Association about the content of the original entry, state:

- 'In DLA and AA [attendance allowance] it is the mobility and care needs resulting from the disabling condition rather than the diagnosis that are paramount. However, as regards eligibility for the higher rate of the mobility component the person must be suffering from a physical disablement so that the person is either unable to walk or virtually unable to walk.' (12.2.4)

- 'There is a wide variation between individuals in the nature and sever-ity of symptoms. These can include muscle pain and exhaustion when attending to normal functions such as washing or dressing, and can be accompanied by a variety of symptoms affecting balance, concen-tration and sleep disturbance. In more severe cases the symptoms can persist for several years, and in a small minority of people there may be total dependency.' (12.3.4)

- [Care Needs] 'There may be wide day-to-day variation in the sever-ity of symptoms. It is necessary to discover what a person can do on a bad day as well as a good day, and to establish how often each type of day occurs. A satisfactory level of physical and mental activity is one which can be sustained day after day without leading to a pro-longed increase in symptoms, and not the amount managed only on a good day.' (12.5.1)

- 'Whilst attending to bodily functions may take longer than normal, the majority of people with CFS appear to manage these unaided most of the time. Matters such as food preparation, shopping and household tasks may appear to cause problems for people with CFS. In those who have been immobile for long periods, physical help from another person may be required. A few people may be bed or wheelchair bound and may need help with personal care and to trans-fer on and off toilets, etc. In a minority there is severe disablement and a state of high dependency.' (12.5.2).

- 'Objective studies of muscle function may fail to reveal abnormal fatigue or weakness. However, when muscle weakness is clinically evident, this may indicate secondary disuse atrophy (wasting), and is an indicator of likely care needs. Severe fatigue in the absence of any objective evidence of muscle wasting or weakness does not neces-sarily imply a definite and exclusively psychological cause. Further-more, in individual cases, causes for severe fatigue which have not yet been diagnosed may be present.' (12.5.3)

- [Mobility Needs] 'The majority of those with CFS are mobile, although they may walk rather more slowly than normal. The diffi-culty in walking is the result of fatigue, but may also be in part, due to muscle pain, loss of balance, or weakness of muscles resulting from disuse . . . Muscle symptoms adversely affecting mobility may con-tinue beyond the actual period of exercise. Physical disability may be influenced by the psychological state of the person. In those with the severest disability there is an increased likelihood of treatable psychological disorders and mental health problems.' (12.6.1)

- [Duration of Need] 'There is a wide variation in both severity and duration of the illness . . . Of those with established CFS, the majority can be expected to show a substantial improvement over time. There are others in whom the symptoms of fatigue last for much longer and may pursue a relapsing course. The persistence of fatigue may occur both in severe and milder forms of the condition. (12.7.1)

The importance of this official statement in relation to claiming DLA is that it makes clear that the DSS (a) recognises ME/CFS to be a genuine and disabling illness, (b) accepts that some people will require a great deal of help with personal care and (c) acknowledges the existence of mobility problems, which may have both physical and psychological causes (i.e. a higher rate mobility component cannot be refused simply on the grounds that the DSS has decided that ME/CFS is a purely psychological illness).

Once awarded, DLA can continue for a fixed period, sometimes even for life. The minimum length of an award is six months.

*Reviews and appeals* If you disagree with an AO decision you can ask for a review, but this must be done within three months of being notified. A review procedure is likely to involve the DSS obtaining further medical information or arranging a medical examination. If you remain in dispute following a review you can appeal against it, but once again this has to be done within three months of notification. A Social Security Appeal Tribunal can examine non-disability issues. A Disability Appeal Tribunal, which consists of a lawyer as chair and two other members, one of whom is a doctor, examines questions of disability. As with incapacity benefit appeals (see pages 379–80) it's important to do all you can to increase your chances of success by consulting experts and even looking up relevant case law.

*'Passporting' to other useful benefits* Once DLA has been granted it can act as a passport to many other benefits. Among the most useful are the various premiums included in the assessment for income support, housing benefit, etc, and:

| | |
|---|---|
| • exemption from road tax | (higher rate mobility) |
| • motability | (higher rate mobility) |
| • Orange parking badge | (higher rate mobility) |
| • a home energy efficiency scheme grant | (lower rate mobility) |
| • 80% disablement for SDA | (higher rate care) |

## Disability Working Allowance (DWA)

This is a benefit which is paid on top of low earnings or self-employed earnings to anyone with a disability that causes disadvantages when it comes to obtaining employment. DWA is tax free but is means tested in a similar way to family credit. One of the key aims of DWA is to encourage people who are already receiving incapacity benefit (ICB) or severe disablement allowance (SDA) to try to return to some form of work. And, under a special two-year link rule, it should be possible to return to claiming these benefits on the same terms as before.

DWA can be claimed by anyone who:

- is aged 16 or over
- is (or will be) working, on average, for 16 or more hours per week as an employee or self-employed.
- has a 'physical or mental disability which puts [them] at a disadvantage in getting a job' (the 'disability' test)
- has been receiving one of a range of qualifying benefits at any time in the eight weeks before making a claim (these include ICB and SDA)
- has savings or capital below £16,000 (1998/9)
- is earning a weekly sum which is within the means-tested limit

*Making a claim* If *all* the above conditions are met, a claim can be made on form DWA1. This can be obtained from the Benefit Enquiry Line on freephone 0800 882200. Decisions about DWA eligibility are made by an Adjudicating Officer (AO) based at the DWA unit in Preston. Each award lasts for 26 weeks, regardless of any change in your circumstances. You can then make another claim for renewal.

*Financial considerations* The amount of DWA you could receive depends on a number of variables, including your income, capital and working hours. Your family situation is also taken into account, particularly whether you are single, have a partner, and have any dependent children. If your normal weekly income is below or the same as what the DSS calculate to be your 'applicable amount', then you should receive the maximum payment possible. If your normal weekly income is above the applicable amount, then your DWA payment will be reduced proportionately.

The Disability Alliance has pointed out the importance of carefully checking to see whether you are actually going to be better off financially from stopping existing benefits and switching to DWA. For example, you could earn up to £48 per week (1998/9) in 'therapeutic earnings' on top of any existing ICB or SDA payments. Consequently, it could still be better to carry on claiming these benefits and doing a limited amount of work rather than switching to DWA.

If you are uncertain about the relative advantages and disadvantages of DWA, talk over your situation with someone from a welfare rights advice centre. Officials at local DSS offices and Jobcentres have also been trained in how to deal with DWA 'better off' calculations.

*Reviews and appeals* If you disagree with the AO's decision, you can request a review within three months of receiving it. A different AO will then examine your claim. DWA will be replaced by a new Disabled Person's Tax Credit in October 1999.

## Attendance Allowance (AA)

This is a tax-free benefit for people over the age of 65 who are severely disabled, either physically or mentally. AA is designed to provide financial help for personal care needs or supervision. You don't actually have to be getting help at the time you apply, what counts is your *need* for such help. You can also apply if you live alone and don't have a carer in the house. AA is not means tested and there are no National Insurance contributions required. It can usually be paid in addition to other benefits, including state retirement pension, income support and severe disablement allowance.

The rules for qualifying are very similar to those already described for the disability living allowance care component at the middle or higher rate. To initiate a claim, phone the Benefit Enquiry line on 0800 882200 and ask for an attendance allowance pack (DS2). Section 2 of this claim pack contains a lengthy self-assessment questionnaire (again, see the section on applying for DLA), and a form for your own doctor to complete. This should provide the Adjudication Officer with enough information on which to make a decision. If this isn't possible, the DSS may request a further report from your doctor or a medical examination.

Attendance allowance can be awarded for life or for a fixed period. If you disagree with any decisions made by the DSS you can ask for a review, but this must be made within three months of being notified. Further appeals can be made to either a Disability Appeal Tribunal or Social Security Appeal Tribunal, depending on the problem.

## Invalid Care Allowance (ICA)

This is a benefit for anyone under the age of 65 who regularly has to spend at least 35 hours per week looking after a severely disabled person who receives one of these three benefits:

- DLA care component at the middle or higher rate
- attendance allowance at either rate
- constant attendance allowance.

ICA is not means tested and does not depend on previous National Insurance contributions. It is, however, taxable and if you still work, then you must not earn more than £50 per week after any allowance expenses are deducted.

Claim on form DS700, obtainable from a local DSS office. The Invalid Care Allowance Unit (Palatine House, Lancaster Road, Preston, Lancashire, PR1 1NS) will then send a written decision. If refused, you can appeal to a Social Security Appeal Tribunal.

ICA also acts as a passport to a number of other benefits, including a carer premium used in the assessment of housing benefit, etc. You will also receive Class 1 National Insurance contribution credits.

## Home Responsibilities Protection (HRP)

This benefit is designed to protect your basic pension rights (and widows' benefits) when not paying National Insurance contributions due to the fact that you have to look after someone at home without receiving an invalid care allowance.

You can qualify for HRP provided you meet one of these criteria:

- you spend at least 35 hours per week looking after someone who receives attendance allowance, DLA care component at the middle or higher rate or constant attendance allowance for 48 or more weeks in a year
- you receive income support in order to stay at home to care for a disabled person
- you receive child benefit for a child under 16.

To apply for HRP, obtain form CF411 from a local DSS office.

## Independent Living (1993) Fund (ILF)

This is a government-funded but independent and discretionary trust fund, governed by a Board of Trustees. The ILF works in partnership with local authorities to provide 'joint care packages' combining services from the local authority with cash payments from the fund. The aim is to help severely disabled people on low incomes lead independent lives in the community. To date, I know of very few people with ME/CFS who are making use of the ILF, but it could well be an extremely valuable source of help if you satisfy the numerous qualifying criteria.

To qualify for help from the fund an applicant would normally have to meet *all* the following criteria:

- severe disability along with a need for extensive help in order to maintain an independent life in the community
- age at least 16 and under 66
- receive (or plan to receive) services to the value of £200 (1998/9) a week from your local authority
- have care needs whose total cost to the fund and local authority are not more than £500 per week (1998/9)

- receive income support payments or have a level of income at or around income support level
- have less than £8,000 in capital.
- live alone or with people who are unable to meet care needs
- have care needs that are stable
- receive a disability living allowance higher rate care component.

*Applying for help from the ILF* First, contact your local authority Social Services Department and ask for a social worker to come and carry out an assessment of your current care needs. If the social worker agrees to support your application, the fund will then arrange for a joint visit with their visiting social worker. Once the fund's Trustees have agreed on a claim, a cash award of up to £300 per week can be made. The Director of the ILF is able to review the decision if you are in any way dissatisfied (see Useful Addresses, page 416).

## Income Support (IS)

This is a means-tested benefit which doesn't depend on National Insurance contributions. It's intended to provide basic living expenses, so if you don't seem to have enough money coming in from your sickness or disability benefits, do check to see if you might be eligible for IS.

There are six principal qualifying criteria:

- you must be aged 16 or over
- you must *not* be in full time, non-advanced education
- you must *not* be working for 16 hours or more per week
- your partner must *not* be working for 24 hours or more per week
- your capital (as well as any belonging to a partner) must *not* exceed £8,000
- you must belong to one of the specific groups of people who are eligible to receive IS. Relevant examples include being incapable of work due to ill health, aged over 60 or acting as a carer.

If you can pass *all* these hurdles, then you may qualify for IS, provided your weekly income is less than what the DSS calls your 'applicable amount' – the sum which they consider you need to live on. Anyone who is claiming other sickness or disability benefits (e.g. disability living allowance, disability working allowance, incapacity benefit) may well find that they qualify for additional premiums, some of which can be quite substantial.

To initiate an IS claim contact your local DSS office or post office and ask for form SP1 (for pensioners) or A1 (others). If your claim is refused, ask the DSS for form A124, which will explain how they worked out the calculations. You can also ask for a full written explanation of the reason for refusal. Appeals against IS decisions can be made to a Social Security Appeal Tribunal, but this must be done within three months.

## Family Credit (FC)

This is a means-tested benefit for people who are working on low wages and having to bring up children. It is paid in addition to the family's normal weekly income and each award will normally last for a period of 26 weeks. Family credit can also act as a passport to other benefits, including free prescriptions, dental treatment, fares to hospital and vouchers for glasses. However, if you are eligible for a disability working allowance, depending on circumstances, you could get a lot more on this benefit than on family credit.

There are four key qualifying criteria for eligibility to family credit:

- you, or your partner, must normally be working for 16 or more hours per week
- you, or your partner, must be responsible for a child who lives with you
- you and your partner must not have savings or capital of over £8,000
- your income must be within a set limit, which varies according to family circumstances.

Family credit is worked out by comparing your net income to what is known as the 'applicable amount' for your particular circumstances. If your net income is higher than the applicable amount, then 70% of your extra net income is deducted from the maximum family credit for your circumstances.

You can obtain a family credit claim pack by phoning the Family Credit Helpline on 01253 500050, or by contacting a local DSS office. Appeals against any aspect of a family credit decision can be made to a Social Security Appeal Tribunal.

Family credit will be replaced by the Working Families Tax Credit in October 1988 – a new benefit which guarantees families a basic income of £180 per week provided one member is in full-time employment.

## Housing Benefit (HB)

This benefit helps people to pay their rent. In most cases it is organised by local authorities. To qualify for HB you will have to meet *all* the following conditions:

- you are not excluded from having HB (e.g. because you live with a landlord who is a close relative)
- you are liable to pay rent on your normal home
- your capital is no more than £16,000

- you are on income support, or income-based job seeker's allowance, or have a fairly low income.

## Council Tax Benefit (CTB)

This is a benefit which helps people on low incomes to pay their council tax. To qualify for CBT you will need to satisfy *all* the following conditions:

- you are not excluded from having CBT (e.g. being a full-time student unless classified as having a disability)
- you are liable to pay council tax on your normal home
- your capital is no greater than £16,000
- you are receiving income support or income-based job seeker's allowance or have a fairly low income.

Your local citizens' advice bureau should have detailed information on housing benefit and council tax benefit.

## Council tax: the disability reduction scheme

You may be able to claim what is called a disability reduction if you or any other resident in the house is 'substantially and permanently disabled'. This can apply to an adult or child of any age, even if they are not related to you.

To qualify for this reduction you must satisfy one of these three criteria:

- you have a second bathroom or kitchen needed by the disabled person
- you have a room (other than a bathroom, kitchen or toilet) needed by and predominantly used by the disabled person
- you have enough space in your house for the disabled person to use a wheelchair which they need for indoor purposes

There is no specific definition as to what counts as 'substantially and permanently disabled' in relation to this benefit, but it clearly implies that a substantial degree of disablement is necessary.

If you do qualify for a disability reduction, then your council tax bill is reduced to the amount normally paid for a house in the valuation band below your own.

Applications have to be made on a standard form from the local authority. The person who pays the council tax (not necessarily the disabled person) has to make the application.

Appeals against any decision should be made to the local authority, then to the Valuation Tribunal (England and Wales) or Valuation Appeal

Committee (Scotland).

People who are 'severely mentally impaired' (i.e. have a severe impairment of intelligence or social functioning which appears to be permanent and are also entitled to one of the main disability benefits), along with certain groups of carers, may be eligible for other types of financial help with council tax payments. The exact rules are complex, so it's worth obtaining expert advice.

## The Social Fund

If you are faced with an exceptional expense which you suddenly find difficult to pay from regular income, you may be able to obtain a payment from the social fund. Any grant will be reduced if you or your partner have savings above £500 (or £1,000 if you or your partner are aged 60 or more).

During a period of exceptionally cold weather, you could qualify for a *cold weather payment* so long as you receive income support with a disability premium or severe disability premium.

You may also be eligible for a *community care grant*. These grants are given to help vulnerable people on income support to live as independent a life as possible within the community. They are not repayable.

If you are on income support and need help to spread the cost of more expensive high priority items such as essential household equipment, you might be eligible for a *budgeting loan*. These loans are interest free but repayable.

Whether or not you are receiving income support you may need a *crisis loan* to help pay for living expenses or something you require urgently. These loans are interest free and repayable. They are intended for people who have no other way of meeting their needs in an emergency.

To claim any of the above social fund benefits you will need to obtain an appropriate form from your local DSS office. DSS guidance to social fund officers states that high priority should be given to applicants who have restricted mobility or suffer from chronic physical/mental illnesses.

## Vaccine Damage Payments

This scheme provides a tax-free lump sum of £30,000 to people who are severely disabled as a result of vaccination. In view of the fact that vaccines can, occasionally, trigger a case of ME/CFS (see pages 35–7), it would appear that some sufferers may be eligible for such payments.

A number of important qualifying criteria apply to this scheme. The most important ones are:

- Disablement has to clearly be the result of vaccination against diphtheria, tetanus, whooping cough, polio, measles, mumps, rubella, TB or haemophilus influenza type b (Hib).
- Vaccination must have been carried out in the UK (with the exception of members of the armed forces serving overseas) either when the claimant was under the age of 18 (except for rubella and polio) or at a time of an outbreak of the relevant infection.
- Claims must be made within six years of the vaccination.
- Disablement must be assessed as being 80% or above (the same sort of level as is required for a severe disablement allowance).

Claim forms and an information leaflet (HB3) can be obtained from the Vaccine Damage Payments Unit, Palatine House, Lancaster Road, Preston PR1 1HB. If a claim is refused, you can then ask for a review of the decision by an Independent Vaccine Damage tribunal. Legal advice for work leading up to the hearing might be eligible for the Green Form scheme should you decide to involve a solicitor. A further appeal to the Secretary of State may be allowed in some circumstances.

## VAT concessions

Anyone who is substantially disabled may be eligible for various types of VAT exemption – see leaflet 701/7/94, *VAT Relief for People with Disabilities*, available from your local VAT enquiries office (in the phone book under 'Customs and Excise').

*N.B. Regulations regarding eligibility for the various social security benefits included in this chapter are constantly changing, and the capital limits are often linked to the rate of inflation. If you feel that you may be able to claim one of these benefits, or wish to appeal against the DSS, do check carefully that you have the most up-to-date information to hand.*

# Useful Publications on DSS Benefits

*Disability Rights Handbook* is the most comprehensive publication available on all the different benefits described in this chapter. It also covers appeal procedures in detail and is thoroughly updated in April each year. Published by the Disability Alliance – see Useful Addresses, page 414.
*After Age 16 What Next?* contains details of services and benefits for young disabled people. Published by the Family Fund, PO Box 50, York, YO1 2ZX.
Disability Living Allowance – a guide and checklist explains more about DLA and how to fill in the claim form. Available from the Disability Alliance, price £3.

*Your Rights 1998–99* is a guide to money benefits for older people. Published by Age Concern England, 1268 London Road, London SW16 4ER.

*Youthaid's Guide to Training and Benefits for Young People* is available from the Child Poverty Action Group, 1–5 Bath Street, London EC1V 9PY.

*Leaflets* You can obtain leaflets on all the various benefits described in this chapter from your local DSS office or by ordering them from:

DSS Stationary Office
The Causeway
Oldham Broadway Business Park
Chadderton
Oldham
OL9 9XD

# PART 4
# APPENDICES

# Useful Names and Addresses

## The ME Association

This is a particularly important source of information, advice and support. The Association was formed in 1976 and now has nearly 10,000 members. Patrons include HRH the Duke of Kent, Sir Harry Secombe and Louie Ramsay (daughter of the late Dr Melvin Ramsay). The Very Reverend Michael Mayne, former Dean of Westminster Abbey, is one of the Association's Presidential group of advisers.

The Association is run by elected Trustees and organised into a large number of locally based groups. There are also a number of full-time paid staff at the office in Essex, who deal with an ever increasing amount of queries from members, doctors and journalists – in fact anyone wanting to know more about ME/CFS.

The Association is actively involved with all aspects of the illness and includes:

- An education and information department dealing with day-to-day enquiries as well as the distribution of literature to doctors, sufferers and carers. A specially produced booklet – *Guidelines for the Care of Patients* – is available for health professionals.
- A welfare department providing advice on DSS benefits, employment and all the practical problems associated with disability.
- A 'listening ear' service run by trained volunteers enabling members to ring up and talk a problem over with someone who is not only understanding, but may be able to offer practical advice as well.
- The organisation of special interest groups (e.g. children/young people with ME/CFS).
- Sponsoring research at various university departments into both the cause(s) and management of ME/CFS.
- A Scientific and Medical Advisory Panel consisting of experts in the areas of neurology, virology, immunology, paediatrics, pharmacology and psychiatry. These doctors are available to advise on research grants and other medical matters as they arise.
- Close and regular contact with government departments and

Members of Parliament on matters of concern, especially benefits and research funding.
* Helping journalists from national newspapers, radio and television with background information in order to achieve a more balanced and positive presentation of the illness.

The Association holds an Annual General Meeting in London each year at which research workers are invited to present and discuss their findings.

Membership currently costs £15 per annum; this includes four issues each year of their journal *Perspectives*. Overseas membership costs £20 (Europe inc. Eire) or £25 (rest of the world). Overseas subscriptions should be paid by banker's draft or sterling cheque. For further information contact:

ME Association
4 Corringham Road
Stanford le Hope
Essex
SS17 0AH

Tel: 01375 642466
Fax: 01375 360256

ME Association, Northern Ireland Region
Bryson House
28 Bedford Street
Belfast
BT2 7FE

Tel/Fax: 01232 439831

ME Association, Scottish Region
52 St Enoch Square
Glasgow
G1 4AA

Tel: 0141-204 3822

## Action for ME

This is a registered medical charity offering support and information to sufferers and their carers as well as employers, medical and education professionals and welfare benefits workers. The charity was founded in 1987 after ME sufferer Sue Finlay wrote an article about her illness in the

*Observer* newspaper. Incredibly, the article prompted a response of 15,000 letters, highlighting the lack of information and support available at that time. Recognising the need for a strong, campaigning support organisation which could also disseminate information, Sue founded Action for ME. Novelist Clare Francis, herself an ME sufferer, became the founding president, a role she was to hold for ten years.

Action for ME is a membership organisation with a subscription of £15 per annum. Membership services include factsheets, books and telephone advice on therapies and welfare benefits. A counselling line is available and the charity also operates a network of local support groups throughout the UK. Members receive three issues each year of *InterAction*, a magazine containing information on the illness and research updates.

For further information contact:

Action for ME
PO Box 1302
Wells
Somerset
BA5 1YE

Tel: 01749 670799
Fax: 01749 679895

## CHROME (Case History Research on ME)

This organisation was established in 1994 to identify severely disabled ME sufferers in the UK and, using detailed questionnaires, to monitor their illness over a ten-year period. Data from this study will supplement medical research in several important ways, and for the first time a detailed picture of how ME affects the most severe cases will be available.

In addition to monitoring severely affected applicants, CHROME has worked to develop links with the research community. Members have participated in conferences, established a team of distinguished specialist advisers and contributed to academic journals.

For further information contact:

CHROME
3 Britannia Road
London
SW6 2HJ

Tel and fax: 0171-736 3511

## The National ME Centre and Centre for Fatigue Syndromes

This important facility was originally created out of a support group set up by Dr Betty Dowsett in 1990 at Harold Wood Hospital in Essex. In 1992, charitable status was granted and Trustees appointed with the aim of developing a unique and comprehensive set of out-patient and in-patient services for people with ME/CFS.

Professor Leslie Findley, a consultant neurologist, acts as the Chief Medical Advisor and runs clinics with the assistance of occupational therapists, other health professionals and volunteers. Well over 2,000 people with ME/CFS have so far been seen at the centre, and waiting lists continue to grow.

The Trustees are currently aiming to raise £1 million in order to purchase a suitable building to house out-patient services and research activities.

For further information contact:

Ms Karen Walsh
Administrator
National ME Centre
Disablement Services Centre
Harold Wood Hospital
Gubbins Lane
Harold Wood
Romford
Essex
RM3 0BE

Tel: 01708 378050

## Persistent Virus Disease Research Foundation

This charity was launched by the late Hugh Faulkner in 1993 with the aim of stimulating and funding research. The name Persistent Viral Disease was chosen in preference to ME/CFS to help differentiate the condition from the many other causes of chronic fatigue.

Since 1993, the foundation has funded a large number of research studies, including work on persisting enteroviral infection, parvovirus infection and the effects of viral infection on the function of muscle mitochondria.

For further information contact:

The Persistent Virus Disease Research Foundation
4 One Tree Lane
Beaconsfield
Bucks
HP9 2BU

Tel: 01494 674769

# Westcare

This is a registered charity which provides professional services relating to ME/CFS. The main services are:

- *An information service* – leaflets and books are available.
- *A telephone advice and counselling service* provided by a professional counsellor. Appointments are booked in advance.
- *A clinic* in Bristol – individual consultations are provided by professional advisers/counsellors, who offer acceptance and reassurance, information about the illness, advice about management and counselling. No charges are made, but donations are requested.
- *A home counselling service* – available to people with ME/CFS in Bristol.
- *Residential rehabilitation courses* – week-long courses are held at a comfortable venue near Bristol. Staff on these courses include doctors, occupational therapists, nutritionists and counsellors. The aim of the courses is to help in self-management of the illness and to aid improvement or recovery. Many participants are fully funded by the NHS.
- *Workshops for doctors and health professionals* – dealing with the practical management of ME/CFS.
- Co-ordination of the *National Task Force on CFS/ME* – an independent scientifically based body which produced a landmark report in 1994 (available from Westcare at £9.95). Further reports are being prepared.

For further information contact:

Westcare
155 Whiteladies Road
Clifton
Bristol
BS8 2RF

Tel: 0117 9239341
Fax: 0117 9239347

# Overseas Organisations

Similar self-help support groups are also operating in various other countries:

## *America*

CFIDS Association
PO Box 220398
Charlotte, NC 28222–0389

Tel: 00 1 800 (toll free in USA) 442 3437

The National CFIDS Foundation
103 Aletha Road
Needham, MA 02192

Tel: 00 1 781 449 3535

## *Australia*

**Australian Capital Territory**
ME/CFS Society ACT
C/– S.H.O.U.T. Office
PO Box 717
Mawson, ACT 2607

Tel: (02) 6290 1984

**New South Wales**
ME/CFS Society of NSW Inc.
Royal South Sydney Community Health Centre
Joynton Avenue
Zetland, NSW 2017

Tel: (02) 9439 6026
Fax: (02) 9382 8160

**Northern Territory**
Darwin ME/CFS Society
C/– PO Box 1062
Palmerston, NT 0831

Tel: (08) 9323 503

**Queensland**
ME/Chronic Fatigue Syndrome Society of Queensland
Street address: 134 St Paul's Terrace
Spring Hill, QLD 4000

Postal address: PO Box 938
Fortitude Valley, QLD 4006

Tel: (07) 3832 9744
Fax: (07) 3832 9755

**South Australia and the Northern Territory**
ME/CFS Society (SA) Inc.
GPO Box 383
Adelaide, SA 5001

Tel: (08) 8266 5833
Fax: (08) 8362 7316

**Victoria and Tasmania**
ME/CFS Society of Victoria
23 Livingstone Close
Burwood, Victoria 3125

Tel/Fax: (03) 9888 8798

**Western Australia**
WISH (Western Institute of Self-Help)
335–337 Pier Street
PO Box 8140, Perth Business Centre
Perth, WA 6849

Tel: (08) 9228 4488

*Belgium*

ME Vereniging
Mrs A. Vertommen
Dorp 73
3221 Nieuwrode

Tel/Fax: (016) 5709 83

*Canada*

ME Canada
246 Queen Street
Suite 400
Ottawa
Ontario, K1P 5E4

Tel: (613) 563 7514
Fax: (613) 567 0614

## Denmark

Danish ME/CFS Association
Rådhustorvet 1,2
DK–3520 Farum

Tel: (45) 44 95 97 00
Fax: (45) 44 95 97 74

## Germany

CFS/CFIDS Self Help Group
Ms Elke Uhlisch
Lubener Weg 3
D–53119 Bonn

## The Irish Republic

Irish ME Support Group
PO Box 3075
Dublin 2

Tel: (01) 235 0965

## Italy

CFS Associazione Italiana
Segreteria: Via Moimacco 20
33100 Udine

## The Netherlands

ME Stichting
PO Box 57436
NL–1040 BH Amsterdam

Tel: (31) 20 6895162
Fax: (31) 20 6188578

## New Zealand

ANZMES
PO Box 36 307
Northcote
Auckland 1309

## Norway

Norges ME Forening
Mrs E. Piro: Eiksveien 96A
1345 Østeras

### South Africa

MEASA (ME Association of South Africa)
PO Box 1802
Umhlanga Rocks
4320
Kwa Zulu Natal

### Switzerland

Swiss ME/CFS Support Group
Mrs F. Moser
Gasse 31
CH–2553 Safnern

# List of Useful Addresses A–Z

Please note that where an organisation uses the words 'British' or 'National' in its title, the address will be listed under the name of the subject it is involved with. So, the British Allergy Foundation can be found under A – Allergy. Where several organisations are involved in one subject (e.g. acupuncture, pensions), they are all listed under that topic.

*Please remember to enclose a large SAE when writing to any of these organisations, as they are likely to have limited financial resources.*

Special addresses relevant to Northern Ireland, Scotland and Wales are listed separately at the end of this section.

### Acupuncture

British Medical Acupuncture Society
Newton House
Newton Lane
Whitley, Warrington
Cheshire
WΛ4 4JA

Tel: 01925 730727
Medically qualified acupuncturists.

British Acupuncture Council
Park House
206–208 Latimer Road
London W10 6RE

Tel: 0181–964 0222

## Alexander Technique

Alexander Technique, The Society of Teachers of
20 London House
266 Fulham Road
London SW10 9EL

Tel: 0171–351 0828

## Allergies

The British Allergy Foundation
Deepdene House
30 Bellgrove Road
Welling
Kent DA16 3BY

Tel: 0181–303 8583

For written information send a cheque for £10 made payable to the BAF
and state the nature of the allergy. This donation will also cover membership and a quarterly magazine. Their *Allergy Helpline* on 0181 303
8583 operates from 10 a.m. to 3 p.m. Monday to Friday.

## Alternative and complementary medicine

The British Holistic Medical Association
Royal Shrewsbury Hospital South
Shrewsbury
Shropshire
SY3 8XF

Tel: 01743 261 155

The Amarant Trust
1st Floor
Sycamore House
5 Sycamore Street
London EC1Y 0SR

Tel: 0171–608 3222

Information and advice on menopausal symptoms, including the use of
hormone replacement therapy (HRT).

The Institute for Complementary Medicine
PO Box 194
London SE16 1QZ
Tel: 0171–237 5165

## *Aromatherapy*

International Federation of Aromatherapists
2–4 Chiswick High Road
London W4 1TH

Tel: 0181–742 2605

## *Bach Flower Remedies*

Dr Edward Bach Centre
Mount Vernon
Bauers Lane
Brightwell cum Sotwell
Wallingford
Oxon OX10 0PZ

Tel: 01491 834678

## *Back pain*

National Back Pain Association
16 Elmtree Road
Teddington
Middlesex
TW11 8ST

Tel: 0181–977 5474

Leaflets and cassettes on how to cope with back pain.

## *Carers organisations*

Black Carers Support Group
Annie Wood Resource Centre
129 Alma Way
Lozells
Birmingham B19 2LS

Tel: 0121–554 7137

Provides information and puts black carers in touch with one another.

Carers National Association
20–25 Glasshouse Yard
London EC1A 4JS

Tel: 0171–490 8818; Advice: 0345 573369

Information and support to people caring for relatives and friends who, because of illness or disability, cannot manage without help.

Crossroads Care Attendant Schemes
10 Regent Place
Rugby
Warwickshire
CV21 2PN

Tel: 01788 573653

The Holiday Care Service
2nd Floor
Imperial Buildings, Victoria Road
Horley
Surrey RH6 7PZ

Tel: 01293 774535

Charity that provides information on specialist holidays available to disabled people and their carers. Publishes holiday brochures and other guides.

The Princess Royal Trust for Carers
Head Office
142 Minories
London EC3N 1LB

Tel: 0171–480 7788

Information, support and practical help for carers through its network of Carers Centres – 42 at present. The trust aims to have a centre in every social services area in the UK.

The Winged Fellowship
Angel House
20–32 Pentonville Road
London N1 9XD

Tel: 0171–833 2594

Provides respite care and holidays for disabled people so that their carers can have time to themselves. Disabled people can holiday on their own or with a full-time carer.

## Children

Advisory Centre for Education (ACE)
1b Aberdeen Studios
22 Highbury Grove
London N5 2DQ

Publishes books and information sheets on all aspects of education, including legal problems. A telephone advice line (0171–354 8321) is available.

The Association of Parents of Vaccine Damaged Children
78 Campden Road
Shipston on Stour
Warwickshire
CV36 4DH

Tel: 01608 661595

Children in Hospital – Action for Sick Children
Argyle House
29–31 Euston Road
London NW1 2SD

Tel: 0171–833 2041
The Family Welfare Association
501–505 Kingsland Road
London E8 4AU

Tel: 0171–254 6251

Professional counselling service for families in distress. Ten local branches in the UK.

Invalid Children's Aid Nationwide
Barbican Citygate
1–3 Dufferin Street
London EC1Y 8NA

Tel: 0171–374 4422

Help and advice for parents with problems associated with disabled children. Will advise on educational difficulties.

Parentability
Alexandra House
Oldham Terrace
Acton
London W3 6NH

Tel: 0181–992 2616

Group within the National Childbirth Trust which supports parents with
disabilities.

## Chinese Medicine

Register of Traditional Chinese Medicine
PO Box 400
Wembley
Middlesex HA9 9NZ

Tel: 0171–224 0803

## Chiropractic

The British Chiropractic Association
Blagrave House
17 Blagrave Street
Reading Berkshire
RG1 1QB

Tel: 0118 950 5950

## Citizens' Advice Bureau

The National Association of Citizens' Advice Bureaux
Myddleton House
115–123 Pentonville Road
London N1 9LZ

Tel: 0171–833 2181

For details of local branches see the phone book.

## Counselling

The British Association of Counselling
1 Regent Place
Rugby
Warwickshire CV21 2PJ

Tel: 01788 578328

Registered charity with a code of ethics for counsellors.

**Capital Radio Helpline**
Euston Tower
London NW1 3DR

Tel: 0171–484 4000

A confidential off-air advice and information service for people in London. Experienced counsellors try to advise or signpost on any sort of problem, or put you in touch with a relevant organisation.

## *Disability Organisations*

**The Centre for Accessible Environments**
60 Gainsford Street
London SE1 2NY

Tel: 0171–357 8182

Information service on practical design of buildings accessible to the disabled.

**DIAL (Disablement Information and Advice Lines) UK**
St Catherine's Hospital
Tickhill Road
Balby
Doncaster DN4 8QN
Tel: 01302 310123

Free confidential information and advice on a variety of issues concerning disabled people. Over 80 branches throughout the UK. Consult your phone book for local branches.

**Disability Alliance**
Universal House
88–94 Wentworth Street
London E1 7SA

Tel: 0171–247 8776 (administration)
0171–247 8763 (Social Security helpline)

Pressure group which campaigns on benefit issues. Publishes the *Disability Rights Handbook*, an invaluable source of information through the DSS benefits maze. Also carries out research into financial problems associated with disability.

The Disability Information Trust
Mary Marlborough Lodge
Nuffield Orthopaedic Centre
Headington
Oxford
OX3 7LD

Tel: 01865 227592

Publishes a series of useful booklets on various aspects of disability.

The Disabled Living Centres Council
1st Floor
Winchester House
11 Cranmer Road
London SW9 6EJ

Tel: 0171–820 0567

Co-ordinates the work of Disabled Living Centres (DLCs).

*Disabled Living Centres*
| | |
|---|---|
| Aberdeen | 01224 685247 |
| Aylesbury | 01296 315066 |
| Beckenham | 0181–663 3345 |
| Belfast | 01232 669501 |
| Birmingham | 0121–643 0980 |
| Bristol | 0117 9653651 |
| Cardiff | 01222 566281 |
| Carmarthen | 01267 241743 |
| Dunstable | 01582 470900 |
| Edinburgh | 0131–537 9190 |
| Elgin | 01343 551339 |
| Exeter | 01392 259260 |
| Grangemouth | 01324 504311 |
| Hillingdon | 01895 233691 |
| Huddersfield | 01484 223000 |
| Hull | 01482 676117 |
| Inverness | 01463 704293 |
| Leeds | 0113 2793140 |
| Leicester | 0116 2700515 |
| Lewes | 01273 472860 |
| Liverpool | 0151–298 2055 |
| London | 0171–289 6111 |
| Lowestoft | 01502 405454 |

| | |
|---|---|
| Macclesfield | 01625 661740 |
| Manchester | 0161–832 3678 |
| Middlesborough | 01642 827471 |
| Newcastle-upon-Tyne | 0191–284 0480 |
| Nottingham | 0115 9420391 |
| Oxford | 01865 798723 |
| Paisley | 0141–887 0597 |
| Papworth Everard | 01480 830495 |
| Portsmouth | 01705 737174 |
| Semington (Wiltshire) | 01380 871007 |
| Shrewsbury | 01743 444599 |
| Southampton | 01703 796631 |
| St Andrew's | 01334 412606 |
| Stamford (Lincolnshire) | 01780 480599 |
| Stockport | 0161–419 4476 |
| Swansea | 01792 580161 |
| Swindon | 01793 643966 |
| Welwyn Garden City | 01707 324581 |

DLCs provide information and advice on a large number of practical aids which are available for the disabled. They are generally open Monday to Friday from 9 a.m. to 5 p.m., by appointment. A telephone/letter enquiry service is also available.

Disablement Income Group (DIG)
Unit 5
Archway Business Centre
19–23 Wedmore Street
London N19 4RZ

Tel: 0171–263 3981

Operates advisory service on DSS benefits. Several publications – list on request.

The Independent Living Fund
PO Box 183
Nottingham
NG8 3RD

Tel: 0115 9428191

Opportunities for People with Disabilities
1 Bank Buildings
Princes Street
London EC2R 8EU

Tel: 0171–726 4961

RADAR (The Royal Association for Disability and Rehabilitation)
12 City Forum
250 City Road
London EC1V 8AF

Tel: 0171–250 3222

Umbrella organisation giving advice on all matters related to disability: access, holidays (publishes useful guides), housing, mobility, welfare and employment. Large number of publications and leaflets.

REMAP (Rehabilitation Engineering Movement Advisory Panel)
J. J. Wright, National Organiser
Hazeldene
Ightham
Sevenoaks
Kent TN15 9AD

Tel: 01732 883818

Makes or adapts aids for disabled people when these are not commercially available.

## Dyslexia

The Dyslexia Institute
133 Gresham Road
Staines
Middlesex
TW18 2AJ
Tel: 01784 463851
National network of 25 centres offering advice, teaching and assessment.

## Dysphasia

Action for Dysphasic Adults
Canterbury House
Royal Street
London SE1 7LL

Tel: 0171–261 9572

Information and advice for people with dysphasia (speech problems).

## Government departments

The Department for Education and Employment, Disability Services
Rockingham House
123 West Street
Sheffield S1 4ER

Tel: 0114 275 6997

The Department of Social Security
The Adelphi
1–11 John Adam Street
London WC2N 6HT

Tel: 0171–692 8000

The Department of Transport, Mobility Unit
1–11 Great Minster House
76 Marsham Street
London SW1P 4DR

Tel: 0171–271 5252

## Healing

The National Federation of Spiritual Healers
Old Manor Farm Studio
Church Street
Sunbury-on-Thames
Middlesex
TW16 6RG

Tel: 01932 783164

## *Health information*

The Association of Community Health Councils for England and Wales
Earlsmead House
30 Drayton Park
London N5 1PB

Tel: 0171–609 8405

There are over 200 CHCs in England and Wales. You can find out where
your local CHC is by looking under 'Community' in the phone book.

The College of Health
St Margaret's House
21 Old Ford Road
London E2 9PL

Tel: 0181–983 1225

Aims to improve self-care and self-help groups through proper use of
NHS facilities and alternative therapies. Publishes a wide range of useful
leaflets. Healthline service has over 350 tapes which can be played over
the phone.

The British Red Cross Society
9 Grosvenor Crescent
London SW1X 7EJ

Tel: 0171–235 5454

For local branches see the phone book.

Freephone NHS Health Information Service
Call free on 0800 665544 for information (but not advice) on all aspects
of health care, disability issues, welfare benefits, NHS complaints and
services.

The General Medical Council
44 Hallam Street
London W1N 6AE

Tel: 0171–580 7642

The Health Service Ombudsman
Millbank Tower
Millbank
London SW1P 4QP

Tel: 0171–217 4051

(Scotland and Wales have their own HSO – see address section at the end of this chapter.)

Healthwatch (formerly Campaign Against Health Fraud)
Box CAHF
London WC1N 3XX

Tel: 01483 503106

Healthwatch campaigns and promotes good practice in the assessment and testing of treatments, whether 'orthodox' or 'alternative'. Membership costs £16 per year.

OP Information Network
Heathfield Farmhouse
Callington
Cornwall PL17 7HP

Tel: 01579 384492

The Patients' Association
PO Box 935
Harrow
Middlesex HA1 3YJ

Tel: Helpline 0181 423 8999

Advice and information on any aspect of health care. Can assist in resolving complaints against doctors and hospitals. Campaigns for better monitoring of drugs and their side-effects and allowing patients more access to all aspects of medical information.

## Herbalists

The National Institute of Medical Herbalists
56 Longbrook Street
Exeter EX4 6AH

Tel: 01392 426022

Register of qualified herbalists.

## *Homoeopathy*

The British Homoeopathy Association
27a Devonshire Street
London W1N 1RJ

Tel: 0171–935 2163

Maintains a membership of individual practitioners in homoeopathy and provides an information service. Also has an up-to-date reference library on homoeopathic medicines.

The Society of Homoeopaths
2 Artisan Road
Northampton
NN1 4HU

Tel: 01604 621400

For details of non-medically qualified homoeopaths.

### Homoeopathic hospitals and clinics (NHS)

These can be found in Bristol, Glasgow, Liverpool, London and Tunbridge Wells. For more information, send an SAE to:

The Faculty of Homeopathy and Homeopathic Trust
15 Clerkenwell Close
London EC1R 0AA

Tel: 0171–566 7800

The Royal London Homeopathic Hospital can be contacted on 0171–833 7276 for information on how your GP can arrange for a referral.

### Homoeopathic medicines

Ainsworths Homoeopathic Pharmacy
36 New Cavendish Street
London W1M 7LH

Tel: 0171–935 5330

Homoeopathic medicines can be prescribed on the NHS, but they are not usually too expensive to purchase without a prescription.

## Hypnosis

The British Society of Medical and Dental Hypnotists
Mrs Anne Valentine
Flat 23
Broadfield Heights
53–59 Broadfields Avenue
Edgeware, Middlesex HA8 8PF

Tel: 0181–905 4342

## Insurance disputes

The Insurance Ombudsman
City Gate One
135 Park Street
London SE1 9EA

Tel: 0171–928 7600

The Personal Insurance Arbitration Service
24 Angel Gate
City Road
London EC1V 2RS

Tel: 0171–837 4483

## Interests and activities

The Association of Swimming Therapy
26 Stone Grove
Edgware
Middlesex HA8 7UA

Tel: 0181–958 1642

The National Trust
36 Queen Anne's Gate
London SW1H 9AS

Tel: 0171–222 9251

The Open University
The Regional Disability Co-ordinator
Room 001
East Perry
Milton Keynes MK7 6AA

Tel: 01908 653442

The Society for Horticultural Therapy
Goulds Ground, Vallis Way
Frome
Somerset BA11 3DW

Tel: 01373 464782

Advice service for disabled gardeners.

## *Irritable Bowel Syndrome*

The Irritable Bowel Syndrome Network
Northern General Hospital
Sheffield
S5 7AU

Tel: 0114 261 1531

## *Legal advice*

Action for Victims of Medical Accidents (AVMA)
Bank Chambers
1 London Road
Forest Hill
London SE23 3TP

Tel: 0181–686 8333

Advises people who feel that something has gone wrong with their medical treatment and refers them to appropriate solicitors.

The Disability Law Service
2nd Floor North
High Holborn House
52–54 High Holborn
London WC1V 6RL

Tel: 0171–831 8031

Legal advice and information for disabled people.

The Law Centres Federation
Duchess House
18–19 Warren Street
London W1P 5DB

Tel: 0171–387 8570

Information on local law centres.

The Law Society
114 Chancery Lane
London WC2A 1PL

Tel: 0171–320 5793

Liberty (formerly The National Council for Civil Liberties)
21 Tabard Street
London SE1 4LA

Tel: 0171–403 3888

## Liver problems

The British Liver Trust
Central House
Central Avenue
Ransomes Europark
Ipswich IP3 9QG

Tel: 01473 276326

## Lupus

Lupus UK
PO Box 999
Romford
Essex RM1 1DW

Tel: 01708 731251

## Medical identification

Medic – Alert Foundation
1 Bridge Wharf
156 Caledonian Road
London N1 9RD

Tel: 0171–833 3034

Identification scheme for people suffering from hidden conditions. Produces bracelets/medallions with 24-hour telephone number of its office, which keeps details of your personal medical history.

## *Mental health*

Depression Alliance
35 Westminster Bridge Road
London SE1 7JB

Tel: 0171–633 -557

Self-help information for people with depression and their families.

MIND (The National Association for Mental Health)
Granta House
15–19 Broadway
Stratford
London E15 4BQ
Tel: 0181–519 2122

0345 660163 (Information Line)

Campaigning group on a range of issues related to mental health. Publishes booklets and leaflets on a variety of issues concerned with psychiatric illness. Has a legal department which will help with mental health problems requiring this sort of advice, e.g. compulsory admission to a psychiatric hospital. Numerous local groups as well – see the phone book for details.

Panic/No Panic
93 Brands Farm Way
Randlay
Telford
Shropshire TF3 2JQ

Tel: 01952 590545 (Helpline service)

Information and advice on panic attacks, phobias and anxiety disorders.

The Royal College of Psychiatrists
17 Belgrave Square
London SW1X 8PG

Tel: 0171–235 2351

Publications and information on all aspects of mental health.

## SAD

The Seasonal Affective Disorder Association
PO Box 989
Steyning BN44 3HG
Tel: 0181–969 7028

Samaritans
10 The Grove
Slough
Berkshire
SL1 1QP

Tel: 0345 909090
Confidential advice over the phone for anyone in despair. For local branches see the phone book.

## Migraine

The Migraine Action Association
178a High Road
Byfleet
West Byfleet
Surrey
KT14 7ED

Tel: 01932 352468

Information and support for sufferers

The Migraine Trust
45 Great Ormond Street
London WC1N 3HD
Tel: 0171–831 4818
Information, advice and research into migraine.

## Mobility

Banstead Mobility Centre
Damson Way
Fountain Drive
Carshalton
Surrey
SM5 4NR

Tel: 0181–770 1151

The British Association of Wheelchair Distributors
1 Webbs Court
Buckhurst Avenue
Sevenoaks
Kent
TN13 1LZ

Tel: 01732 458868

Details of private wheelchair distributors.

The Disabled Drivers' Association
Ashwellthorpe
Norwich
Norfolk
NR16 1EX

Tel: 01508 489449

Self-help group aiming to help disabled motorists.

The Disabled Drivers' Motor Club
Cottingham Way
Thrapston
Northamptonshire
NN14 4PL

Tel: 01832 734724

Advice on mobility problems, conversions, insurance, foreign travel, etc, in relation to driving a car.

London Transport -- Unit for Disabled Passengers
55 Broadway
London SW1H 0BD

Tel: 0171–918 3312

The Mobility Information Service
Unit 2a
Atcham Estate
Upton Magna
Shrewsbury
SY4 4UG

Tel: 01743 761889

Motability
Goodman House
Station Approach
Harlow
Essex CM20 2ET

Tel: 01279 635666

Motability Advice and Vehicle Information Service (MAVIS)
Department of Transport
Transport and Road Research Laboratory
Crowthorne
Berkshire
RG11 6AU

Tel: 01344 661 000

The National Federation of Shopmobility
85 High Street
Worcester
WR1 2ET

Tel: 01905 617761

See phone book for details of local Shopmobility schemes.

The Orange Badge Network
52 High Street
Blackheath
Rowley Regis
West Midlands
B65 0EH
Tel: 0121–561 3265

Represents rights and needs of orange badge holders.

*Narcolepsy*

The Narcolepsy Association
1 Brook Street
Stoke-on-Trent
ST4 1JN

Tel: 01273 832725

## Naturopathy

The General Council and Register of Naturopaths
Goswell House
2 Goswell Road
Street
Somerset
BA16 0JG

Tel: 01458 840072

## Osteopathy

The Osteopathic Information Service
Premier House
10 Greycoat Place
London SW1P 1SB

Tel: 0171–799 2559

Provides information on osteopathy and keeps a list of osteopaths.

## Osteoporosis

The National Osteoporosis Society
PO Box 10
Radstock
Bath BA3 3YB

Tel: 01761 471771

## Pain relief

The Pain Society
9 Bedford Square
London WC1B 3RA

Tel: 0171–636 2750

Information on the management of chronic pain and availability of pain clinics.

## Pension disputes

The Occupational Pensions Advisory Service (OPAS)
11 Belgrave Road
London SW1V 1RB

Tel: 0171–233 8080

The Pensions Ombudsman
11 Belgrave Road
London SW1V 1RB

Tel: 0171–834 9144

When requiring advice or complaining about a decision relating to an occupational pension try OPAS first.

## Physiotherapists

For details of chartered physiotherapists working in private practice contact: 01702 392124.

## Polio

The British Polio Fellowship
Unit A
Eagle Office Centre
The Runway, South Ruislip
Middlesex HA4 6SE

Tel: 0181 842 4999

## Premenstrual tension

The National Association for Premenstrual Tension
PO Box 72
Sevenoaks
Kent
TN13 1XQ

Tel: 01732 741709

## Raynaud's syndrome

The Raynaud's and Scleroderma Association Trust
112 Crewe Road
Alsager
Cheshire
ST7 2JA

Tel: 01270 872776

Information and practical advice on coping with Raynaud's syndrome (cold hands and feet).

### Reflexology

Association of Reflexologists
27 Old Gloucester Street
London WC1N 3XX

Tel: 0870 567 3320

### Relationships

RELATE (formerly The Marriage Guidance Council)
Herbert Gray College
Little Church Street
Rugby
Warwickshire
CV21 3AP

Tel: 01788 573241

For local branches see the phone book.

SPOD (The Association to Aid Sexual and Personal Relationships of People with a Disability)
286 Camden Road
London N7 0BJ

Tel: 0171–607 8851
Information and advice on sexuality and disability. Can put you in touch with experienced sexual counsellors.

### Relaxation

Relaxation for Living
Foxhills
30 Victoria Avenue
Shanklin
Isle of Wight PO37 6LS

Tel: 01983 868166

Information on relaxation techniques and courses.

### Research
Linbury Trust
9 Red Lion Court
London EC4A 3EB

Tel: 0171–410 0330

Major source of funding for research into ME/CFS.

*Self-help*
Lifeskills
60 Wimpole Street
London W1M 7DE

Tel: 01823 451771

Produces a variety of self-help cassette tapes.

*Sjögren's syndrome*
The British Sjögren's Syndrome Association
Unit 1
Manor Workshops
Wall Lane, West End
Nailsea, Bristol BS48 2DD

Tel: 01275 854215

## Sleep

The British Snoring and Sleep Association
The Steps
How Lane
Chipstead
Surrey CR5 3LT

Tel: 01737 557997

Information and advice about sleep apnoea, sleep disturbance and snoring.

## Tinnitus

The British Tinnitus Association
4th Floor
White Building
Fitzalian Square
Sheffield S1 2AZ

Tel: 0114 2796600

Information and counselling on all aspects of tinnitus (ringing in the ears).

## *Volunteers*

Community Service Volunteers
237 Pentonville Road
London N1 9NJ

Tel: 0171–278 6601

Source of volunteer help to enable those with disabilities to lead a more independent life at home or in residential care.

The National Association of Volunteer Bureaux
New Oxford House
16 Waterloo Street
Birmingham B2 5UG

Tel: 0121–633 4555

Addresses of local volunteer bureaux can be found in the phone book.

## *Northern Ireland*

The ME Association
See listing on page 400.

The Association for Mental Health, Northern Ireland
80 University Street
Belfast BT7 1HE

Tel: 01232 237937 (Advice line: Mon.–Fri. 2 p.m.–4 p.m.; Tues. 6 p.m.–8 p.m.)
Information and advice on all aspects of mental illness.

The Carers National Association
Northern Ireland Regional Office ·
113 University Street
Belfast BT7 1HP

Tel: 01232 439843

Crossroads Care Attendant Schemes
7a Regent Street
Newtownards
Co. Down BT23 4AB

Tel: 01247 814455

Branches throughout the province. The headquarters will be able to pass on the relevant address and phone number.

Disability Action
2 Annadale Avenue
Belfast BT7 3JR

Tel: 01232 491011

Forum for over 130 organisations in Northern Ireland concerned with all forms of disability. Offers an information and training service, driving assessment and mobility information.

The Independent Tribunal Service, Northern Ireland
6th Floor, Cleaver House
3 Donegal Square North
Belfast BT1 5GA

Tel: 01232 539900

The Labour Relations Agency
2/8 Gordon Street
Belfast BT1 2LG

Tel: 01232 321442

Useful agency for anyone experiencing problems with employment, especially where there is no trade union to help with advice.

The Social Security Agency
Head Office
Castlecourt Complex
Royal Avenue
Belfast BT1 1DF

Tel: 01232 336000

Deals with all aspects of the benefits system.

## Scotland

The ME Association
See listing on page 400.

Crossroads Care Attendant Schemes
24 George Square
Glasgow G2 1EG

Tel: 0141–226 3793

Respite relief for carers.

The Department of Social Security
Central Office for Scotland
Argyle House
3 Lady Lawson Street
Edinburgh EH3 0XY

Tel: 0131–229 9191

DIAL (Disablement Information and Advice Lines) Scotland
Braid House
Labrador Avenue
Howden
Lothian EH54 6BU

Tel: 01506 433468

For information on local DIAL groups in Scotland.

Disability Scotland
5 Shandwick Place
Edinburgh EH2 4RG

Tel: 0131–229 8632

Information on all aspects of disability.

Disablement Income Group Scotland
5 Quayside Street
Edinburgh EH6 6EJ

Tel: 0131–555 2811

The Law Society of Scotland
26 Drumsheugh Gardens
Edinburgh EH3 7YR

Tel: 0131–226 7411

Provides details of Scottish solicitors.

The Red Cross, Scottish Branch
204 Bath Street
Glasgow G2 4HL

Tel: 0141–332 9591

The Scottish Association for Mental Health
Cumbrae House
15 Carnton Court
Glasgow G5 9JP

Tel: 0131–229 9687

Independent voluntary organisation dealing with all aspects of mental illness in Scotland

## Wales

Action Aid for the Disabled
Griffin Street
Newport
Gwent
NP9 1GL

Tel: 01633 258212

Information, advice, tribunal representation, counselling service.

Cardiff Law Centre
15 Splott Road
Splott
Cardiff
CF2 2BU

Tel: 01222 498117

DIAL (Disablement Information and Advice Lines)
Llan Harry (01443 237937)
Swansea (01792 588322)

Disability Wales
Llys lfor
Crescent Road
Caerphilly
Mid Glamorgan
CF83 1XL

Tel: 01222 887325

Information and campaigning organisation.

**Disablement Welfare Rights**
2 Glanrafon
Bangor
Gwynedd
LL57 1LH
Tel: 01248 352227

MIND, Cymru/Wales
23 St Mary Street
Cardiff
CF1 2AA

Tel: 0345 660163 (Information line 9.15 a.m.–4.45 p.m. Mon.–Fri.)

Information and advice on mental health services.

# Further Sources of Information

## Books

In addition to a vast range of self-help guidebooks, many of which provide uncritical support for treatments of no proven value, there are several books aimed at those who require more detailed information on the medical and scientific aspects of ME/CFS. These tend to take the form of multi-author textbooks, whereby 'experts' on various aspects of ME/CFS contribute review chapters on their own areas of interest (e.g. epidemiology, immunology, virology).

The two books that I most frequently refer to for information are an account of a three-day symposium on ME/CFS which was held at the CIBA Foundation in London in 1992 (Bock, G. R. and Wheelan, J., *Chronic Fatigue Syndrome*, CIBA Foundation Symposium 173, John Wiley, Chichester, 1993) and a more recent overall review from America (Straus, S., *Chronic Fatigue Syndrome*, Marcel Dekker, New York, 1994). The account of the CIBA meeting is unique in that it includes the text of discussions which took place between doctors who have very different opinions on the various topics under discussion. Stephen Straus's book contains some extremely detailed reviews on symptoms, virology and immunology, and is essential reading if you want to follow up these particular aspects of ME/CFS. Anyone who wishes to consult a book with more of a psychiatric bias should read *Chronic Fatigue and its Syndromes* by Simon Wessely, Mathew Hotopf and Michael Sharpe (Oxford University Press, Oxford, 1998).

I would also recommend:
*Chronic Fatigue Syndrome* by Yehuda and Mostofsky (Plenum Press, New York, 1997).
*CFIDS: A Disease of a Thousand Names* by Dr David Bell (D. Pollard, USA, 1991) – written by an American paediatrician who has looked after a large number of children with ME/CFS.
*Betrayal of the Brain* by Dr Jay Goldstein (Haworth Press, New York, 1996) – if you want to read some rather more lateral thinking on the subject.

There are three other books which are also well worth a read:
*Myalgic Encephalomyelitis and Postviral Fatigue States: The Saga of Royal Free Disease* by Dr Melvin Ramsay (Gower Medical Publishing, London, 1988) provides an excellent historical account of the numerous outbreaks of this illness which have occurred throughout the world since 1934. Copies are available from the UK ME Association.

*A Year Lost and Found* by the Very Reverend Michael Mayne, formerly Dean of Westminster (Darton, Longman and Todd, London) is a personal account of living with the illness.

*Osler's Webb* by the journalist Hilary Johnson (Crown Publications, New York, 1996) is a highly controversial account of issues surrounding ME/CFS in America.

## Regular Publications

You can obtain up-to-date information on research activity into ME/CFS from the following publications:

*Journal of Chronic Fatigue Syndrome* Published quarterly by Haworth Medical Press, 10 Alice Street, Binghamton, NY 13904–1580, USA.
Tel: 800 Haworth (429 6784) in USA & Canada or (607) 722 5857 outside USA/Canada.
Fax: 800 895 0582 in USA & Canada or (607) 722 6362 outside USA & Canada.

The only medical journal which is devoted to papers covering original research and practical management of ME/CFS.

*Medline Update on Chronic Fatigue Syndromes* Published quarterly by Health Care Information Service, (part of the British Library)
Publications Department, Science Reference and Information Services, 25 Southampton Buildings, London WC3A 1AW.
Tel: 0171–412 7469, Fax: 0171–412 7947
Annual subscription: £24 in European Union countries; £29 elsewhere
Brief abstracts from papers and correspondence relating to ME/CFS which has appeared worldwide in reputable medical journals during the previous few months. *An invaluable source of information.*

## Special Reports

*CFS: Report of a joint working group of the Royal Colleges of Physicians, Psychiatrists and General Practitioners* (October 1996). This report, was described by an editorial in *The Lancet* was being 'haphazardly set-up, biased, and inconclusive, and of little help to patients or their physicians'. Despite an emphasis on psychological explanations and treatments, it will continue to have a major effect on how the medical profession and some sections of the media view ME/CFS. Available from the Royal College of Physicians, 11 St Andrew's Place, London NW1 4LE; price £10.

*Report from the National Task Force on Chronic Fatigue Syndrome, Post Viral Fatigue Syndrome, Myalgic Encephalomyelitis* (September 1994). An extremely useful report produced by a multidisciplinary group of medical experts. Particularly helpful sections on management and service provision. Available from the charity Westcare (see page 403); price £6.95.

Separate Task Force reports are also available on *Chronic Fatigue Syndrome in Children and Young People* and *NHS Services for People with Chronic Fatigue Syndrome.*

*CFS: Clinical Practice Guidelines on the evaluation of prolonged fatigue and the diagnosis of Chronic Fatigue Syndrome* This report was produced by a working group convened by the Royal Australian College of Physicians and published in 1998 after a considerable amount of debate regarding its recommendations and conclusions.

# The Internet

A vast amount of information on ME/CFS is available via the Internet. Unfortunately, searching the Web can easily produce some very misleading information when it comes to ME/CFS. Sites are being created by people with no understanding of medical or scientific data, resulting in research findings being misinterpreted and new forms of treatment being advocated which have not been properly assessed or tested for safety. You also need to remember that a link from one Web site to another doesn't necessarily mean that the information being provided has the endorsement of the initiating site.

A good starting-point for medical information is the search engine Achoo. This has more than 7,000 entries, many of which link into other similar sites. One of the key sites for information on ME/CFS is: http://www.cais.net/cfs-news

Other ME/CFS sites include:
- The American Association for Chronic Fatigue Syndrome, which includes an extensive bibliography:
  http://weber.u.washington.edu~/dedra/aacfsl.html
- The CFIDS Association (publishers of the *CFIDS Chronicle*): http://cfids.org/cfids
- Cheney Clinic Information Service (information on all forms of treat-

ment from the US): http://www.fnmedcenter.com/ccis
- Centre for Disease Control and Prevention (USA):
  http://www.cdc.gov
- National Institute of Allergy and Infectious Diseases (USA):
  http://www.niaid.nih.gov
- *CFS News* is an irregularly published newsletter by Roger Burns in
  the USA: http://www.cais.net/cfs-news/cfs-news htm

Medical journals with Home Pages include:
- *The British Medical Journal:* http://www.bmj.com/bjm/
- *The Lancet*: http://www.thelancet.com
- *The Journal of the American Medical Association*:
  http://www.ama.assn.org/public/journals/jama/jamahome.htm

Although you may be fascinated by the latest details on research or treatment to be made available via the Internet, your doctor is likely to take a
far more sceptical view of this source of information.

# References

## *How to obtain medical references*

Medical journal references, which are frequently quoted throughout this
book, are from publications which shouldn't be too hard to find in any
good medical library (all large hospitals will have such a library but
access to the general public isn't always allowed). There is no 'embargo'
on the general public obtaining this sort of information if they decide to
do so. However, some doctors are still very opposed to patients reading
scientific literature on their own illness, as they feel (with some justification) that there is a real danger of the data being misinterpreted or
misused. Sadly, a significant minority of doctors still don't like the idea
of patients being better informed about particular conditions than the
medical profession!

If you want to obtain a copy of one of the listed references, phone your
local public library librarian and ask if this can be done – librarians are
usually very obliging and may even locate the more obscure references.
You'll have to pay a small fee, but it shouldn't be excessive. If your local
library can't help, then it's still worth contacting your local hospital
librarian to see if you could come in and make a copy.

Unfortunately, if you go into a library and try to look up ME or CFS
in one of the large medical textbooks, the chances are that you won't find
anything of help. Much of the information contained in standard textbooks covering neurology, infectious diseases or general medicine is
either out of date, inadequate or inaccurate. If your doctor claims that he

can't find anything about ME/CFS in his medical textbooks, this is the reason why!

# Chapter 1: Names, Definitions and Numbers

## Diagnostic criteria

1 Fukada, K., *et al.*, 'The chronic fatigue syndrome: a comprehensive approach to its definition and study', *Annals of Internal Medicine*, 1994, 121, 953–9. Correspondence: 1995, 123, 74–6.

2 Holmes, G., *et al.*, 'Chronic fatigue syndrome: a working case definition', *Annals of Internal Medicine*, 1988, 108, 387–9.

3 Katon, W. and Russo, J., 'Chronic fatigue syndrome criteria – a critique of the requirement for multiple physical symptoms', *Archives of Internal Medicine*, 1992, 152, 1604–9. Editorial on 1569–70.

4 Komaroff, A. L., *et al.*, 'An examination of the working case definition of chronic fatigue syndrome', *American Journal of Medicine*, 1996, 100, 56–64.

5 Lloyd, A. R., *et al.*, 'What is myalgic encephalomyelitis?' *Lancet*, 1988, 1, 1286–7.

6 Sharpe, M. C., *et al.*, 'A report – chronic fatigue syndrome: guidelines for research', *Journal of the Royal Society of Medicine*, 1991, 84 118–21.

## Epidemiology

7 Bates, D. W., *et al.*, 'Prevalence of fatigue and chronic fatigue syndrome in a Primary Care Practice', *Archives of Internal Medicine*, 1993, 153, 2759–65.

8 Buchwald, D., *et al.*, 'Frequency of "Chronic Active Epstein-Barr Virus Infection" in a general medical practice', *Journal of the American Medical Association*, 1987, 257, 2303–7.

9 Buchwald, D., *et al.*, 'Gender differences in patients with chronic fatigue syndrome', *Journal of General Internal Medicine*, 1994, 9, 397–401.

10 Buchwald, D., *et al.*, 'Chronic fatigue and the chronic fatigue syndrome: prevalence in a Pacific Northwest Health Care System', *Annals of Internal Medicine*, 1995, 123, 81–8.

11 Cathebras, P., *et al.*, 'Fatigue in primary care: prevalence, psychiatric comorbidity, illness behaviour and outcome', *Journal of General Internal Medicine*, 1992, 7, 276–86.

12 David, A., *et al.*, 'Tired, weak or in need of a rest: fatigue among general practice attenders', *British Medical Journal*, 1990, 301, 1109–22.

13 Dowsett, E. G., *et al.*, 'Myalgic encephalomyelitis – a persistent enteroviral infection?' *Postgraduate Medical Journal*, 1990, 66, 526–30.

14 Euba, R., *et al.*, 'A comparison of the characteristics of chronic fatigue syndrome in primary and tertiary care', *British Journal of Psychiatry*, 1996, 168, 121–6.

15 Hickie, I., *et al.*, 'Socio-demographic, psychiatric and medical correlates of fatigue in primary care', *Medical Journal of Australia*, 1996, 164, 585–8.

16 Hinds, G. M. E., 'A retrospective study of the chronic fatigue syndrome', *Proceedings of the Royal College of Physicians of Edinburgh*, 1993, 23, 10–14.

17 Ho-Yen, D. O. and McNamara, I., 'General Practitioners' experience of chronic fatigue syndrome', *British Journal of General Practice*, 1991, 41, 324–6.

18 Jason, L. A., *et al.*, 'Estimating rates of chronic fatigue syndrome from a community-based sample: a pilot study', *American Journal of Community Psychology*, 1995, 23, 557–68.

19 Kroenke, K., *et al.*, 'Chronic fatigue in primary care: prevalence, patient characteristics and outcome', *Journal of the American Medical Association*, 1988, 260, 929–34.

20 Lawrie, S. and Pelosi, A., 'Chronic fatigue syndrome in the community: prevalence and associations', *British Journal of Psychiatry*, 1995, 166, 793–7.

21 Levine, P. H., 'Epidemiologic advances in chronic fatigue syndrome', *Journal of Psychiatric Research*, 1997, 31, 7–18.

22 Lewis, G. and Wessely, S., 'The epidemiology of fatigue: more questions than answers', *Journal of Epidemiology and Community Health*, 1992, 46, 92–7.

23 Lloyd, A. R., *et al.*, 'Prevalence of chronic fatigue syndrome in an Australian population', *Medical Journal of Australia*, 1990, 153, 522–8.

24 McDonald, E., *et al.*, 'Chronic fatigue in general practice attenders', *Psychological Medicine*, 1993, 23, 987–98.

25 Minowa, M. and Jiamo, M., 'Descriptive epidemiology of chronic fatigue syndrome based on a nationwide survey in Japan', *Journal of Epidemiology*, 1996, 6, 75–80.

26 Price, R. K., *et al.*, 'Estimating the prevalence of chronic fatigue syndrome and associated symptoms in the community', *Public Health Reports*, 1992, 107, 514–22.

27 Wessely, S., 'The epidemiology of chronic fatigue syndrome', *Epidemiology Review*, 1995, 17, 139–51.

28 Wessely, S., *et al.*, 'The prevalence and morbidity of chronic fatigue

and chronic fatigue syndrome: a prospective primary care study', *American Journal of Public Health*, 1997, 87, 1449–55.

# Chapter 2: The History of ME/CFS in Different Parts of the World

29 Acheson, E. D., 'The clinical syndrome variously called benign myalgic encephalomyelitis, Iceland disease and epidemic neuromyasthenia', *American Journal of Medicine*, 1959, 26, 569–95.

30 Barnes, D., 'Mystery disease at Lake Tahoe challenges virologists and clinicians', *Science*, 1986, 234, 541.

31 Beard, G., 'Neurasthenia, or nervous exhaustion', *Boston Medical and Surgical Journal*, 1869, 3, 217–20.

32 Field, E. J., 'Darwin's illness', *Lancet*, 1990, 336, 826.

33 Gillam, A. G., 'Epidemiological study of an epidemic diagnosed as poliomyelitis occurring amongst the personnel of Los Angeles County General Hospital during the summer of 1934', *Public Health Bulletin* no. 240, April 1938.

34 Henderson, D. A. and Shelokov, A., 'Epidemic neuromyasthenia: clinical syndrome?' *New England Journal of Medicine*, 1959, 260, 757–64.

35 Hyde, B. and Bergmann, S., 'Akureyri disease (myalgic encephalomyelitis), forty years on', *Lancet*, 1988, 1192.

36 Leading article: 'A new clinical entity?' *Lancet*, 1956, i, 789.

37 Levine, P. H., *et al.*, 'Epidemic neuromyasthenia and chronic fatigue syndrome in West Otago, New Zealand', *Archives of Internal Medicine*, 1997, 157, 750–4.

38 Manningham, R., *The symptoms, nature, causes and cure of the febricula or little fever; commonly called the nervous or hysteric fever; the fever on the spirits; vapours, hypo or spleen*, second edition, J. Robertson, London, 1750, 52–3.

39 Maros, K. A., 'Portrait of a plague', *Medical Journal of Australia*, 1991, 155, 132.

40 McEvedy, C. P. and Beard, A. W., 'Royal Free Epidemic of 1955 – a reconsideration', *British Medical Journal*, 1970, 1, 7–11.

41 Medical Staff of the Royal Free Hospital, 'An outbreak of encephalomyelitis in the Royal Free Hospital Group, London, in 1955', *British Medical Journal*, 1957, 2, 895–904.

42 Pellew, R. A. A., 'A clinical description of a disease resembling poliomyelitis seen in Adelaide', *Medical Journal of Australia*, 1951, 1, 944–6.

43 Poore, M., *et al.*, 'An unexplained illness in West Otago', *New Zealand Medical Journal*, 1984, 97, 351.

44 Ramsay, A. M., 'Epidemic neuromyasthenia (1955–1978)', *Postgraduate Medical Journal*, 1978, 54, 718.

45 Sigurdsson, B., *et al.*, 'A disease epidemic in Iceland simulating poliomyelitis', *American Journal of Hygiene*, 1950, 52, 222–38.

46 Young, D. A. B., 'Florence Nightingale's fever', *British Medical Journal*, 1995, 311, 1697–9.

47 Young, D. A. B., 'The illnesses of Elizabeth Barrett Browning', *British Medical Journal*, 1989, 298, 439–43.

## Chapter 3: What Causes ME/CFS?

48 Delage, G., *et al.*, 'Report of a working group on the possible relationship between hepatitis B vaccination and chronic fatigue syndrome', *Canadian Medical Association Journal*, 1993, 149, 314–16.

49 Hall, G. H., *et al.*, 'Increased illness experience preceding chronic fatigue syndrome: a case control study', *Journal of the Royal College of Physicians*, 1998, 32, 44–8. Correspondence: 274

50 Hanin, I., 'The Gulf War, stress and a leaky blood–brain barrier', *Nature Medicine*, 1996, 2, 1307–8; see also pages 1382–5.

51 Hotopf, M., *et al.*, 'Chronic fatigue and psychiatric morbidity following viral meningitis: a controlled study', *Journal of Neurology, Neurosurgery and Psychiatry*, 1996, 60, 495–503.

52 Keller, R. H., *et al.*, 'Association between HLA class 11 antigens and the chronic fatigue syndrome', *Clinical Infectious Diseases*, 1994, 18 (suppl. 1), S154–S156.

53 MacDonald, K. L., *et al.*, 'A case-control study to assess possible triggers and cofactors in chronic fatigue syndrome', *American Journal of Medicine*, 1996, 100, 548–554.

54 Salit, I. E., 'Precipitating factors for the chronic fatigue syndrome', *Journal of Psychiatric Research*, 1997, 31, 59–65.

55 Wessely, S., *et al.*, 'Postinfectious fatigue: prospective cohort study in primary care', *Lancet*, 1995, 345, 1333–8. Correspondence: 346, 47–8 & 449.

56 White, P. D., 'The relationship between infection and fatigue', *Journal of Psychosomatic Research*, 1997, 43, 345–50.

57 Wood, B. and Wessely, S., 'Personality and social attitudes in chronic fatigue syndrome', *Psychosomatic Medicine*, 1998.

## Chapter 4 and 5: The Cardinal Symptoms and Secondary Problems

58 Hickie, I., *et al.*, 'Can the chronic fatigue syndrome be defined by distinct clinical features?' *Psychological Medicine*, 1995, 25, 925–35.

## Problems with balance

59  Ash-Bernal, R., *et al.*, 'Vestibular function test anomalies in patients with chronic fatigue syndrome', *Acta Otolaryngol*, 1995, 115, 9–17.

## Co-ordination

60  Boda, W. L., *et al.*, 'Gait abnormalities in chronic fatigue syndrome', *Journal of Neurological Sciences*, 1995, 131, 156–61.

## Eyes

61  Macintyre, A., 'Post-viral fatigue and the eye', *Optician*, 1994, 207, 26.

62  Potaznick, W. and Kozol, N., 'Ocular manifestations of chronic fatigue and immune dysfunction syndrome', *Optometry and Vision Science*, 1992, 69, 811–14.

## Irritable bowel symptomatology

63  Chua, A., *et al.*, 'Central serotonin receptors and delayed gastric emptying in non-ulcer dyspepsia', *British Medical Journal*, 1992, 305, 280–2.

64  Gomborone, J. E., *et al.*, 'Prevalence of irritable bowel syndrome in chronic fatigue', *Journal of the Royal College of Physicians*, 1996, 30, 512–13.

65  Hadjivassiliou, M., *et al.*, 'Does cryptic gluten sensitivity play a part in neurological illness?' *Lancet*, 1996, 347, 369–71.

## Hypoglycaemia

66  Riley, M. S., *et al.*, 'Aerobic work capacity with patients with chronic fatigue syndrome', *British Medical Journal*, 1990, 301, 953–6.

## Osteoporosis

67  Hoskin, L., *et al.*, 'Bone mineral density in pre-menopausal nulliparous women with chronic fatigue syndrome compared with age, weight matched controls', *Journal of Bone and Mineral Research*, 1997, 12, S228.

## Pre-menstrual syndrome

68  Studd, J. and Panay, N., 'Chronic fatigue syndrome', *Lancet*, 1996, 348, 1384.

## Pain in the joints

69  Hurst, N. P., *et al.*, 'Coxsackie B infection and arthritis', *British Medical Journal*, 1983, 286, 605.

## Respiratory problems

70 Delorenzo, F., *et al.*, 'Lung function test findings in patients with chronic fatigue syndrome', *Australian and New Zealand Journal of Medicine*, 1996, 26, 563–4.

## Weight changes

71 Park, R. J., *et al.*, 'Post-viral onset of anorexia nervosa', *British Journal of Psychiatry*, 1995, 166, 386–9.

# Chapter 6: Other Causes of Chronic Fatigue

72 Ayres, J. G., *et al.*, 'Protracted fatigue and debility after Q fever', *Lancet*, 1996, 347, 978–9.

73 Ayres, J. G., *et al.*, 'Post-infection fatigue syndrome following Q fever', *Quarterly Journal of Medicine*, 1998, 91, 105–13.

74 Berelowitz, G. J., *et al.*, 'Post-hepatitis syndrome revisited', *Journal of Viral Hepatitis*, 1995, 2, 133–8.

75 Calabrese, L. H., *et al.*, 'Chronic fatigue syndrome and a disorder resembling Sjögren's Syndrome: preliminary report', *Clinical Infectious Diseases*, 1994, 18, (supp. 1) S28–S32.

76 Cleary, K. J. and White, P. D., 'Gilbert's and chronic fatigue syndromes in men', *Lancet*, 1993, 341, 842.

77 Critchley, E. M. R., *et al.*, 'Outbreak of botulism in North West England and Wales, June 1989', *Lancet*, 1989, ii, 849–53.

78 Critchley, E. M. R., *et al.*, 'Botulism and Gulf War Syndrome', *Lancet*, 1996, 347, 1561.

79 Eltumi, M., *et al.*, 'Protracted fatigue and debility after acute Q fever', *Lancet*, 1996, 347, 978–9.

80 Gompels, M. M. and Spickett, G. P., 'Chronic fatigue, arthralgia and malaise', *Annals of the Rheumatic Diseases*, 1996, 55, 502–3.

81 Hadjivassiliou, *et al.*, 'Neuromuscular disorder as a presenting feature of coeliac disease', *Journal of Neurology, Neurosurgery and Psychiatry*, 1997, 63, 770–5.

82 Hurel, S. R., *et al.*, 'Patients with a self-diagnosis of myalgic encephalomyelitis', *British Medical Journal*, 1995, 311, 329.

83 Jacobsen, S. K., *et al.*, 'Chronic parvovirus B19 infection resulting in chronic fatigue syndrome: case history and review', *Clinical Infectious Diseases*, 1997, 24, 6, 1048–51.

84 Marmion, B. P., *et al.*, 'Protracted debility and fatigue after Q fever', *Lancet*, 1996, 347, 977–8.

85 Martin, W. J., 'Cytomegalovirus-related sequence in an atypical cytopathic virus repeatedly isolated from a patient with chronic fatigue syndrome', *American Journal of Pathology*, 1994, 145,

440–51.

86 Mesch, U., *et al.*, 'Lead poisoning masquerading as chronic fatigue syndrome', *Lancet*, 1996, 347, 1193.

87 Poser, C. M., 'Misdiagnosis of multiple sclerosis and beta-interferon', *Lancet*, 1997, 349, 1916.

88 Valesini, G., *et al.*, 'Gilbert's Syndrome and chronic fatigue syndrome', *Lancet*, 1993, 341, 1162–3.

## Conditions which overlap with ME/CFS: athletic overtraining, ciguatera poisoning and fibromyalgia

89 Budgett, R., 'The overtraining syndrome', *British Medical Journal*, 1994, 309, 465–8.

90 Fitzcharles, M.-A. and Esdaile, J. M., 'The over-diagnosis of fibromyalgia syndrome', *American Journal of Medicine*, 1997, 103, 44–50.

91 Ledingham, J., *et al.*, 'Primary fibromyalgia syndrome – an outcome study', *British Journal of Rheumatology*, 1993, 32, 139–42.

92 Maffulli, N., *et al.*, 'Post-viral fatigue syndrome: a longitudinal assessment in varsity athletes', *Journal of Sports Medicine and Physical Fitness*, 1993, 33, 392–9.

93 Pearn, J. H., 'Chronic fatigue syndrome: chronic ciguatera poisoning as a differential diagnosis', *Medical Journal of Australia*, 1997, 166, 309–10.

## Gulf War Syndrome/Gulf War illnesses

94 Haley, R., *et al.*, 'Is there a Gulf War Syndrome? Searching for syndromes by factor analysis of symptoms', *Journal of the American Medical Association*, 1997, 277, 215–22.

95 Haley, R., *et al.*, 'Self-reported exposure to neurotoxic chemical combinations in the Gulf War', *Journal of the American Medical Association*, 1997, 277, 231–7.

96 Haley, R., *et al.*, 'Evaluation of neurologic function in Gulf War veterans: a blinded case-control study', *Journal of the American Medical Association*, 1997, 277, 223–30.

97 Jamal, G. A., *et al.*, 'The "Gulf War Syndrome". Is there evidence of dysfunction in the nervous system?' *Journal of Neurology, Neurosurgery and Psychiatry*, 1996, 60, 449–51.

98 Persian Gulf Veterans Co-ordinating Board, 'Unexplained illnesses among Desert Storm veterans', *Archives of Internal Medicine*, 1995, 155, 262–8.

99 Rook, G. A. W. and Zumla, A., 'Gulf War Syndrome: Is it due to a systemic shift in cytokine balance towards a Th2 profile?' *Lancet*, 1997, 349, 1831–3.

100 The Iowa Persian Gulf Study Group, 'Self-reported illness and health status among Gulf War veterans', *Journal of the American Medical Association*, 1997, 277, 238–45.

## Pesticides

101 Ahmed, G. M. and Davies, D. R., 'Chronic organophosphate exposure: towards the definition of a neuropsychiatric syndrome', *Journal of Nutritional and Environmental Medicine*, 1997, 7, 169–76.

102 Behan, P. O. and Haniffah, B. A. G., 'Chronic fatigue syndrome: a possible delayed hazard of pesticide exposure', *Clinical Infectious Diseases*, 1994, 18 (Suppl. 1), S54.

103 Behan, P. O., 'Chronic fatigue syndrome as a delayed reaction to low-dose organophosphate exposure', *Journal of Nutritional and Environmental Medicine*, 1996, 6, 341–50.

104 Corrigan, F. M., *et al.*, 'Neurasthenic fatigue, chemical sensitivity and GABAa receptor toxins', *Medical Hypotheses*, 1994, 43, 195–200.

105 Davies, D. R., 'Organophosphates, affective disorders and suicide', *Journal of Nutritional and Environmental Medicine*, 1994, 5, 367–74.

106 Good, J. L., *et al.*, 'Pathophysiological studies of neuromuscular function in subacute organophosphate poisoning induced by phosmet', *Journal of Neurology, Neurosurgery and Psychiatry*, 1993, 56, 290–4.

107 O'Malley, 'Clinical evaluation of pesticide exposure and poisonings', *Lancet*, 1997, 349, 1161–6.

108 Newcombe, D. S., 'Immune surveillance, organophosphate exposure and lymphomagenesis', *Lancet*, 1992, 339, 539–41.

109 Rosenstock, L., *et al.*, 'Chronic central nervous system effects of acute organophosphate pesticide intoxication', *Lancet*, 1991, 338, 223–7.

110 Shepherd, C. B., 'Organophosphate pesticides – cause for concern?' *Practitioner*, 1993, 237, 212–14.

111 Steenland, K., 'Chronic neurological effects of organophosphate pesticides', *British Medical Journal*, 1996, 312, 1312–13.

112 Stephens, R., *et al.*, 'Neuropsychological effects of long-term exposure to organophosphates in sheep dip', *Lancet*, 1995, 345, 1135–9.

## Post-polio syndrome

113 Bruno, R. L., *et al.*, 'Polioencephalitis, stress and the aetiology of Post-Polio Sequelae', *Orthopaedics*, 1991, 14, 1269–76.

114 Bruno, R. L., *et al.*, 'Pathophysiology of a central cause of Post-Polio Fatigue', *Annals of the New York Academy of Science*, 1995, 753, 257–75.

115 Chetwynd, J., *et al.*, 'Post-Polio Syndrome in New Zealand: a survey

of 700 polio survivors', *New Zealand Medical Journal*, 1993, 106, 406–8.

116 Dalakas, M. C., *et al.*, 'A long term follow up study of patients with post poliomyelitis neuro-muscular symptoms', *New England Journal of Medicine*, 1986, 314, 959–63.

117 Packer, T. L., *et al.*, 'Activity and Post-Polio Fatigue', *Orthopaedics*, 1991, 14, 1223.

118 Trojan, D. A., *et al.*, 'Anticholinesterase-responsive neuromuscular junction transmission defects in post-poliomyelitis fatigue', *Journal of Neurological Sciences*, 1993, 114, 170–7.

# Chapter 7: Quality of Life, Disability Assessment and Recovery from ME/CFS

## *Functional Assessment (quality of life)*

119 Buchwald, D., *et al.*, 'Functional status in patients with chronic fatigue syndrome, other fatiguing illnesses, and healthy individuals', *American Journal of Medicine*, 1996, 101, 364–70.

120 Komaroff, A. L., *et al.*, 'Health status in patients with chronic fatigue syndrome and in the general population and disease comparison groups', *American Journal of Medicine*, 1996, 101, 281–90.

121 Schweitzer, R., *et al.*, 'Quality of life in chronic fatigue syndrome', *Social Science Medicine*, 1995, 41, 1367–72.

## *Prognosis*

122 Aylward, M., 'Government's expert group has reached consensus on prognosis of chronic fatigue syndrome', *British Medical Journal*, 1996, 313, 885.

123 Bombardier, C. H. and Buchwald, D., 'Outcome and prognosis of patients with chronic fatigue and chronic fatigue syndrome', *Archives of Internal Medicine*, 1995, 155, 2105–10.

124 Dowsett, E. G., *et al.*, 'Myalgic encephalomyelitis – a persistent enteroviral infection?' *Postgraduate Medical Journal*, 1990, 66, 526–30.

125 Hinds, G. M. E., *et al.*, 'A retrospective study of the chronic fatigue syndrome. Proceedings of the Royal College of Physicians of Edinburgh', 1993, 23, 10–14.

126 Joyce, J., *et al.*, 'The prognosis of chronic fatigue and chronic fatigue syndrome: a systematic review', *Quarterly Journal of Medicine*, 1997, 90, 223–33. Correspondence: 723–5.

127 Ray, C., *et al.*, 'Coping and other predictors of outcome in chronic fatigue syndrome: a 1-year follow-up', *Journal of Psychosomatic*

*Research*, 1997, 43, 405–15.

128  Sharpe, M. C., *et al.*, 'Follow up of patients presenting with fatigue to an infectious diseases clinic', *British Medical Journal*, 1992, 305, 147–52.

129  Vercoulen, J. H. M. M., *et al.*, 'Prognosis in chronic fatigue syndrome: a prospective study on the natural course', *Journal of Neurology, Neurosurgery and Psychiatry*, 1996, 60, 489–94.

130  Wilson, A., *et al.*, 'Longitudinal study of outcome of chronic fatigue syndrome', *British Medical Journal*, 1994, 308, 756–9.

# Chapter 8: Current Research

## *General reviews*

131  Behan, P. O., *et al.*, 'The post-viral fatigue syndrome – an analysis of the findings in 50 cases', *Journal of Infection*, 1985, 10, 211–22.

132  Behan, P. O. and Behan, W. M. H., 'Post-viral fatigue syndrome', *CRC Critical Reviews in Neurobiology*, 1988, 4, 157–78.

133  David, A., *et al.*, 'Post-viral fatigue syndrome – time for a new approach', *British Medical Journal*, 1988, 296, 696–9.

134  David, A., *et al.*, 'Chronic fatigue syndrome: signs of a new approach', *British Journal of Hospital Medicine*, 1991, 45, 158–63.

135  Demitrack, M. A. and Greden, J. F., 'Chronic fatigue syndrome: the need for an integrative approach', *Biological Psychiatry*, 1991, 30, 747–52.

136  Dickinson, C. J., 'Chronic fatigue syndrome – aetiological aspects', *European Journal of Clinical Investigation*, 1997, 27, 257–67.

137  Dowsett, E. G., *et al.*, 'Myalgic encephalomyelitis – a persistent enteroviral infection?' *Postgraduate Medical Journal*, 1990, 66, 526–30.

138  Lloyd, A. R., *et al.*, 'What is myalgic encephalomyelitis?' *Lancet*, 1988, I, 1286–7.

139  Moutschen, M., *et al.*, 'Pathogenic tracks in fatigue syndromes', *Acta Clinica Belgica*, 1994, 49, 274–89.

140  Shepherd, C. B., 'Myalgic encephalomyelitis – is it a real disease?' *The Practitioner*, 1989, 223, 41–6.

141  Weir, W. R. C., 'the post-viral fatigue syndrome', *The Royal Society of Medicine – Current Medical Literature: Infectious Diseases*, 1992, 6, 3–6.

142  Wessely, S., 'Old wine in new bottles: neurasthenia and "ME"', *Psychological Medicine*, 1990, 20, 35–53.

## The autonomic nervous system

143 Bou-Holaigah, I., *et al.*, 'The relationship between neurally mediated hypotension and the chronic fatigue syndrome', *Journal of the American Medical Association*, 1995, 274, 961–7. Correspondence: 1996, 275, 359–60.

144 Cordero, D. L., *et al.*, 'Decreased vagal power during treadmill walking in patients with chronic fatigue syndrome', *Clinical Autonomic Research*, 1996, 6, 329–33.

145 De Lorenzo, F., *et al.*, 'Possible relationship between chronic fatigue and postural tachycardia syndromes', *Clinical Autonomic Research*, 1996, 6, 263–4.

146 De Lorenzo, F., *et al.*, 'Pathogenesis and management of delayed orthostatic hypotension in patients with chronic fatigue syndrome', *Clinical Autonomic Research*, 1997, 7, 185–90.

147 Freeman, R. and Komaroff, A. L., 'Does the chronic fatigue syndrome involve the autonomic nervous system?' *American Journal of Medicine*, 1997, 102, 357–64.

148 Rowe, C., *et al.*, 'Is neurally mediated hypotension an unrecognised cause of chronic fatigue?' *Lancet*, 1995, 345, 623–4. Correspondence: 1995, 345, 1112–13.

149 Sisto, S. A., *et al.*, 'Vagal tone is reduced during paced breathing in patients with chronic fatigue syndrome', *Clinical Autonomic Research*, 1995, 5, 139–43.

150 Yataco, A., *et al.*, 'Comparison of heart rate variability in patients with chronic fatigue syndrome', *Clinical Autonomic Research*, 1997, 7, 293–7.

## Brain and nervous system

151 Ash-Bernal, R., *et al.*, 'Vestibular function test anomalies in patients with chronic fatigue syndrome', *Acta Otolaryngol* (Stockh.), 1995, 115, 9–17.

152 Boda, W. L., *et al.*, 'Gait abnormalities in chronic fatigue syndrome', *Journal of Neurological Sciences*, 1995, 131, 156–61.

153 Brouwer, B. and Packer, T., 'Corticospinal excitability in patients diagnosed with chronic fatigue syndrome', *Muscle and Nerve*, 1994, 17, 1210–12.

154 Prasher, D., *et al.*, 'Sensory and cognitive event-related potentials in myalgic encephalomyelitis', *Journal of Neurology, Neurosurgery and Psychiatry*, 1990, 53, 247–53.

## The hypothalamus and hormonal control

155 Allain, T. J., *et al.*, 'Changes in growth hormone, insulin, insulin-like growth factors (IGFs), and IGF-binding protein-1 in chronic fatigue

syndrome', *Biological Psychiatry*, 1997, 41, 567–73.

156 Bakheit, A. M. O., *et al.*, 'Possible upregulation of hypothalamic 5 – hydroxytryptamine receptors in patients with post-viral fatigue syndrome', *British Medical Journal*, 1992, 304, 1010–12.

157 Bakheit, A. M. O., *et al.*, 'Abnormal arginine-vasopressin secretion and water metabolism in patients with post-viral fatigue syndrome', *Acta Neurologica Scandinavia*, 1993, 87, 234–8.

158 Bearn, J. A., *et al.*, 'Neuroendocrine responses to D-fenfluramine and insulin-induced hypoglycaemia in chronic fatigue syndrome', *Biological Psychiatry*, 1995, 37, 245–52.

159 Bennett, A. L., *et al.*, 'Somatomedin C (insulin-like growth factor 1) levels in patients with chronic fatigue syndrome', *Journal of Psychiatric Research*, 1997, 31, 91–6.

160 Buchwald, D., *et al.*, 'Insulin-like growth factor-1 (somatomedin C) levels in chronic fatigue syndrome and fibromyalgia', *Journal of Rheumatology*, 1996, 23, 739–42.

161 Cleare, A., *et al.*, 'Contrasting neuroendocrine responses in depression and chronic fatigue syndrome', *Journal of Affective Disorders*, 1995, 35, 283–9.

162 Demitrack, M. A., *et al.*, 'Evidence for impaired activation of the hypothalamic-pituitary–adrenal axis in patients with chronic fatigue syndrome', *Journal of Endocrinology and Metabolism*, 1991, 73, 1224–34.

163 Demitrack, M. A., 'Chronic fatigue syndrome: a disease of the hypothalamic-pituitary–adrenal axis?' (Editorial), *Annals of Medicine*, 1994, 26, 1–5.

164 Demitrack, M. A., 'Neuroendocrine correlates of chronic fatigue syndrome: a brief review', *Journal of Psychiatric Research*, 1997, 31, 69–82.

165 Dinan, T. G., *et al.*, 'Blunted serotonin-mediated activation of the hypothalamic-pituitary–adrenal axis in chronic fatigue syndrome', *Psychoneuroendocrinology*, 1997, 22, 261–7.

166 Goldberg, M., 'High androgen levels in chronic fatigue patients', *Journal of Clinical Endocrinology and Metabolism*, 1995, 80, 3390–1.

167 Leese, G., *et al.*, 'Short-term night-shift working mimics pituitary–adrenocortical dysfunction of chronic fatigue syndrome', *Journal of Clinical Endocrinology and Metabolism*, 1996, 81, 1867–70.

168 Majeed, T., *et al.*, 'Defective dexamethasone induced growth hormone release in chronic fatigue syndrome: evidence for glucocorticoid receptor resistance and lack of plasticity?' *Journal of the Irish Colleges of Physicians and Surgeons*, 1995, 1, 20–4.

169 Mitchell, A. and O'Keane, V., 'Steroids and depression', *British*

*Medical Journal*, 1998, 316, 244–5.

170 Poteliakhoff, A., 'Adrenocortical activity and some clinical findings in acute and chronic fatigue', *Journal of Psychosomatic Research*, 1982, 25, 91–5.

171 Scott, L. C. and Dinan, T. G., 'Urinary free cortisol excretion in chronic fatigue syndrome, major depression and in healthy controls', *Journal of Affective Disorders*, 1998, 47, 49–54.

172 Sharpe, M., *et al.*, 'Increased prolactin response to buspirone in chronic fatigue syndrome', *Journal of Affective Disorders*, 1996, 41, 71–6.

173 Sharpe, M., *et al.*, 'Increased brain serotonin function in men with chronic fatigue syndrome', *British Medical Journal*, 1997, 315, 164–5.

174 Strickland, P., *et al.*, 'A comparison of salivary cortisol in chronic fatigue syndrome, community depression and healthy controls', *Journal of Affective Disorders*, 1998, 47, 191–4.

175 Studd, J. and Panay, N., 'Chronic fatigue syndrome', *Lancet*, 1996, 348, 1384.

176 Ur, E., *et al.*, 'The effect of metyrapone on the pituitary adrenal axis in depression: relation to dexamethasone suppresser status', *Neuroendocrinology*, 1992, 56, 533–5.

177 Wood, B., *et al.*, 'Salivary cortisol profiles in chronic fatigue syndrome', *Biological Psychiatry*, 1998, 37, 1–4.

178 Yatham, L. N., *et al.*, 'Neuroendocrine assessment of serotonin function in chronic fatigue syndrome', *Canadian Journal of Psychiatry*, 1995, 40, 92–6.

## *Immunology*

179 Ablashi, D. V., *et al.*, 'A chronic "post-infectious" fatigue syndrome associated with benign lymphoproliferation, B-cell proliferation and active replication of human herpes virus 6', *Journal of Clinical Investigation*, 1990, 10, 335–44.

180 Aoki, T., *et al.*, 'Low natural killer syndrome: clinical and immunological features', *National Immunological Cell Growth Regulations*, 1987, 6, 116–28.

181 Behan, P. O., *et al.*, 'The post-viral fatigue syndrome – an analysis of the findings in 50 cases', *Journal of Infection*, 1985, 10, 211–22.

182 Bennett, A. L., *et al.*, 'Immunoglobulin subclass levels in chronic fatigue syndrome', *Journal of Clinical Immunology*, 1996, 16, 315–20.

183 Bennett, A. L., *et al.*, 'Elevation of bioactive transforming growth factor-beta in serum from patients with chronic fatigue syndrome', *Journal of Clinical Immunology*, 1997, 17, 160–6.

184 Buchwald, D., *et al.*, 'A chronic illness characterised by fatigue,

neurologic and immunologic disorders and active human herpes virus type 6 infection', *Annals of Internal Medicine*, 1992, 116, 103–13.

185 Buchwald, D., *et al.*, 'Markers of inflammation and immune activation in chronic fatigue and chronic fatigue syndrome', *Journal of Rheumatology*, 1997, 24, 372–6.

186 Caligiuri, M., *et al.*, 'Phenotypic and functional deficiency of natural killer cells in patients with chronic fatigue syndrome', *Journal of Immunology*, 1987, 139, 3306–13.

187 Cannon, J. G., *et al.*, 'Interleukin-1 beta, interleukin-1 receptor antagonist, and soluble interleukin-1 receptor type 11 secretion in chronic fatigue syndrome', *Journal of Clinical Immunology*, 1997, 17, 253–61.

188 Chao, C. C., *et al.*, 'Serum neopterin and interleukin 6 levels in chronic fatigue syndrome', *Journal of Infectious Diseases*, 1990, 162, 1412–13.

189 Chao, C. C., *et al.*, 'Altered cytokine release in peripheral blood mononuclear cell cultures from patients with the chronic fatigue syndrome', *Cytokine*, 1991, 3, 292–8.

190 Cheney, P. R., *et al.*, 'Interleukin-2 and the chronic fatigue syndrome', *Annals of Internal Medicine*, 1989, 110, 321.

191 Gupta, S., *et al.*, 'Cytokine production by adherent and non-adherent mononuclear cells in chronic fatigue syndrome', *Journal of Psychiatric Research*, 1997, 31, 149–56.

192 Ho-Yen, D. O., *et al.*, 'Myalgic encephalomyelitis and alpha-interferon' (letter), *Lancet*, 1988, i, 125.

193 Ho-Yen, D. O., *et al.*, 'Natural killer cells and the post-viral fatigue syndrome', *Scandinavian Journal of Infectious Diseases*, 1991, 23, 711–16.

194 Klimas, N. G., *et al.*, 'Immunologic abnormalities in chronic fatigue syndrome', *Journal of Clinical Microbiology*, 1990, 28, 1403–10.

195 Landay, A., *et al.*, 'Chronic fatigue syndrome: clinical condition associated with immune activation', *Lancet*, 1991, 338, 707–11.

196 Lever, A. M. L., *et al.*, 'Interferon production in post-viral fatigue syndrome', *Lancet*, 1988, 2, 101.

197 Linde, A., *et al.*, 'IgG subclass deficiency and chronic fatigue syndrome', *Lancet*, 1988, 1, 885–6.

198 Linde, A., *et al.*, 'Serum levels of lymphokine and soluble cellular receptors in primary Epstein-Barr infections in patients with chronic fatigue syndrome', *Journal of Infectious Diseases*, 1992, 165, 994–1000.

199 Lloyd, A. R., *et al.*, 'Immunological abnormalities in the chronic fatigue syndrome', *Medical Journal of Australia*, 1989, 151, 122–4.

200 Lloyd, A. R., *et al.*, 'Cytokine levels in serum and cerebrospinal fluid in patients with chronic fatigue syndrome and control subjects', *Journal of Infectious Diseases*, 1991, 164, 1023–4.

201 Lloyd, A. R., *et al.*, 'Cell-mediated immunity in patients with chronic fatigue syndrome, healthy control subjects and patients with major depression', *Clinical Experimental Immunology*, 1992, 87, 76–9.

202 Lloyd, A. R., *et al.*, 'Immune function in chronic fatigue syndrome and depression: implications for understanding these disorders and for therapy', *Clinical Immunotherapy*, 1994, 2, 84–8.

203 Lusso, P., *et al.*, 'Infection of natural killer cells by human herpesvirus type 6', *Nature*, 1993, 362, 458–62.

204 Mawle, A., *et al.*, 'Immune responses associated with chronic fatigue syndrome: a case-control study', *Journal of Infectious Diseases*, 1997, 175, 136–41.

205 McDonald, E. M., *et al.*, 'Interferons as mediators of psychiatric morbidity', *Lancet*, 1987, ii, 1175–8.

206 Milton, J. D., *et al.*, 'Immune responsiveness in chronic fatigue syndrome', *Postgraduate Medical Journal*, 1991, 67, 532–7.

207 Morrison, L. J. A., *et al.*, 'Changes in natural killer cell phenotype in patients with post-viral fatigue syndrome', *Clinical and Experimental Immunology*, 1991, 83, 441–6.

208 Morte, S., *et al.*, 'Gamma-interferon and chronic fatigue syndrome', *Lancet*, 1988, 2, 623–4.

209 Morte, S., *et al.*, 'Production of interleukin-1 in peripheral blood mononuclear cells in patients with chronic fatigue syndrome', *Journal of Infectious Diseases*, 1989, 152, 362.

210 Murdoch, J. C., 'Cell-mediated immunity in patients with myalgic encephalomyelitis syndrome', *New Zealand Medical Journal*, 1988, 101, 511–12.

211 Natelson, B. H., *et al.*, 'Frequency of deviant immunological test values in chronic fatigue syndrome patients', *Clinical and Diagnostic Laboratory Immunology*, 1995, 2, 238–40.

212 Peakman, M., *et al.*, 'Clinical improvement in chronic fatigue syndrome is not associated with lymphocyte subsets of function or activation', *Clinical Immunology and Immunopathology*, 1997, 82, 83–91.

213 Penttila, I. A., 'Cytokine dysregulation in post Q fever debility and fatigue syndrome', *Quarterly Journal of Medicine*.

214 Peterson, P. K., *et al.*, 'Effects of mild exercise on cytokines and cerebral blood flow in chronic fatigue syndrome patients', *Clinical Diagnostic Laboratory Immunology*, 1994, 1, 222–36.

215 Read, R., *et al.*, 'IgG1 subclass deficiency in patients with chronic fatigue syndrome', *Lancet*, 1988, 1, 241–2.

216 Rook, G. A. W. and Zumla, A., 'Gulf War Syndrome: Is it due to a sys-

temic shift in cytokine balance towards a Th2 profile?' *Lancet*, 1997, 349, 1831–3.

217 Straus, S. E., *et al.*, 'Circulating lymphokine levels in the chronic fatigue syndrome' (letter), *Journal of Infectious Diseases*, 1989, 160, 1085–6.

218 Straus, S. E., *et al.*, 'Lymphocyte phenotype and function in the chronic fatigue syndrome', *Journal of Clinical Immunology*, 1993, 13, 30–40.

219 Subira, M. L., *et al.*, 'Deficient display of CD3 on lymphocytes of patients with chronic fatigue syndrome', *Journal of Infectious Diseases*, 1989, 160, 165–6.

220 Swanink, C. M. A., *et al.*, 'Lymphocyte subsets, apoptosis and cytokines in patients with chronic fatigue syndrome', *Journal of Infectious Diseases*, 1996, 173, 460–3.

221 Tirelli, U., *et al.*, 'Immunological abnormalities in patients with chronic fatigue syndrome', *Scandinavian Journal of Immunology*, 1994, 40, 601–8.

222 Vojdani, A., *et al.*, 'Elevated apoptotic cell population in patients with chronic fatigue syndrome: the pivotal role of protein kinase RNA', *Journal of Internal Medicine*, 1997, 242, 465–78.

223 Von Mikecz, A., *et al.*, 'High frequency of autoantibodies of insoluble cellular antigens in patients with chronic fatigue syndrome', *Arthritis and Rheumatology*, 1997, 40, 295–305.

224 Wakefield, D., *et al.*, 'Immunoglobulin subclass abnormalities in patients with chronic fatigue syndrome', *Paediatric Infectious Disease Journal*, 1990, 9, S50–S53.

## Muscle

225 Arnold, D. L., *et al.*, 'Excessive intracellular acidosis of skeletal muscle on exercise in a patient with a post-viral/exhaustion fatigue syndrome', *Lancet*, 1994, 1, 1367–9.

226 Barnes, P. R. J., *et al.*, 'Skeletal muscle bioenergetics in the chronic fatigue syndrome', *Journal of Neurology, Neurosurgery and Psychiatry*, 1993, 56, 679–83.

227 Behan, W. M. H., *et al.*, 'Mitochondrial abnormalities in the post-viral fatigue syndrome', *Acta Neuropathologica*, 1991, 83, 61–5.

228 Byrne, E., *et al.*, 'Chronic fatigue and myalgia syndrome: mitochondrial and glycolytic studies in skeletal muscle', *Journal of Neurology, Neurosurgery and Psychiatry*, 1987, 50, 743–6.

229 Connolly, S., *et al.*, 'Chronic fatigue: electromyographic and neuropathological evaluation', *Journal of Neurology*, 1993, 240 (7), 435–8 and *Journal of Neurology, Neurosurgery and Psychiatry*, 1994, 57, 1157 (letter).

230 Djaldetti, R., *et al.*, 'Fatigue in multiple sclerosis compared with chronic fatigue syndrome', *Neurology*, 1996, 46, 632–5.

231 Gibson, H., *et al.*, 'Exercise performance and fatiguability in patients with chronic fatigue syndrome', *Journal of Neurology, Neurosurgery and Psychiatry*, 1993, 56, 993–8.

232 Grau, J. M., *et al.*, 'Chronic fatigue syndrome: studies on skeletal muscle', *Clinical Neuropathology*, 1992, 11, 329–32.

233 Jamal, G. A. and Hansen, S., 'Post-viral fatigue syndrome: evidence for underlying organic disturbance in the muscle fibre', *European Neurology*, 1989, 29, 273–6.

234 Kent-Braun, J., *et al.*, 'Central basis of muscle fatigue in chronic fatigue syndrome', *Neurology*, 1993, 43, 125–31.

235 Kuratsune, H., *et al.*, 'Acylcarnitine deficiency in chronic fatigue syndrome', *Clinical Infectious Diseases*, 1994, 18 (Suppl. 1), 62–7.

236 Lane, R. J. M., *et al.*, 'A double-blind, placebo-controlled, crossover study of verapamil in exertional muscle pain', *Muscle and Nerve*, 1986, 9, 635–41.

237 Lane, R. J. M., *et al.*, 'Exercise responses and psychiatric disorder in chronic fatigue syndrome', *British Medical Journal*, 1995, 311, 544–5.

238 Lloyd, A. R., *et al.*, 'Muscle strength, endurance and recovery in the post-infection fatigue syndrome', *Journal of Neurology, Neurosurgery and Psychiatry*, 1988, 51, 1316–22.

239 Lloyd, A. R., 'Muscle and brain: chronic fatigue syndrome', *Medical Journal of Australia*, 1990, 153, 530–4.

240 Lloyd, A. R., *et al.*, 'Muscle performance, voluntary activation, twitch properties and perceived effort in normal subjects and patients with chronic fatigue syndrome', *Brain*, 1991, 114, 85–9.

241 Lodi, R. L., *et al.*, 'Chronic fatigue syndrome and skeletal muscle mitochondrial function', *Muscle and Nerve*, 1997, 20, 765–6.

242 Majeed, T., *et al.*, 'Abnormalities of carnitine metabolism in chronic fatigue syndrome', *European Journal of Neurology*, 1995, 2, 425–8.

243 McCully, K. K., *et al.*, 'Reduced oxidative muscle metabolism in chronic fatigue syndrome', *Muscle and Nerve*, 1996, 19, 621–5.

244 Pacy, P. J., *et al.*, 'Post-absorptive whole body leucine kinetics and quadriceps muscle protein synthesis rate (MPSR) in the post-viral syndrome', *Clinical Science*, 1988, 75 (suppl. 19) 36–7.

245 Plioplys, A. and Plioplys, S., 'Electron-microscopic investigation of muscle mitochondria and chronic fatigue syndrome', *Neuropsychobiology*, 1995, 32, 175–81.

246 Plioplys, A. V., 'Anti-muscle and anti-CNS circulating antibodies in chronic fatigue syndrome', *Neurology*, 1997, 48, 1717–19.

247 Preedy, V. R., *et al.*, 'Biochemical and muscle studies in patients

with acute onset post-viral fatigue syndrome', *Journal of Clinical Pathology*, 1993, 46, 722–6.

248 Riley, M. S., *et al.*, 'Aerobic work capacity in patients with chronic fatigue syndrome', *British Medical Journal*, 1990, 301, 953–6.

249 Roberts, L. and Byrne, E., 'Single fibre EMG studies in chronic fatigue syndrome: a reappraisal', *Journal of Neurology, Neurosurgery and Psychiatry*, 1994, 57, 375–6.

250 Rutherford, O. and White, P., 'Human quadriceps strength and fatiguability in patients with post-viral fatigue', *Journal of Neurology, Neurosurgery and Psychiatry*, 1991, 54, 961–4.

251 Stokes, M. J., *et al.*, 'Normal muscle strength and fatiguability in patients with effort syndromes', *British Medical Journal*, 1988, 297, 1014–17. Correspondence 1610–11; 298, 1521–22 and 1711–12.

252 Teahon, K., *et al.*, 'Clinical studies of the post-viral fatigue syndrome with special reference to skeletal muscle function', *Clinical Science*, 1988, 75, 45.

253 Walton, J., 'Diffuse exercise-induced muscle pain of undetermined cause relieved by verapamil', *Lancet*, 1981, i, 993.

254 Wassif, W. S., *et al.*, 'Use of dynamic tests of muscle function and histomorphometry of quadriceps muscle biopsies in the investigation of patients with chronic alcohol misuse and chronic fatigue syndrome', *Annals of Clinical Biochemistry*, 1994, 31, 462–8.

255 Wong, R., *et al.*, 'Skeletal muscle metabolism in the chronic fatigue syndrome', *Chest*, 1992, 102, 1716–22.

256 Yonge, R. P., 'Magnetic resonance muscle studies: implications for psychiatry', *Journal of the Royal Society of Medicine*, 1988, 81, 322–6.

357 Zhang, C., *et al.*, 'Unusual pattern of mitochondrial DNA deletions in skeletal muscle of an adult with chronic fatigue syndrome', *Human Molecular Genetics*, 1995, 4, 751–4.

## Neuroimaging (MRI and SPECT scans)

258 Buchwald, D., *et al.*, 'A chronic illness characterised by fatigue, neurologic and immunologic disorders and active human herpesvirus type 6 infection', *Annals of Internal Medicine*, 1992, 116, 103–13.

259 Cope, H., *et al.*, 'Cognitive functioning and magnetic resonance imaging in chronic fatigue', *'British Journal of Psychiatry*, 1995, 167, 86–94.

260 Cope, H. and David, A., 'Neuroimaging in chronic fatigue syndrome', *Journal of Neurology, Neurosurgery and Psychiatry*, 1996, 60, 471–3.

261 Costa, D., *et al.*, 'Brainstem perfusion is impaired in patients with myalgic encephalomyelitis/chronic fatigue syndrome', *Quarterly*

*Journal of Medicine*, 1995, 88, 767–73.

262 Daugherty, S., *et al.*, 'Chronic fatigue syndrome in Northern Nevada', *Reviews of Infectious Diseases*, 1991, 13 (suppl. 1) S39–44.

263 Fishler, B., *et al.*, 'Comparison of 99m HMPAO SPECT scan between chronic fatigue syndrome, major depression and healthy controls: an exploratory study of clinical correlates of regional cerebral blood flow', *Neuropsychobiology*, 1996, 34, 175–83.

264 Golberg, M. J., *et al.*, 'NeuroSPECT findings in children with chronic fatigue syndrome', *Journal of Chronic Fatigue Syndrome*, 1997, 3, 61–8.

265 Greco, A., *et al.*, 'Brain MR in chronic fatigue syndrome', *American Journal of Neuroradiology*, 1997, 18, 1265–9.

266 Ichise, M., *et al.*, 'Assessment of regional cerebral perfusion by $^{99}Tc^m$ – HMPAO SPECT in chronic fatigue syndrome', *Nuclear Medicine Communications*, 1992, 13, 767–72.

267 Natelson, B. H., *et al.*, 'A controlled study of brain magnetic resonance imaging in patients with the chronic fatigue syndrome', *Journal of the Neurological Sciences*, 1993, 120, 213–17.

268 Patterson, J. *et al.*, 'SPECT brain imagining in chronic fatigue syndrome', *Reviews of Immunology and Immunopharmacology*, 1995, 15, 53–8.

269 Schwartz, R. B., *et al.*, 'Detection of intracranial abnormalities in patients with chronic fatigue syndrome: comparison of MR imaging and SPECT', *American Journal of Roentgenlogy*, 1994, 162, 935–41.

270 Schwartz, R. B., *et al.*, 'SPECT imaging of the brain: comparison of findings in patients with chronic fatigue syndrome, AIDS dementia complex and major unipolar depression', *American Journal of Roentgenology*, 1994, 162, 943–51.

271 Simon, T. R., *et al.*, 'Chronic fatigue syndrome: flow and functional abnormalities seen with SPECT', *Radiology*, 1991, 181, S173.

272 Tavio, M., *et al.*, 'Brain positron emission tomography (PET) in chronic fatigue syndrome: a useful tool for differential diagnosis', American Association for Chronic Fatigue Syndrome: Research Conference, San Francisco, 1996.

## Neurotransmitter abnormalities

273 Chaudhuri, A., *et al.*, 'Chronic fatigue syndrome: a disorder of central cholinergic transmission', *Journal of Chronic Fatigue Syndrome*, 1997, 3, 3–16.

274 Demitrack, M. A., *et al.*, 'Plasma and cerebrospinal fluid monoamine metabolism in patients with chronic fatigue syndrome: preliminary findings', *Biological Psychiatry*, 1992, 32, 1065–77.

275 Dinan, T. G., *et al.*, 'Blunted serotonin-mediated activation of the

hypothalamic-pituitary–adrenal axis in chronic fatigue syndrome', *Psychoneuroimmunology*, 1997, 4, 261–7.

## Psychological testing

276 Altay, H., *et al.*, 'The neuropsychological dimensions of post infectious neuromyasthenia (chronic fatigue syndrome): a preliminary report', *International Journal of Psychiatric Medicine*, 1990, 20, 141–9.

277 Cope, H., *et al.*, 'Cognitive functioning and magnetic resonance imaging in chronic fatigue', *British Journal of Psychiatry*, 1995, 167, 86–94.

278 DeLuca, J., *et al.*, 'Information processing efficiency in chronic fatigue syndrome and multiple sclerosis', *Archives of Neurology*, 1993, 50, 301–4.

279 DeLuca, J., *et al.*, 'Neuropsychological impairments in chronic fatigue syndrome, multiple sclerosis and depression', *Journal of Neurology, Neurosurgery and Psychiatry*, 1995, 58, 38–43.

280 DeLuca, J., *et al.*, 'Cognitive functioning is impaired in patients with chronic fatigue syndrome devoid of psychiatric disease', *Journal of Neurology, Neurosurgery and Psychiatry*, 1997, 62, 151–5.

281 Gaudino, E. A., *et al.*, 'Post-Lyme syndrome and chronic fatigue syndrome: neuropsychiatric similarities and differences', *Archives of Neurology*, 1997, 54, 1372–6.

282 Grafman, J., *et al.*, 'Analysis of neuropsychological functioning in patients with chronic fatigue syndrome', *Journal of Neurology, Neurosurgery and Psychiatry*, 1993, 56, 684–9.

283 Johnson, S. K., *et al.*, 'Selective impairment of auditory processing in chronic fatigue syndrome: a comparison with multiple sclerosis and healthy controls', *Perceptual and Motor Skills*, 1996, 83, 51–62.

284 Joyce, E., *et al.*, 'Memory, attention and executive function in chronic fatigue syndrome', *Journal of Neurology, Neurosurgery and Psychiatry*, 1996, 60, 495–503.

285 Kane, R. L., *et al.*, 'Neuropsychological and psychological functioning in chronic fatigue syndrome', *Neuropsychiatry and Neuropsychological Behavioural Neurology*, 1997, 10, 25–31.

286 Krupp, L. B., *et al.*, 'Cognitive functioning and depression in patients with chronic fatigue syndrome and multiple sclerosis', *Archives of Neurology*, 1994, 51, 705–10.

287 McDonald, E., *et al.*, 'Cognitive impairment in patients with chronic fatigue: a preliminary study', *Journal of Neurology, Neurosurgery and Psychiatry*, 1993, 56, 812–15.

288 Marcel, B., *et al.*, 'Cognitive defects in patients with chronic fatigue syndrome', *Biological Psychiatry*, 1996, 40, 535–41.

289 Marshall, P., *et al.*, 'An assessment of cognitive function and mood in chronic fatigue syndrome', *Biological Psychiatry*, 1996, 39, 199–206.

290 Michiels, V., *et al.*, 'Cognitive functioning in patients with chronic fatigue syndrome', *Journal of Experimental Neuropsychology*, 1996, 18, 666–77.

291 Moss-Morris, R., *et al.*, 'Neuropsychological deficits in chronic fatigue syndrome: artefact or reality?', *Journal of Neurology, Neurosurgery, Psychiatry*, 1996, 60, 474–7.

292 Ray, C., *et al.*, 'Quality of attention in chronic fatigue syndrome: subjective reports of everyday attention and cognitive difficulty, and performance on tasks of focused attention,' *British Journal of Clinical Psychology*, 1993, 32, 357–64.

293 Riccio, M., *et al.*, 'Neuropsychological and psychiatric abnormalities in myalgic encephalomyelitis: a preliminary report', *British Journal of Clinical Psychology*, 1992, 31, 111–20.

294 Sandman, C. A., *et al.*, 'Memory deficits associated with chronic fatigue immune dysfunction syndrome', *Biological Psychiatry*, 1993, 33, 618–23.

295 Scheffers, M. K., *et al.*, 'Attention and short-term memory in chronic fatigue syndrome patients – an even-related potential analysis', *Neurology*, 1992, 42, 1667–75.

296 Schmaling, K., *et al.*, 'Cognitive functioning in chronic fatigue syndrome and depression: a preliminary comparison', *Psychosomatic Medicine*, 1994, 56, 383–8.

297 Smith, A., 'Cognitive changes in myalgic encephalomyelitis', in Jenkins, R. and Mowbray, J. F., (eds), *Post-viral Fatigue Syndrome*, Wiley, New York, 1991, 179–94.

298 Smith, A., *et al.*, 'Behavioural problems associated with the chronic fatigue syndrome', *British Journal of Psychology*, 1993, 84 (pt 3), 411–23.

299 Tiersky, L. A., *et al.*, 'Neuropsychology of chronic fatigue syndrome: a critical review', *Journal of Clinical and Experimental Neuropsychology*, 1997, 19, 560–86.

300 Vollmer-Conna, U., *et al.*, 'Cognitive defects in patients suffering from chronic fatigue syndrome, acute infective illness or depression', *British Journal of Psychiatry*, 1997, 171, 377–81.

301 Wearden, A. and Appleby, L., 'Cognitive performance and complaints of cognitive impairment in chronic fatigue syndrome', *Psychological Medicine*, 1997, 27, 81–90.

302 Wearden, A. and Appleby, L., 'Research on cognitive complaints and cognitive functioning in patients with chronic fatigue syndrome: what conclusions can we draw?' *Journal of Psychosomatic*

*Research*, 1996, 41, 197–211.

## Sleep

303 Arendt, J., 'Melatonin', *British Medical Journal*, 1996, 312, 1242–3.

304 Attenburrow, M. E. J., *et al.*, 'Case-controlled study of evening melatonin concentration in primary insomnia', *British Medical Journal*, 1996, 1263–4.

305 Bonn, D., 'Melatonin's multifarious marvels: miracle or myth?' *Lancet*, 1996, 347, 184.

306 Krupp, L. B., *et al.*, 'Sleep disturbance in chronic fatigue syndrome', *Journal of Psychosomatic Research*, 1993, 37, 325–31.

307 Moldofsky, H., 'Non-restorative sleep and symptoms after a febrile illness in patients with fibrositis and chronic fatigue syndromes', *Journal of Rheumatology*, 1989, (suppl. 19), 16, 150–3.

308 Morriss, R. K., *et al.*, 'Abnormalities in sleep in patients with chronic fatigue syndrome', *British Medical Journal*, 1993, 306, 1161–4.

309 Morriss, R. K., *et al.*, 'The relation of sleep difficulties to fatigue, mood and disability in chronic fatigue syndrome', *Journal of Psychosomatic Research*, 1997, 42, 597–605.

310 Sharpley, A., *et al.*, 'Do patients with "pure" chronic fatigue syndrome (neurasthenia) have abnormal sleep?' *Psychosomatic Medicine*, 1997, 59, 592–6.

311 Whelton, C. L., *et al.*, 'Sleep, Epstein-Barr virus infection, musculoskeletal pain and depressive symptoms in chronic fatigue syndrome', *Journal of Rheumatology*, 1992, 19, 939–43.

## Virology: general

312 Buchwald, D., *et al.*, 'Viral sequences in patients with chronic fatigue syndrome', *Journal of Medical Virology*, 1996, 50, 25–30.

313 Gow, J. W., *et al.*, 'Borna virus disease in chronic fatigue syndrome', *Neurological Infections and Epidemiology*, 1997, 2.

314 Martin, W. J. and Glass, R. T., 'Acute encephalopathy induced in cats with a stealth virus isolated from a patient with chronic fatigue syndrome', *Pathology*, 1995, 63, 115–18.

315 Mawle, A. C., *et al.*, 'Seroepidemiology of chronic fatigue syndrome', *Clinical Infectious Diseases*, 1995, 21, 1386–9.

316 Nakaya, T., *et al.*, 'Demonstration of Borna disease virus RNA in peripheral blood mononuclear cells derived from Japanese patients with chronic fatigue syndrome', *FEBS* (letters), 1996, 378, 145–9.

317 Oldstone, M. B. A., *et al.*, 'Alterations of acetylcholine enzymes in neuroblastoma cells persistently infected with lymphocytic choriomeningitis virus', *Journal of Cell Physiology*, 1977, 91, 459–72.

318 Oldstone, M. B. A., 'Viruses can cause disease in the absence of

morphological evidence of cell injury: implications for uncovering new diseases in the future', *Journal of Infectious Diseases*, 1989, 159, 384–9.

## Virology: enteroviruses

319 Archard, L. C., *et al.*, 'Post-viral fatigue syndrome: persistence of enterovirus RNA in muscle and elevated creatine kinase', *Journal of the Royal Society of Medicine*, 1988, 81, 326–9.

320 Bell, E. J., *et al.*, 'Coxsackie B viruses and myalgic encephalomyelitis', *Journal of the Royal Society of Medicine*, 1988, 81, 329–31.

321 Bowles, N. E., *et al.*, 'Persistence of enterovirus RNA in muscle biopsy samples suggests that some cases of chronic fatigue syndrome result from a previous inflammatory viral myopathy', *Journal of Medicine*, 1993, 24, 145–60.

322 Calder, B. D. and Warnock, P. J., 'Coxsackie B infection in a Scottish general practice', *Journal of the Royal College of General Practitioners*, 1984, 34, 15–19.

323 Calder, B. D., *et al.*, 'Coxsackie B viruses and post-viral syndrome: a prospective study in general practice', *Journal of the Royal College of General Practitioners*, 1987, 37, 11–14.

324 Clements, G. B., *et al.*, 'Detection of enterovirus-specific RNA in serum: the relationship to chronic fatigue', *Journal of Medical Virology*, 1995, 45, 156–61.

325 Cunningham, L., *et al.*, 'Persistence of enteroviral RNA in chronic fatigue syndrome is associated with the abnormal production of equal amounts of positive and negative strands of enteroviral RNA', *Journal of General Virology*, 1990, 71, 1399–402.

326 Fegan, K. G., *et al.*, 'Myalgic encephalomyelitis – report of an epidemic', *Journal of the Royal College of General Practitioners*, 1983, 33, 335–7.

327 Galbraith, D. N., *et al.*, 'Phylogenic analysis of short enteroviral sequences from patients with chronic fatigue syndrome', *Journal of General Virology*, 1995, 75, 1701–7.

328 Galbraith, D. N., *et al.*, 'Evidence for enteroviral persistence in humans', *Journal of General Virology*, 1997, 78, 307–12.

329 Gow, J. W., *et al.*, 'Enteroviral sequences detected by polymerase chain reaction in muscle of patients with post-viral fatigue syndrome', *British Medical Journal*, 1991, 302, 692–6.

330 Gow, J. W., *et al.*, 'Studies on enterovirus in patients with chronic fatigue syndrome', *Clinical Infectious Diseases*, 1994, 18 (suppl. 1), 126–9.

331 McArdle, A., *et al.*, 'Investigation by polymerase chain reaction of enteroviral infection in patients with chronic fatigue syndrome',

*Clinical Science*, 1996, 90, 295–300.

332 McGarry, F., *et al.*, 'Enterovirus in chronic fatigue syndrome', *Annals of Internal Medicine*, 1994, 120, 972–3.

333 Melchers, W., *et al.*, 'There is no evidence for persistent enterovirus infections in chronic medical conditions in humans', *Reviews in Medical Virology*, 1994, 4, 235–43.

334 Miller, N. A., *et al.*, 'Antibody to Coxsackie B virus in diagnosing post-viral fatigue syndrome', *British Medical Journal*, 1991, 302, 140–3.

335 Muir, P. and Archard, L. C., 'There is evidence for persistent enterovirus infections in chronic medical conditions in humans', *Reviews in Medical Virology*, 1994, 4, 245–50.

336 Nairn, C., *et al.*, 'Comparison of Coxsackie B neutralisation and enteroviral PCR in chronic fatigue patients', *Journal of Medical Virology*, 1995, 46, 310–13.

337 Swanink, C. M. A., *et al.*, 'Enteroviruses and the chronic fatigue syndrome', *Clinical Infectious Diseases*, 1994, 19, 980–4.

338 Vedhara, K., *et al.*, 'Consequences of live polio virus vaccine administration in chronic fatigue syndrome', *Journal of Neuroimmunology*, 1997, 75, 183–95.

339 Yousef, G. E., *et al.*, 'Chronic enterovirus infection in patients with post-viral fatigue syndrome', *Lancet*, 1988, 1, 146–7.

## Virology: Epstein-Barr virus (glandular fever/infectious mononucleosis) and other herpes viruses

340 Buchwald, D., *et al.*, 'Frequency of "chronic active Epstein-Barr" virus infection in a general practice', *Journal of the American Medical Association*, 1987, 257, 2303–7.

341 Hamblin, T. J., *et al.*, 'Immunological reason for ill health after infectious mononucleosis', *British Medical Journal*, 1983, 287, 85–8.

342 Hellinger, W. C., *et al.*, 'Chronic fatigue syndrome and the diagnostic utility of antibody to Epstein-Barr virus early antigen', *Journal of the American Medical Association*, 1988, 260, 971–3.

343 Holmes, G. P., *et al.*, 'A cluster of patients with a chronic mononucleosis-like syndrome: is Epstein-Barr virus the cause?' *Journal of the American Medical Association*, 1987, 259, 2297–302.

344 Jones, J. F., *et al.*, 'Evidence for active Epstein-Barr virus infection in patients with persistent, unexplained illness: elevated anti-early antigen antibodies', *Annals of Internal Medicine*, 1985, 102, 1–7.

345 Jones, J. F., *et al.*, 'Antibodies to Epstein-Barr specific DNAse and DNA polymerase in the chronic fatigue syndrome', *Archives of Internal Medicine*, 1988, 148, 1957–60.

346 Josephs, S. F., *et al.*, 'HHV-6 reactivation in chronic fatigue syn-

drome', *Lancet*, 1991, 337, 1346–7.

347 Manian, F. A., 'Simultaneous measurement of antibodies to Epstein-Barr virus, human herpes virus 6, herpes simplex virus types 1 and 2 and 14 enteroviruses in chronic fatigue syndrome: is there evidence of activation of a non-specific polyclonal response?' *Clinical Infectious Diseases*, 1994, 19, 448–53.

348 Natelson, B. H., *et al.*, 'High titres of anti Epstein-Barr virus DNA polymerase are found in patients with severe fatiguing illness', *Journal of Medical Virology*, 1994, 42, 42–6.

349 Straus, S. E., *et al.*, 'Persisting illness and fatigue in adults with evidence of Epstein-Barr virus infection', *Annals of Internal Medicine*, 1985, 102, 7–16.

350 Straus, S. E., 'The chronic mononucleosis syndrome', *Journal of Infectious Diseases*, 1988, 157, 404–12.

351 Sumaya, C., 'Serologic and virologic epidemiology of Epstein-Barr virus: relevance to chronic fatigue syndrome', *Reviews of Infectious Diseases*, 1991, (suppl. 1), 13, S19–S25.

352 White, P. D., *et al.*, 'The existence of a fatigue syndrome after glandular fever', *Psychological Medicine*, 1995, 25, 907–16.

353 White, P. D., *et al.*, 'The validity and reliability of the fatigue syndrome that follows glandular fever', *Psychological Medicine*, 1995, 25, 917–24.

## Virology: retroviruses

354 De Freitas, E., *et al.*, 'Retroviral sequences related to human T-lymphotrophic virus type II in patients with chronic fatigue immune dysfunction syndrome', *Proceedings of the National Academy of Sciences (USA)*, 1991, 81, 2922–6.

355 Gow, J. W., *et al.*, 'Search for retrovirus in the chronic fatigue syndrome', *Journal of Clinical Pathology*, 1992, 45, 1058–61.

356 Gunn, W. J., *et al.*, 'Inability of retroviral tests to identify persons with chronic fatigue syndrome', *MMWR*, 1992, 42, 183–90.

357 Khan, A. S., *et al.*, 'Assessment of a retroviral sequence and other possible risk factors for chronic fatigue syndrome in adults', *Annals of Internal Medicine*, 1993, 188, 241–5.

## Other types of research into ME/CFS

358 Chaudhuri, A., *et al.*, 'Arguments for a role of abnormal ionophore function in chronic fatigue syndrome' in Yehuda and Mostofsky (eds), *Chronic Fatigue Syndrome*, Plenum Press, New York, 1997, 119–30.

359 Dworkin, H. J., *et al.*, 'Abnormal left ventricular myocardial dynamics in eleven patients with chronic fatigue syndrome',

*Clinical Nuclear Medicine*, 1994, 19, 675–7.

360 Lerner, A. M., *et al.*, 'Repetitively negative changing T waves at 24-h electrocardiographic monitors in patients with the chronic fatigue syndrome', *Chest*, 1993, 104, 1417–21.

361 Lieberman, J. and Bell, D. S., 'Serum angiotensin-converting enzyme as a marker for the chronic fatigue immune dysfunction syndrome: a comparison to serum angiotensin-converting enzyme in sarcoidosis', *American Journal of Medicine*, 1993, 95, 407–12.

362 McGregor, N. R., *et al.*, 'Preliminary determination of a molecular basis to chronic fatigue syndrome', *Biochemical and Molecular Medicine*, 1996, 57, 73–80.

363 McGregor, N. R., *et al.*, 'Preliminary determination of the association between symptom expression and urinary metabolites in subjects with chronic fatigue syndrome', *Biochemical and Molecular Medicine*, 1996, 58, 85–92.

364 Regland, B., *et al.*, 'Increased concentrations of homocysteine in the cerebrospinal fluid in patients with fibromyalgia and chronic fatigue syndrome', *Scandinavian Journal of Rheumatology*, 1997, 26, 301–7.

365 Suhadolnik, R. J., *et al.*, 'Upregulation of the 2-5A synthetase/Rnase L antiviral pathway associated with chronic fatigue syndrome', *Clinical Infectious Diseases*, 1994, 18 (suppl. 1), 96–104.

366 Suhadolnik, R., *et al.*, 'Biochemical evidence for a novel low molecular weight 2-5A dependent RNase L in chronic fatigue syndrome', *Journal of Interferon and Cytokine Research*, 1997, 17, 377–85.

# Chapter 9: ME/CFS and your Doctor

## *Blood tests*

367 Bates, D. W., *et al.*, 'Clinical laboratory test findings in patients with chronic fatigue syndrome', *Archives of Internal Medicine*, 1995, 155, 97–193.

368 Buchwald, D., *et al.*, 'Review of laboratory findings in patients with chronic fatigue syndrome', *Reviews of Infectious Diseases*, 1991, 13 (suppl. 1), S12–18.

369 Burnet, R. B., *et al.*, 'Chronic fatigue syndrome: is total body potassium important?' *Medical Journal of Australia*, 1996, 164, 384.

370 Cleary, K. J. and White, P. D., 'Gilbert's and chronic fatigue syndromes in men', *Lancet*, 1993, 341, 842.

371 Valesini, G., *et al.*, 'Gilbert's syndrome and chronic fatigue syndrome', *Lancet*, 1993, 341, 1162–3.

# Chapter 10: Drug Treatments

372 Adolphe, A. B., 'Chronic fatigue syndrome: possible effective treatment with nifedipine', *American Journal of Medicine*, 1988, 85, 892.

373 Aoki, T., *et al.*, 'Low natural killer cell syndrome: clinical and immunological features', *Natural Immunological Cell Growth Regulation*, 1987, 6, 116–28.

374 Baschetti, R., 'Chronic fatigue syndrome and liquorice', *New Zealand Journal of Medicine*, 1995, 108, 156–7.

375 Behan, P., *et al.*, 'A pilot study of sertraline for the treatment of chronic fatigue syndrome', *Clinical Infectious Diseases*, 1994, 18 (suppl. 1), S111.

376 Behan, P. O., *et al.*, 'Effect of high doses of essential fatty acids on the post-viral fatigue syndrome', *Acta Neurologica Scandinavia*, 1990, 82, 209–16.

377 Behan, P. O. and Behan, W. M. H., 'Post-viral fatigue syndrome', *CRC Critical Reviews in Neurobiology*, 1988, 4, 157–78.

378 Bendahan, D., *et al.*, 'P$^{31}$ NMR spectroscopy and ergometer exercise test as evidence for muscle oxidative performance improvement with coenzyme Q in mitochondrial myopathies', Neurology, 1992, 42, 1203–8.

379 Bou-Holaigah, I., *et al.*, 'The relationship between neurally mediated hypotension and the chronic fatigue syndrome', *Journal of the American Medical Association*, 1996, 274, 961–7.

380 Bowman, M. A., *et al.*, 'Use of amantadine for chronic fatigue syndrome', *Archives of Internal Medicine*, 1997, 157, 1264–5.

381 Brook, M. G., *et al.*, 'Interferon-alpha therapy for patients with chronic fatigue syndrome', *Journal of Infectious Diseases*, 1993, 168, 791–2.

382 Chaudhuri, A., *et al.*, 'Chronic fatigue syndrome: a disorder of central cholinergic transmission', *Journal of Chronic Fatigue Syndrome*, 1997, 3, 3–16.

383 Cox, I. M., *et al.*, 'Red blood cell magnesium and chronic fatigue syndrome', *Lancet*, 1991, 337, 757–60. See also letters on pages 1094–5 (Wessely, Young and Trimble, Richmond, Shepherd): 1295 (Cox *et al.*, Davies, Walden): 338, 66 (Gantz): 1992, 340, 124–5 (Claque *et al.*): 426 (Howard *et al.*).

384 Goldberg, M., 'High androgen levels in chronic fatigue patients', *Journal of Clinical Endocrinology and Metabolism*, 1995, 80, 3390–1.

385 Goodnick, P. J., *et al.*, 'Bupropion treatment of fluoxetine-resistant chronic fatigue syndrome', *Biological Psychiatry*, 1992, 32, 834–8.

386 Goodnick, P. J., 'Treatment of chronic fatigue syndrome with venlafaxine', *American Journal of Psychiatry*, 1996, 153, 294.

387 Hickie, I,. *et al.*, 'Immunological and psychological dysfunction in patients receiving immunotherapy for chronic fatigue syndrome', *Australian and New Zealand Journal of Psychiatry*, 1992, 26, 249–56.

388 Hickie, I., *et al.*, 'A randomised, double-blind, placebo-controlled trial of moclobemide in patients with chronic fatigue syndrome', *British Journal of Psychiatry*, 1998.

389 Lane, R. J. M., 'A double-blind, placebo-controlled, crossover study of verapamil in exertional muscle pain', *Muscle and Nerve*, 1986, 9, 635–41.

390 Lerner, A. M., *et al.*, 'New cardiomyopathy: pilot study on intravenous ganciclovir in a subset of the chronic fatigue syndrome', *Infectious Diseases in Clinical Practice*, 1997, 6, 110–17.

391 Lloyd, A. R., *et al.*, 'A double-blind, placebo-controlled trial of intravenous immunoglobulin therapy in patients with chronic fatigue syndrome', *American Journal of Medicine*, 1990, 89, 561–8.

392 Lloyd, A. R., *et al.*, 'Immunologic and psychologic therapy for patients with chronic fatigue syndrome: a double-blind, placebo-controlled trial', *American Journal of Medicine*, 1993, 94, 197–203. Correspondence: 1995, 98, 419–22.

393 McBride, S. J. and McCluskey, D. R., 'Treatment of chronic fatigue syndrome', *British Medical Bulletin*, 1991, 47, 895–907.

394 Natelson, B. H., *et al.*, 'Randomised, double blind, controlled placebo-phase in trial of low dose phenelzine in the chronic fatigue syndrome', *Psychopharmacology*, 1996, 124, 226–30.

395 Peterson, P. K., *et al.*, 'A controlled trial of intravenous immunoglobulin G in chronic fatigue syndrome', *American Journal of Medicine*, 1990, 89, 554–60.

396 Plioplys, A. V. and Plioplys, S., 'Meeting the frustrations of chronic fatigue syndrome', *Hospital Practice*, 1997, 35, 16–23.

397 Plioplys, A. V. and Plioplys, S., 'Amantadine and L-carnitine treatment of chronic fatigue syndrome', *Neuropsychobiology*, 1997, 35, 16–23.

398 Rowe, K. S., 'Double-blind randomised controlled trial to assess the efficacy of intravenous gammaglobulin for the management of chronic fatigue syndrome in adolescents', *Journal of Psychiatric Research*, 1997, 31, 133–47.

399 See, D. M. and Tilles, J. G., 'Alpha-interferon treatment of patients with chronic fatigue syndrome', *Immunological Investigations*, 1996, 25, 153–64.

400 Skinner, G. R. B., *et al.*, 'Thyroxine should be tried in clinically hypothyroid but biochemically euthyroid patients', *British Medical Journal*, 1997, 314, 1764. Correspondence: 1997, 315, 491.

401 Skolnick, A. A., 'Scientific verdict still out on DHEA', *Journal of the*

*American Medical Association*, 1996, 276, 1365–7.

402 Snorrason, E., *et al.*, 'Trial of a selective acetylcholinesterase inhibitor, galanthamine hydrobromide, in the treatment of chronic fatigue syndrome', *Journal of Chronic Fatigue Syndrome*, 1996, 2, 35–54.

403 Steinberg, P., *et al.*, 'Double-blind, placebo-controlled study of the efficacy of oral terfenadine in the treatment of chronic fatigue syndrome', *Journal of Allergy and Clinical Immunology*, 1996, 97, 119–26.

404 Straus, S. E., *et al.*, 'Acyclovir treatment of the chronic fatigue syndrome: lack of efficacy in a placebo-controlled trial', *New England Journal of Medicine*, 1988, 319, 1692–8.

405 Strayer, D. R., *et al.*, 'A controlled clinical trial with a specifically configured RNA drug, poly (1). Poly ($C_{12}U$) in chronic fatigue syndrome', *Clinical Infectious Diseases*, 1994, 18 (suppl. 1), S88–95.

406 Studd, J. and Panay, N., 'Chronic fatigue syndrome', *Lancet*, 1996, 348, 1384.

407 Vercoulen, J., *et al.*, 'Randomized, double-blind, placebo-controlled study of fluoxetine in chronic fatigue syndrome', *Lancet*, 1996, 347, 858–61. Correspondence, 1770–2.

408 Vollmer-Conna, U., *et al.*, 'Intravenous immunoglobulin is ineffective in the treatment of patients with chronic fatigue syndrome', *American Journal of Medicine*, 1997, 103, 38–43.

409 Walton, J., 'Diffuse exercise-induced muscle pain of undetermined cause relieved by verapamil', *Lancet*, 1981, i, 993.

410 White, P. D., *et al.*, 'An open study of the efficacy and adverse effects of moclobemide in patients with the chronic fatigue syndrome', *International Clinical Psychopharmacology*, 1997, 12, 47–52.

411 Wiebe, E., 'Managing patients with chronic fatigue syndrome: a case report', *Canadian Family Physician*, 1996, 42, 2214–17.

# Chapter 11: Self-help

*Exercise*

412 Elliot, D. L., *et al.*, 'Graded exercise testing and chronic fatigue syndrome', *American Journal of Medicine*, 1997, 103, 84–6.

413 Fulcher, K. Y. and White, P. D., 'Randomised controlled trial of graded exercise in patients with chronic fatigue syndrome', *British Medical Journal*, 1997, 314, 1647–52. Correspondence: 315, 947–8.

414 Lapp, C. W., 'Exercise limits in the chronic fatigue syndrome', *American Journal of Medicine*, 1997, 103, 83–4.

415 Sharpe, M. and Wessely, S., 'Putting the rest cure to rest-again',

*British Medical Journal*, 1998, 316, 796.

416 Sisto, S. A., *et al.*, 'Metabolic and cardiovascular effects of a progressive exercise test in patients with chronic fatigue syndrome', *American Journal of Medicine*, 1996, 100, 634–40.

# Chapter 12: Mind and Body

## *General psychiatry*

417 Blakely, A. A., *et al.*, 'Psychiatric symptoms, personality and ways of coping in chronic fatigue syndrome', *Psychological Medicine*, 1991, 21, 347–62.

418 Buchwald, D., *et al.*, 'Screening for psychiatric disorders in chronic fatigue and chronic fatigue syndrome', *Journal of Psychosomatic Research*, 1997, 42, 87–94.

419 Chalder, T., *et al.*, 'Chronic fatigue in the community: a question of attribution', *Psychological Medicine*, 1996, 26, 791–800.

420 Cope, H., *et al.*, '"Maybe it's a virus?": beliefs about viruses, symptom attributional style and psychological health', *Journal of Psychosomatic Research*, 1994, 38, 89–98.

421 Cope, H., *et al.*, 'Psychological risk factors for chronic fatigue and chronic fatigue syndrome following presumed viral illness: a case-controlled study', *Psychological Medicine*, 1996, 26, 1197–209.

422 Farmer, A., *et al.*, 'Neurasthenia revisited: ICD1O and DSM-111-R psychiatric syndromes in chronic fatigue patients and comparison subjects', *British Journal of Psychiatry*, 1995, 167, 503–6.

423 Farmer, A., *et al.*, 'Screening for psychiatric morbidity in subjects presenting with chronic fatigue syndrome', *British Journal of Psychiatry*, 1996, 168, 354–8.

424 Gold, D., *et al.*, 'Chronic fatigue: a prospective clinical and virological study', *Journal of the American Medical Association*, 1990, 264, 48–53.

425 Hickie, I., *et al.*, 'The psychiatric status of patients with the chronic fatigue syndrome', *British Journal of Psychiatry*, 1990, 154, 534–40.

426 Jason, L. A., *et al.*, 'Politics, science and the emergence of a new disease: the case of chronic fatigue syndrome', *American Psychologist*, 1997, 52, 973–83.

427 Johnson, S., *et al.*, 'Assessing somatisation disorder in the chronic fatigue syndrome', *Psychosomatic Medicine*, 1996, 58, 50–7.

428 Johnson, S., *et al.*, 'Personality dimensions in the chronic fatigue syndrome: a comparison with multiple sclerosis and depression', *Journal of Psychiatric Research*, 1996, 30, 9–20.

429 Johnson, S., *et al.*, 'Depression in fatiguing illness: comparing

patients with chronic fatigue syndrome, multiple sclerosis and depression', *Journal of Affective Disorder*.

430 Katon, W., *et al.*, 'Psychiatric illness in patients with chronic fatigue and rheumatoid arthritis', *Journal of General Internal Medicine*, 1991, 6, 277–85.

431 Kendall, R., 'Chronic fatigue, viruses and depression', *Lancet*, 1991, 337, 160–2. Correspondence: 564–5.

432 Kruesi, M., *et al.*, 'Psychiatric diagnoses in patients who have chronic fatigue syndrome', *Journal of Clinical Psychiatry*, 1989, 50, 53–6.

433 Lane, T. J., *et al.*, 'Depression and somatisation in the chronic fatigue syndrome', *American Journal of Medicine*, 1991, 91, 335–44.

434 Manu, P., *et al.*, 'The mental health of patients with a chief complaint of chronic fatigue: a prospective evaluation and follow-up', *Archives of Internal Medicine*, 1988, 148, 2213–17.

435 Manu, P., *et al.*, 'Somatisation disorder in patients with chronic fatigue syndrome', *Psychosomatics*, 1989, 30, 388–95.

436 Petrie, K., *et al.*, 'The impact of catastrophic beliefs on functioning in chronic fatigue syndrome', *Journal of Psychosomatic Research*, 1995, 39, 31–7.

437 Powell, R,. *et al.*, 'Attributions and self-esteem in depression and chronic fatigue syndromes', *Journal of Psychosomatic Research*, 1990, 34, 665–73.

438 Ray, C., 'Chronic fatigue syndrome and depression: conceptual and methodological ambiguities', *Psychological Medicine*, 1991, 21, 1–9.

439 Ray, C., *et al.*, 'Coping with chronic fatigue syndrome: illness responses and their relationship with fatigue, functional impairment and emotional status', *Psychological Medicine*, 1995, 25, 937–45.

440 Shanks, M. F. and Ho-Yen, D. O., 'A clinical study of chronic fatigue syndrome', *British Journal of Psychiatry*, 1995, 166, 798–801.

441 Taerk, G. S., *et al.*, 'Depression in patients with neuromyasthenia (benign myalgic encephalomyelitis)', *International Journal of Psychiatry*, 1987, 17, 49–56.

442 Wessely, S., 'Myalgic encephalomyelitis – a warning' (discussion paper), *Journal of the Royal Society of Medicine*, 1989, 82, 215–17.

443 Wessely, S. and Powell, R., 'Fatigue syndromes: a comparison of chronic "post-viral" fatigue with neuromuscular and affective disorders', *Journal of Neurology, Neurosurgery and Psychiatry*, 1989, 52, 940–8.

444 Wessely, S., *et al.*, 'Psychological symptoms, somatic symptoms and psychiatric disorder in chronic fatigue and chronic fatigue syndrome: a prospective study in primary care', *American Journal of Psychiatry*, 1996, 153, 1050–9.

445 Wessely, S., 'Chronic fatigue syndrome: a 20th century illness?' *Scandinavian Journal of Work and Environmental Health*, 1997, 23, S17–34.

446 Wood, G., *et al.*, 'A comparative psychiatric assessment of patients with chronic fatigue syndrome and muscle disease', *Psychological Medicine*, 1991, 21, 619–28.

447 Yeomans, J. D. I. and Conway, S. P., 'Biopsychosocial aspects of chronic fatigue syndrome', *Journal of Infection*, 1991, 23, 263–9.

## Cognitive behaviour therapy

448 Best, L., *Cognitive Behaviour Therapy in the Treatment of Chronic Fatigue Syndrome*, Wessex Institute of Public Health Medicine, 1996.

449 Bonner, D., *et al.*, 'A follow up study of chronic fatigue syndrome', *Journal of Neurology, Neurosurgery and Psychiatry*, 1994, 57, 617–21.

450 Butler, S., *et al.*, 'Cognitive behaviour therapy in chronic fatigue syndrome', *Journal of Neurology, Neurosurgery and Psychiatry*, 1991, 54, 153–8.

451 Deale, A., *et al.*, 'Cognitive behaviour therapy for the chronic fatigue syndrome: a randomised controlled trial', *American Journal of Psychiatry*, 1997, 154, 408–14.

452 Deale, A., *et al.*, 'Illness beliefs and outcome in chronic fatigue syndrome: do patients need to change their beliefs in order to get better?' *Journal of Psychosomatic Research*, 1998, 45, 77–83.

453 Friedberg, F. and Krupp, L. B., 'A comparison of cognitive behavioural treatment for chronic fatigue syndrome and depression', *Clinical Infectious Diseases*, 1994, 18 (suppl. 1), S105–10.

454 Lloyd, A., *et al.*, 'Immunologic and psychological therapy for patients with chronic fatigue syndrome', *American Journal of Medicine*, 1993, 94, 197–203. Correspondence: 1995, 98, 419–22.

455 Sharpe, M., *et al.*, 'Cognitive behaviour therapy for chronic fatigue syndrome: a randomised controlled trial', *British Medical Journal*, 1996, 312, 22–6.

456 Suraway, C., *et al.*, 'Chronic fatigue syndrome: a cognitive approach', *Behaviour Research Therapy*, 1995, 33, 535–44.

## Hyperventilation

457 Bazelmans, E., *et al.*, 'The chronic fatigue syndrome and hyperventilation', *Journal of Psychosomatic Research*, 1997, 43, 371–7.

458 Dyer, C., 'Cardiologist admits research misconduct', *British Medical Journal*, 1997, 314, 1501.

459 Gardner, W., 'Hyperventilation disorders', *Journal of the Royal Society of Medicine*, 1990, 83, 755–7.

460 Nixon, P. G. F. and Freeman, L. J., 'The "think test": a further technique to elicit hyperventilation', *Journal of the Royal Society of Medicine*, 1988, 81, 277–9.

461 Rosen, S. D., *et al.*, 'Is chronic fatigue syndrome synonymous with effort syndrome?' *Journal of the Royal Society of Medicine*, 1990, 83, 761–4.

462 Saisch, S. G. N., *et al.*, 'Hyperventilation and the chronic fatigue syndrome', *Quarterly Journal of Medicine*, 1994, 87, 63–7.

# Chapter 13: Alternative and Complementary Approaches to the Management of ME/CFS

## Acupuncture

463 Deluze, C., *et al.*, 'Electroacupuncture in fibromyalgia: results of a controlled trial', *British Medical Journal*, 1992, 305, 1249–52.

464 Norheim, A. J. and Fønnebø, V., 'Adverse effects of acupuncture', *Lancet*, 1995, 345, 1576.

## Allergy

465 Olson, G. B., *et al.*, 'Correlation between allergy and persistent Epstein-Barr virus infections in the chronic-active Epstein-Barr virus-infected patients', *Journal of Allergy and Clinical Immunology*, 1986, 78, 308–20.

466 Steinberg, P., *et al.*, 'Double-blind placebo-controlled study of the efficacy of oral terfenadine in the treatment of chronic fatigue syndrome', *Journal of Allergy and Clinical Immunology*, 1996, 97, 119–26.

467 Straus, S. E., *et al.*, 'Allergy and chronic fatigue syndrome', *Journal of Allergy and Clinical Immunology*, 1988, 81, 791–5.

## Candida albicans

468 Bennett, J. E., 'Searching for the yeast connection', *New England Journal of Medicine*, 1990, 323, 1766–7.

469 Cater, R. E., 'Chronic intestinal candidiasis as a possible aetiological factor in the chronic fatigue syndrome', *Medical Hypotheses*, 1995, 44, 507–15.

470 Dismukes, W. E., *et al.*, 'A randomized, double-blind trial of Nystatin therapy for the candidiasis hypersensitivity syndrome', *New England Journal of Medicine*, 1990, 323, 1717–23. Editorial in the same issue on pages 1766–7. Correspondence on pages 1592–4.

471 Middleton, S. J., *et al.*, 'The role of faecal *Candida albicans* in the pathogenesis of food-intolerant irritable bowel syndrome',

*Postgraduate Medical Journal*, 1992, 68, 453–4.

472 Renfro, L., *et al.*, 'Yeast connection among 100 patients with chronic fatigue', *American Journal of Medicine*, 1989, 86, 165–8.

## Chemical sensitivities

473 Fieldler, N. F., *et al.*, 'A controlled comparison of multiple chemical sensitivities and chronic fatigue syndrome', *Psychosomatic Medicine*, 1996, 58, 38–49.

## Dental amalgam removal

474 Barregård, L., *et al.*, 'People with high mercury uptake from their own dental amalgam fillings', *Occupational and Environmental Medicine*, 1995, 52, 124–8.

## Dietary supplementation

475 Cox, I. M., *et al.*, 'Red blood cell magnesium and chronic fatigue syndrome', *Lancet*, 1991, 337, 757–60. Letters on pages 1094–5 (Wessely, Young and Trimble, Richmond, Shepherd): 1295 (Cox *et al.*, Davies, Walden): 338, 66 (Gantz): 1992, 340, 124–5 (Clague *et al.*): 426 (Howard *et al.*).

476 Dalton, K. and Dalton, M. J. T. 'Characteristics of pyridoxine overdose neuropathy syndrome', *Acta Neurologica Scandinavia*, 1987, 76, 8–11.

477 Evans, C. D. H. and Lacey, J. H., 'Toxicity of vitamins – complications of a health movement', *British Medical Journal*, 1986, 292, 509–10.

478 Jacobson, W., *et al.*, 'Serum folate and chronic fatigue syndrome', *Neurology*, 1993, 43, 2645–7, and *Neurology*, 1994, 44, 2214–15 (letter from Schmidley and Hines).

479 Kaslow, J. E., *et al.*, 'Liver extract – folic acid – cyanocobalamin vs placebo for chronic fatigue syndrome', *Archives of Internal Medicine*, 1989, 149, 2501–3.

480 Lewis, J. G., 'Adverse reactions to vitamins', *Adverse Drug Reaction Bulletin*, 1982, 296–9.

## Herbal medicines

481 Baldwin, C. A., *et al.*, 'What pharmacists should know about ginseng', *Pharmaceutical Journal*, 1986, 583–6.

482 Behan, P. O., *et al.*, 'Effect of high doses of essential fatty acids on the post-viral fatigue syndrome', *Acta Neurologica Scandinavica*, 1990, 82, 209–16.

483 De Smet, P. A. G. M. and Nolen, W. A., 'St John's Wort as an antidepressant', *British Medical Journal*, 1996, 313, 241–2.

484 Kleinjnen, J. and Knipschild, P., 'Ginkgo biloba', *Lancet*, 1992, 340, 1136–9.

485 Lewis, J. G., 'Adverse reactions to vitamins', *Adverse Drug Reaction Bulletin*, 1980, 82, 296–9.

486 Leyton, E. and Pross, H., 'Chronic fatigue syndrome: do herbs or homeopathy help?' *Canadian Family Physician*, 1992, 38, 2021–6.

487 Linde, K., *et al.*, 'St John's Wort for depression – an overview and meta-analysis of randomised clinical trials', *British Medical Journal*, 1996, 313, 253–8.

488 MacGregor, F. B., *et al.*, 'Hepatotoxicity of herbal remedies (valerian)', *British Medical Journal*, 1989, 299, 1156–7.

## Homoeopathy

489 Awdry, R., 'Homoeopathy and chronic fatigue – the search for proof', *International Journal of Alternative and Complementary Medicine*, 1996, 14, 12–16.

490 Fisher, P., *et al.*, 'Effect of homoeopathic treatment on fibrositis (primary fibromyalgia)', *British Medical Journal*, 1989, 299, 365–6.

491 Jenkins, M., 'Thoughts on the management of ME', *British Journal of Homoeopathy*, 1989, 78, 6–14.

492 Linde, K., *et al.*, 'Are the clinical effects of homoeopathy placebo effects? A meta-analysis of placebo-controlled trials', *Lancet*, 1997, 350, 834–43. Commentaries on 824 and 825.

## Osteopathy

493 Perrin, R. N., *et al.*, 'An evaluation of the effectiveness of osteopathic treatment on symptoms associated with myalgic encephalomyelitis: a preliminary report', *Journal of Medical Engineering and Technology*, 1998, 22, 1–13.

# Chapter 14: Three Case Histories

## Children and young people with ME/CFS

494 Baetz-Greenwalt, B., *et al.*, 'Chronic fatigue syndrome in children and adolescents: a somatiform disorder often complicated by treatable organic disease', *Clinical Infectious Diseases*, 1993, 17, 571.

495 Bell, D., 'Chronic fatigue syndrome in children', *Journal of Chronic Fatigue Syndrome*, 1995, 1, 9–33.

496 Carter, B,. *et al.*, 'Chronic fatigue in children: illness or disease?' *Paediatrics*, 1993, 90, 163.

497 Carter, B., *et al.*, 'Case control study of chronic fatigue in paediatric patients', *Paediatrics*, 1995, 95, 179–86.

498 Cox, D. and Findley, L., 'Chronic fatigue syndrome in adolescence', *British Journal of Hospital Medicine*, 1994, 51, 614.

499 Dowsett, E. G. and Colby, J., 'Long term sickness absence due to ME/CFS in UK schools: an epidemiological study with medical and educational implications', *Journal of Chronic Fatigue Syndrome*, 197, 3, 29–42.

500 Feder, H., *et al.*, 'Outcome of 48 paediatric patients with chronic fatigue: a clinical experience', *Archives of Family Medicine*, 1994, 3, 1049–55.

501 Franklin, A., *Children with ME: Guidelines for School Doctors and General Practitioners*, ME Association, Essex, 1995.

502 Garralda, M., 'Severe chronic fatigue syndrome in childhood: a discussion of psychopathological mechanisms', *European Journal of Child and Adolescent Psychiatry*, 1992, 1, 111–18.

503 Giannopoulou, J. and Marriott, S., 'Chronic fatigue syndrome or affective disorder? Implications of diagnosis on management', *European Journal of Child and Adolescent Psychiatry*, 1994, 3, 97–100.

504 Graham, H., 'Family interventions in general practice: a case of chronic fatigue', *Journal of Family Therapy*, 1990, 13, 225–30.

505 Harris, F. and Taitz, L., 'Damaging diagnosis of myalgic encephalomyelitis in children', *British Medical Journal*, 1989, 299, 790.

506 Khawaja, S. and Van Boxel, P., 'Chronic fatigue syndrome in children', *Psychiatric Bulletin*, 1998, 22.

507 Lask, B. and Dillon, M. J., 'Post-viral fatigue syndrome', *Archives of Disease in Childhood*, 1990, 65, 1198.

508 Marcovitch, H., 'Managing chronic fatigue syndrome in children', *British Medical Journal*, 1997, 314, 1635–6.

509 Plioplys, A. V., 'Chronic fatigue syndrome should not be diagnosed in children', *Paediatrics*, 1997, 100, 270–1.

510 Richards, J. and Smith, F., 'Chronic fatigue syndrome in children and adolescents: general practitioners' experience of the problem and their views about its treatment', *Psychiatric Bulletin*, 1998.

511 Rikard-Bell, C. and Waters, B., 'Psychosocial management of chronic fatigue syndrome in adolescence', *Australia and New Zealand Psychiatry*, 1992, 26, 64–72.

512 Shepherd, C. B., 'Chronic fatigue syndrome: a joint paediatric-psychiatric approach', *Archives of Disease in Childhood*, 1992, 67, 1410.

513 Sidebotham, P., *et al.*, 'Refractory chronic fatigue syndrome in adolescence', *British Journal of Hospital Medicine*, 1994, 51, 110–12.

514 Smith, M., *et al.*, 'Chronic fatigue syndrome in adolescents', *Paediatrics*, 1991, 88, 195–201.

515 Wachsmuth, J. and MacMillan, H., 'Effective treatment for an ado-

lescent with chronic fatigue syndrome', *Clinical Paediatrics*, 1991, 30, 488–90.

516 Walford, G. A., *et al.*, 'Fatigue, depression and social adjustment in chronic fatigue syndrome', *Archives of Disease in Childhood*, 1993, 68, 384–8.

517 Vereker, M., 'Chronic fatigue syndrome: a joint paediatric-psychiatric approach', *Archives of Disease in Childhood*, 1992, 67, 550–5.

518 Wessely, S., 'Chronic fatigue syndrome in children', *Psychiatric Bulletin*, 1998.

## Chapter 16: ME/CFS and your Job

519 Lloyd, A. R. and Pender, H., 'The economic impact of chronic fatigue syndrome', *Medical Journal of Australia*, 1992, 157, 599–601.

520 Mountstephen, A. and Sharpe, M., 'Chronic fatigue syndrome and occupational health', *Occupational Medicine*, 1997, 47, 217–27.

521 Peel, M., 'Rehabilitation in the post-viral syndrome', *Journal of the Society of Occupational Medicine*, 1988, 38, 44–5.

## Chapter 19: Additional Help and Benefits Available in Britain

522 Finestone, A. J., 'A doctor's dilemma – is a diagnosis disabling or enabling?' *Archives of Internal Medicine*, 1997, 157, 49–50. Correspondence: 157, 2663–4.

523 Woodward, R. V., *et al.*, 'Diagnosis in chronic illness: disabling or enabling – the case of chronic fatigue syndrome', *Journal of the Royal Society of Medicine*, 1995, 88, 325–9.

### Additional References

524 Bennett, R. M., *et al.*, 'A randomised, double-blind, placebo-controlled study of growth hormone in the treatment of fibromyalgia', *American Journal of Medicine*, 1998, 104, 227–31.

525 Christodoulou, C., *et al.,* 'Relation between neuropsychological impairment and functional disability in patients with chronic fatigue syndrome;, *Journal of Neurology, Neurosurgery and Psychiatry*, 1998, 64, 431–4..

526 Deale, A., *et al.*, 'Illness beliefs and treatment outcome in chronic fatigue syndrome', *Journal of Psychosomatic Research*, 1998, 45, 77–83.

527 Ford, H., *et al.*, 'The nature of fatigue in multiple sclerosis', *Journal of Psychosomatic Medicine*, 1998, 45, 33–38.

528 Gregg, V. H., 'Hypnosis in chronic fatigue syndrome', *Journal of the*

*Royal Society of Medicine*, 1997, 90, 682–3.

529 Hassan, I., *et al.*, 'A study of the immunology of the chronic fatigue syndrome: correlation of immunologic paramaters to health dysfunction', *Clinical Immunology and Immunopathology*, 1998, 87, 60–7.

530 Korszun, A., *et al.*, 'Melatonin secretion in temperomandibular disorders, fibromyalgia and chronic fatigue syndrome', *Journal of Dental Research*, 1998, 77, 772 (abs 1128)

531 Lane, R. J. M., et al., 'Heterogenicity in chronic fatigue syndrome: evidence from nuclear magnetic resonance spectroscopy of muscle', *Neuromuscular Disorders*, 1998, 8, 204–9.

532 Lane, R. J. M., *et al.*, 'Muscle fibre characteristics and lactate responses to exercise in chronic fatigue syndrome', *Journal of Neurology, Neurosurgery and Psychiatry 1998*, 64, 362–7.

533 Montague, T. J., *et al.*, 'Cardiac function at rest and with exercise in the chronic fatigue syndrome', Chest, 1989, 95, 779–84

534 Peterson, P. K., *et al.*, 'A preliminary placebo-controlled crossover trial of fludrocortisone for chronic fatigue syndrome', *Archives of Internal Medicine* 1998, 158, 908–14.

535 Rose, M. R. 'Neurological channelopathies', *British Medical Journal*, 1993, 316, 1104–5.

536 Scott, L. V., *et al.*, 'The low dose ACTH test in chronic fatigue syndrome and in health', *Clinical Endocrinology*, 1998, 48, 773–7.

537 Scott, L. V., *et al.*, 'Blunted adrenocorticotrophin and cortisol responses to corticotropin-releasing hormone stimulation in chronic fatigue syndrome', *Acta Psychiatrica Scandinavica*, 1998, 97, 450–7.

538 Sisto, S. A., *et al.*, 'Physical activity before and after exercise in women with chronic fatigue syndrome'. *Quaterly Journal of Medicine*, 1998, 91, 465–73.

539 Stores, G., *et al.*, 'Sleep abnormalities demonstrated by home polysomnography in teenagers with chronic fatigue syndrome', *Journal of Psychosomatic Research*, 1998, 45, 85–91.

540 Troughton, A. H., *et al.*, '99mTc-HMPAO SPECT in chronic fatigue syndrome', *Clinical Radiology*, 1992, 45, 59.

541 Visser, J., *et al.*, 'CD4 T lymphocytes from patients with chronic fatigue sndrome have decreased interferon-gamma production and increased sensitivity to dexamethasone', *Journal of Infectious Diseases*, 1998, 177, 451–4.

542 Wearden, A. J., *et al.*, 'Randomised, double-blind, placebo-controlled treatment trial of fluoxetine and graded exercise for chronic fatigue syndrome', *British Journal of Psychiatry*, 1998, 172, 485–90.

543 Franklin, A. 'How I manage chronic fatigue syndrome', Archives of Disease in Childhood, 1998, 79, 375–378.

544 McKenzie, R., *et al.*, 'Low-dose hydrocortisone for treatment of chronic fatigue syndrome', Journal of the American Medical Association, 1998, 280, 1061–1066.

# Index

YEOVIL COLLEGE
LIBRARY